TRIVENT

PUBLISHING

TRIVENT
medieval

Beyond Cadfael

Medieval Medicine and Medical Medievalism

Edited by

Lucy C. Barnhouse and Winston Black

Medievalism, vol. 2

Beyond Cadfael. Medieval Medicine and Medical Medievalism
Ed. Lucy C. Barnhouse and Winston Black
ISBN 978-615-6405-80-7
Medievalism, vol. 2
Series ed. Karl Christian Alvestad
ISSN 2939-8991
Responsible publisher: Teodora C. Artimon
https://trivent-publishing.eu/66-medievalism

First published in 2023 by Trivent Publishing

Trivent Publishing
1119 Budapest, Etele ut 59–61
Hungary

For more information, visit our website: http://trivent-publishing.eu

TABLE OF CONTENTS

INTRODUCTION

BEYOND CADFAEL: IDENTIFYING AND DEFINING MEDICAL MEDIEVALISM

LUCY C. BARNHOUSE AND WINSTON BLACK

In 1984, a tourist attraction called Shrewsbury Quest opened in the town of the same name in Shropshire, England, located on the grounds of the Abbey of St Peter and St Paul and the parish church of The Holy Cross. Shrewsbury Quest, which closed in 2001, was dedicated to many aspects of the history of medieval Shrewsbury, but its main focus was immersion in the twelfth-century world of Shrewsbury's most famous fictional resident, the monk and herbalist Brother Cadfael.[1] Cadfael is the protagonist of twenty crime novels written by Ellis Peters (the pen name of Edith Pargeter, 1913-1995) and of the television series of thirteen episodes based on the novels, starring Sir Derek Jacobi (ITV, 1994-1998). The novels have been translated into multiple languages and sold tens of millions of copies worldwide. They have also served for many people as an entry into medieval studies and some aspects of medieval medicine, as witnessed by a spate of popular books from the heyday of the television series: *Brother Cadfael's Book of Days, Brother Cadfael's Herb Garden,* and *The Cadfael Companion.*[2] The underlying premise of these and

[1] A description of this attraction, with photographs, is provided at a German fan site for Brother Cadfael, *Die Chroniken des Bruder Cadfael* (also in English), which claims to be "probably the most extensive private Cadfael website" and "approved by Ellis Peters' trustee of estate": www.cadfael.de/html/es-s-quest.html, Accessed May 27, 2022. Special thanks to Dr. Emily Reiner for her additional editorial assistance with this volume.

[2] Robin Whiteman, *Brother Cadfael's Book of Days: The Material and Spiritual Wisdom of a Medieval Crusader-Monk* (London: Headline, 2000); Rob Talbot and Robin Whiteman,

similar books is that the medieval world depicted by Peters, however fictional, is nonetheless a reasonably accurate reflection of a historical reality, one that a fan of Cadfael's adventures can readily enter.

Cadfael is probably the best-known example in the Anglophone world of "medical medievalism": a modern representation of medieval medicine, intended for a popular audience.[3] A Welsh Benedictine monk, Cadfael not only serves as the herbalist and medic for his monastery, but also applies his skills in plant lore and natural observation to solving the shocking number of murders that occur in the town of Shrewsbury and its environs. He is positioned as a liminal figure of "intimate alterity," comfortably at home in an English monastery, but also an outsider as both a Welshman and a long-time resident of the Holy Land.[4] This alterity makes him not only attuned to identifying and tracking important clues but also approachable to a modern audience, who are also sympathetic outsiders to the medieval, monastic setting of the stories.

The first five books in the series of Brother Cadfael novels all open with the crusader-turned-monk in his garden or workshop (both key stops on the Shrewsbury Quest tour), overseeing the work of medieval medicine. The second novel, *One Corpse Too Many*, exemplifies particularly well the tensions inherent in much medievalism, that is, between the vision of the medieval past as one characterized by violence and brutality, and that of the medieval world as characterized by relationships believed lost to modern society: a closeness to God, to nature, and to community. In *One Corpse Too Many*, the violence of twelfth-century England's interregnum and civil war (1138-1153) comes to Shrewsbury and its abbey with the siege of a castle and its disturbing aftermath.[5] It also

Brother Cadfael's Herb Garden: An Illustrated Companion to Medieval Plants and Their Uses (Boston: Bulfinch Press, 1997); *The Cadfael Companion: The World of Brother Cadfael* (New York: Mysterious Press, 1995).

[3] Our definition of the term "medical medievalism" is inspired by—but slightly different—its first application by Zrinka Stahuljak in her monograph *Pornographic Archaeology: Medicine, Medievalism, and the Invention of the French Nation* (Philadelphia: University of Pennsylvania Press, 2013), 3.

[4] The term is from Lesley Jacobs, "Idealized Images of Wales in the Fiction of Edith Pargeter/Ellis Peters," in *Mass Market Medieval: Essays on the Middle Ages in Popular Culture*, ed. David W. Marshall (Jefferson, NC: McFarland & Company, 2007), 90-101, at 91, building on the work of Jeffrey Jerome Cohen on Gerald of Wales in "Hybrids, Monsters, Borderlands," in *The Postcolonial Middle Ages*, ed. Jeffrey Jerome Cohen (New York: Palgrave, 2000), 85-104.

[5] Ellis Peters, *One Corpse Too Many* (London: Macmillan, 1979), 53-57, 79-82, 116, 213.

enables Cadfael to discover the location of a murder. In the 1994 television adaptation of the novel, the plant goosegrass also becomes a visual motif, with Derek Jacobi's Cadfael carefully obtaining and preserving samples of the plant found on the corpse and at the crime scene. This visual motif is easily recognizable from decades of serialized detective shows; here, the sleuth and his clues are made recognizably medieval in appearance but comfortably modern in the context of a crime novel.

But this recognition of the medieval world may be a false one. Goosegrass (or cleavers), while common to Ellis Peters' beloved native Shropshire, was not a particularly popular ingredient in medieval medical texts. The reference work designed to explicate Cadfael's botanical knowledge for readers cites a seventeenth-century herbal in its discussion of the plant.[6] And Cadfael's activities owe much more to the tropes of detective fiction from Poe and Conan Doyle onwards than to his duties as a monastic herbalist, even in the turbulent times of the English interregnum. "If the Middle Ages hadn't existed," Catherine Brown has suggested, "people might have had to invent them, just so that we could safely be non-medieval."[7] This invented Middle Ages is on display as much in the theme park as in the novels and television series. As one reviewer of Shrewsbury Quest remarked, the town of Shrewsbury became the site of "a battle between real history and fictional history."[8] At Shrewsbury Quest visitors could explore replicas of Cadfael's hut and his "physic garden," key scenes from the murder mysteries. Cadfael's medical skills, we read, were learned from Muslims in the Holy Land when he was serving as a soldier there during and after the First Crusade. Readers of the novels understand from this plot element that any useful knowledge in physiology, anatomy, or therapeutics could not be gained

[6] Rob Talbot and Robin Whiteman, *Brother Cadfael's Herb Garden: An Illustrated Companion to Medieval Plants and their Uses* (Boston: Bulfinch Press, 1997), 108-09. Goosegrass (if we can understand this as the modern plant, *Galium aparine* L.) does not occur in any of the most important high medieval herbals, such as Macer Floridus's *De viribus herbarum*, *Circa instans*, or Hildegard of Bingen's *Physica*. For later medieval references to a plant that may be goosegrass or cleavers, see Tony Hunt, *Plant Names of Medieval England* (Woodbridge: D.S. Brewer, 1989), s.v. Galium Aparine, 324.

[7] Catherine Brown, "In the Middle," *Journal of Medieval and Early Modern Studies* 30:3 (2000), 549.

[8] Martha Moffett, "Cadfael's cloister," *South Florida Sun-Sentinel* Jan 1, 1995, www.sun-sentinel.com/news/fl-xpm-1995-01-01-9412270315-story.html, accessed Dec 30, 2021.

in twelfth-century Europe but had to come from a civilization that is portrayed as both timeless and exotic, which serves as a medieval proxy for modern medical skills.[9] When a European gained that sort of knowledge, they could transcend the backwardness of medieval Western Europe and display the skills of a modern medical examiner. Visitors to Shrewsbury Quest co-create a similar anachronism, using clues from Cadfael's rustic hut and herbarium to solve a mystery in the style of a modern investigative detective. This opposition of the medieval and the modern, as Helen Young and Kavita Mudan Finn have recently argued, has been used from the early modern period onwards in service of a modernity imagined as exclusively and inevitably white and European.[10]

The use of the (invented) Middle Ages as a site of imagined contrast with the modern is particularly prevalent in popular culture depictions of medieval medicine. This volume aims to show that medieval medicine occupies multiple and multivalent spaces in the modern imagination. Recent decades have seen particularly robust scholarship on both medieval medicine and popular medievalism, but work uniting these threads of scholarship remains a desideratum. Medieval medicine retains, in the words of several scholars, an "'eye-of-newt' image among the general public,"[11] who often assume (or are told through popular media) that medieval remedies and medical practices were reminiscent of the repulsive and magical ingredients in the Three Witches' bubbling cauldron in Shakespeare's *Macbeth*.

Moralizing and prejudiced attitudes towards disease, moreover, have even been referred to as a kind of "diagnostic medievalism," associated with a mode of understanding and engaging with disease imagined as

---

[9] See Edward Said, *Orientalism* (London: Routledge, 1980), 9-11, for this mode of co-creating 'Europe' and 'the Orient' in the western imagination. See also Robin S. Reich's essay in this volume, "The Fantasy of Medieval Medicine: Orientalizing Experiential and Textual Traditions in the Imagined Medieval Past".

[10] Helen Young and Kavita Mudan Finn, *Global Medievalism* (Cambridge: Cambridge University Press, 2022), 1-4. This valuable work appeared after this volume was in proofs.

[11] Anne van Arsdall, "Rehabilitating Medieval Medicine," in: *Misconceptions About the Middle Ages*, eds. Stephen J. Harris and Bryon L. Grigsby (New York: Routledge, 2007), 135-41; Peregrine Horden, "What's Wrong with Early Medieval Medicine?" *Social History of Medicine* 24 (2011), 24-25; Anne Van Arsdall. "Challenging the 'Eye of Newt' Image of Medieval Medicine" in *The Medieval Hospital and Medical Practice.* ed by Barbara S. Bowers. (Burlington: Ashgate, 2007), 195-204.

distinctively medieval." [12] Especially – but by no means exclusively – since the outbreak of the COVID-19 pandemic, the medieval has appeared as a signifier of inadequate medical knowledge, helplessness in the face of disease, and failures of both imagination and implementation in public health policy.[13] It is widely assumed that medieval people could do nothing—and thus did do nothing—in the face of premodern pandemics like the Black Death of 1346-1353. Contemporary calls to embrace effective countermeasures to COVID-19, including masks, vaccines, and social isolation measures, are routinely depicted as modern innovations that can save us from the implied failures of medieval medicine. At the same time, the plague masks used by some doctors only in the seventeenth century have been hailed as supposedly medieval precursors to modern protective equipment.[14] In the context of widespread personal anxiety and often incoherent public health policy, the alterity of the medieval and the construction of popular medical medievalisms can serve as both exhortation and comfort: this is what should be abandoned; this is what can be transcended. If collective inertia and willful ignorance are understood as 'medieval,' we can reject the ways in which these patterns indict our own societies.

Imagining the historical past and the contemporary moment as basic, opposing facts on either side of a chasm is an all too prevalent conceptual binary.[15] Moreover, this constructed opposition is not unique to the modern period. The practice of medievalism can be viewed as having begun in the Middle Ages itself, with literary narratives inventing a

---

[12] Jessica Chace, "Diagnostic Medievalism: The Case of Leprosy's Stigma," *Disability Studies Quarterly* 39 (2019), https://dsq-sds.org/article/view/6410/5409. Last accessed January 7, 2020.

[13] For an overview of such coverage see Ali Shamekh, Ata Mahmoudpoor, and Sarvin Sanaie, "COVID-19: Is it the black death of the 21st century?" *Health promotion perspectives* 10:3 (2020), 166-167. See also "The Mother of All Pandemics: The State of Black Death Research in the Era of Covid-19," a 2020 webinar sponsored by the Medieval Academy of America, with Winston Black and Lori Jones as moderators, and Monica H. Green as respondent, www.medievalacademy.org/general/custom.asp?page=PandemicWebinar. See also Umberto Eco, "Living in the Middle Ages," in *Travels in Hyperreality* (New York, NY: Harvest Press, 1990), 73-85.

[14] See, for example, Ainsley Hawthorn, "Plague doctors and PPE: Today's gear has nothing on the medical garb of the Renaissance," *CBC News Newfoundland & Labrador* August 23, 2020. www.cbc.ca/news/canada/newfoundland-labrador/renaissance-ppe-plague-doctors-1.5687152

[15] Larry Scanlon, "Introduction," *American Literary History* 22 (2010), 718-719.

chivalric past which contrasts with the authors' own historical moment, itself envisioned as one of decline.[16] With the creation of an imagined Middle Ages came its "ideological conscription"; whether romantic ideal or barbaric other, the Middle Ages are never neutral.[17] Their uses of the Middle Ages, moreover, are notable for their multiplicity and flexibility, and, sometimes, for their syncretism and anachronism.[18] Whereas Regency England or Renaissance Italy may behave in more or less predictable ways as backdrops for historical fictions, the fictional Middle Ages – of Britain, of Baghdad, or even of Westeros in George R.R. Martin's fantasy novels and HBO series – do not. They can be idyllic settings for heroic endeavor and for the "love, truth, and faithfulness" which Thomas Malory lamented in 1485 as lost, part of the "irrecuperable pastness" which is so frequently projected onto the premodern.[19] Such is the power of medievalism that fantasy worlds are often treated as recognizably "medieval," as attested by both academic and popular discourse on *Game of Thrones* and *Lord of the Rings*.[20] Both scholarly and popular definitions of the Middle Ages are "constructed, invented, produced," undermining the frequently critiqued divide between medieval studies and medievalism.[21] The essays in this volume analyze how medical medievalisms are produced, circulated, and debated. As a whole, the volume examines the extent to which such medievalisms "habitually tell the same story of the European Middle Ages," and the

---

16 Tison Pugh and Susan Aronstein, "Introduction: Theorizing America's Medievalisms," in: *The United States of Medievalism*, eds. Tison Pugh and Susan Aronstein (Toronto: University of Toronto Press, 2021), 3-18, at 5. See also Umberto Eco, "Dreaming the Middle Ages," in *Travels in Hyperreality*, 65-67, for the idea of a continuous return of the Middle Ages.

17 Pugh and Aronstein, "Introduction," 5; Young and Finn, *Global Medievalism*, 1.

18 Marcus Bull, *Thinking Medieval: An Introduction to the Study of the Middle Ages* (New York, NY: Palgrave, 2005), 38-39; Louise D'Arcens, "Medievalism: Scope and Complexity," in *The Cambridge Companion to Medievalism*, ed. Louise D'Arcens (Cambridge: Cambridge University Press, 2016), 5-6.

19 Thomas Malory, *Le Morte d'Arthur*, Book XVIII (New York, NY: Heritage Press, 1955), 674; Larry Scanlon, "Introduction," 719; Bull, *Thinking Medieval*, 18-19, 25-26.

20 See for example Jane Chance, ed. *Tolkien the Medievalist* (London: Routledge, 2008); Shiloh Carroll, *Medievalism in A Song of Ice and Fire and A Game of Thrones* (Woodbridge: Boydell and Brewer, 2018); Kavita Mudan Finn, "Game of Thrones is Based in History—Outdated History," *The Public Medievalist*, May 2019, www.publicmedievalist.com/thrones-outdated-history/, accessed April 15, 2022.

21 Fitzpatrick, "The Academy and the Making of Neomedievalism," 14.

ways in which they can complicate or contradict narratives of medieval history in general and the history of medicine in particular.[22]

Many of the contributors to this volume, when explaining to acquaintances that they study medieval medicine, have received the response, "Oh, like Brother Cadfael?" As those exchanges indicate, Cadfael provides a popular locus of understanding that can serve as an entry point to critical analysis of medieval medical history. Yet Cadfael and other figures of medical medievalism have also become an impediment to researching and teaching about medieval medicine. Arguably, Ellis Peters's stories have calcified medieval medicine in the popular imagination: her representation of Anglo-Welsh monastic medicine in the early twelfth century has come to serve as representative of all medieval medicine. Yet medicine changed vastly over the millennium of the Middle Ages and particularly in the century (ca.1150-1250 CE) after the setting of the Cadfael Chronicles. It also differed significantly between geographical regions, social classes, and religious and secular groups, not to mention differing in diagnoses and treatments for specific diseases and specific patients. We can and should complicate matters further by emphasizing that the medicine of medieval Europe is not the medicine of the Islamicate Middle East, of south Asia, or of China and Korea in the same period.[23] While the concept of a 'global Middle Ages' is an inevitably fraught one, our understanding of the medical traditions of each region in the premodern era is enriched by contextualization, comparison, and exploration of difference. This approach is highlighted in the third and final section of this volume, in which the authors pose a series of comparisons about medicine and medievalism between Europe and East Asia and between the Middle Ages and today.

The relationships of medievalism to the formal study of the Middle Ages are many, and these relationships have been changing and

22 Young and Mudan Finn, *Global Medievalism*, 7-10, quoted at 7.

23 On the term 'Islamicate,' coined by the historian Marshall Hodgson (1922-1968), and its historiography, see Fitzroy Morrissey, "The Venture of the Islamicate: The History of a Key Concept in Islamic Intellectual History," 29 July 2021, https://intellectual history.web.ox.ac.uk/article/venture-islamicate-history-keycon cept-islamic-intellectual-history.

diversifying in the twenty-first century.[24] The Middle Ages can sometimes be pretextual: a background for the exploration of ideas with little connection to the mental and physical worlds of the medieval past.[25] But as has been widely noted, the desire for a certain vision of the Middle Ages has driven scholarly as well as popular medievalism.[26] And medieval studies, as an academic field, has come a long way from the skepticism with which nineteenth- and twentieth-century scholars treated amateur medievalism and the study of such medievalism.[27] Though the relationship between the study of medievalism and more traditional medieval studies remains fragile, it has been suggested that increased scholarly attention to medievalism offers rich possibilities at a time when academic support for the study of the Middle Ages themselves is in decline.[28] While the methods of scholarly and amateur medievalism may differ, these modes of pursuing and imagining the Middle Ages are characterized by complex interdependence, as illustrated in the media and medical practices examined by this volume.[29]

Even as scholarship on medievalism and scholarship on medieval medicine have burgeoned simultaneously in medieval studies, they have rarely been in conversation with each other. While many clichés about the Middle Ages – about science and sex, about race and gender, about travel and trade – have been increasingly queried and undermined, popular medical medievalisms remain largely unchanged.[30] Persistently,

---

[24] KellyAnn Fitzpatrick, "The Academy and the Making of Neomedievalism," in: *Neomedievalism, Popular Culture, and the Academy: From Tolkien to Game of Thrones* (Woodbridge: Boydell and Brewer, 2019), 4.

[25] Eco, "Dreaming of the Middle Ages," 68-69.

[26] See, for example, Miri Rubin, *The Middle Ages: A Very Short Introduction* (Oxford: Oxford University Press, 2014), 6-9; D'Arcens, "Medievalism: Scope and Complexity," 1-7.

[27] Kathleen Biddick, *The Shock of Medievalism* (Durham, NC: Duke University Press, 1998), 1-4, discusses both change and continuity in scholarly anxieties.

[28] Fitzpatrick, "The Academy and the Making of Neomedievalism," 6-8.

[29] D'Arcens, "Medievalism: Scope and Complexity," 6, on the "complex history of interdependence" linking scholarly and non-scholarly approaches to the Middle Ages; on the different approaches to method in scholarly and popular medievalism, see Andrew B.R. Elliott, *Remaking the Middle Ages: The Methods of Cinema and History in Portraying the Medieval World* (Jefferson, NC: McFarland and Co., 2011), 9-34.

[30] Andrew Albin et al., eds., *Whose Middle Ages? Teachable Moments for an Ill-Used Past* (New York, NY: Fordham University Press, 2019), for instance, is a valuable collection but contains no essays focused on medicine. Stephen J. Harris and Bryon L. Grigsby, eds.,

too, the Middle Ages are imagined as quintessentially a time of disease. This is an idea found not only in popular culture but in the most essential scholarly works on medieval medicine. Katharine Park, in her foundational essay "Medicine and society in medieval Europe," described the European Middle Ages as "a universe of disease," playing on Jacques Le Goff's own interpretation of the Middle Ages as "a universe of hunger."[31] From leprosy to dysentery, from malaria to tuberculosis, from vitamin deficiencies to intestinal parasites, illness and disease were omnipresent in medieval society, and it is both possible and worthwhile to write a history of disease in the Middle Ages, while rejecting an image of the Middle Ages as uniquely diseased.[32] The premodern identification and modern portrayal of some of these diseases are explored in the first section of this volume, particularly in the essays by Luke Demaitre and Courtney A. Krolikoski.

To write a history of disease in medievalism, however, is a different matter. What diseases are considered stereotypically "medieval"? How and when do they appear in modern contexts and in what sort of media? Is the presence of a disease in a "medieval" movie, game, or novel an example of medical medievalism that reflects conscious thought about healing in the past, or has it been placed there by the authors or creators simply as part of the expected "Dark Ages" scenery? Are these "medieval" diseases actual historical pathologies, fictionalized representations of known diseases, or entirely fictional? A case study may be found in the open-access publication of "a digital cautionary tale" about misidentifying medieval images of disease as representations of the Black Death.[33] This co-authored article contains an edition and translation of primary sources alongside an analysis of images

Misconceptions about the Middle Ages (New York, NY: Routledge, 2001), has only two of its thirty-one essays dedicated to medieval medicine: Van Arsdall, "Rehabilitating Medieval Medicine," 135-41, and Bryon Grigsby, "Medical Misconceptions," 142-50. For a counterexample, see Winston Black, *The Middle Ages: Facts and Fictions* (Santa Barbara, CA: ABC-CLIO, 2019).

[31] Katharine Park, "Medicine and Society in Medieval Europe," in *Medicine in Society: Historical Essays*, ed. Andrew Wear (Cambridge University Press, 1992), 59-90, at 60.

[32] One of the most recent and progressive contributions to this field is *Death and Disease in the Medieval and Early Modern World: Perspectives from Across the Mediterranean and Beyond*, ed. Lori Jones and Nükhet Varlik (Boydell & Brewer, 2022).

[33] Monica H. Green, Kathleen Walker-Meikle, and Wolfgang P. Mueller, "Diagnosis of a 'Plague' Image: A Digital Cautionary Tale," *The Medieval Globe* 1 (2014), 309-325.

representing leprosy and the biblical plague of boils that have been repeatedly misconstrued in modern publications as representing bubonic plague. Three years after its publication, one of the authors was again driven to correct misuse of the latter image.[34] And as recently as 2020, one of the present editors was presented with the biblical image as a depiction of plague, to accompany an essay on the Black Death and COVID-19.[35] It is not enough to correct the misuse of medieval images of disease; we should query why modern audiences continue to interpret images of leprosy as images of plague, even after repeated correction. In that spirit, this collection brings the subfields of medievalism and medieval medicine into conversation with each other, engaging with the imagined oppositions of the medieval and the scientific, and medieval and modern understandings of medical practice. From practical medicine to postage stamps, and from video games to the vocabulary of disease, the topics of the following essays offer a kaleidoscopic view of medieval medicine and its afterlives.

Beyond Cadfael examines both how the practices and understandings of medicine and illness were shaped by cultural contexts in the Middle Ages, and how representations of medieval medicine in popular culture are influenced by popular ideas of the medieval. Popular stereotypes of the medical and the medieval have often been at odds. As François-Olivier Touati and other historians of premodern medicine have observed, the Middle Ages is often imagined as a time essentially characterized by the inescapable prevalence of disease.[36] Medicine, on the other hand, is often conceptualized — particularly in western media — as belonging to the modern, the clinical, and the professional. And yet, as Umberto Eco dryly observed, "Indeed, it seems that people like

[34] Rae Ellen Bichell, "Iconic Plague Images Are Often Not What They Seem," *NPR Goats and Soda*, August 18, 2017, www.npr.org/sections/goatsandsoda/2017/08/18/542435991/those-iconic-images-of-the-plague-thats-not-the-plague, accessed January 15, 2022.

[35] Lucy Barnhouse, email correspondence, November 25, 2020. A compromise was reached in correctly captioning the image for Barnhouse, "The Pestilential Premodern? Going Digital with the Medieval," *EuropeNow*, Dec. 2020, www.europenowjournal.org/2020/12/07/the-pestilential-premodern-going-digital-with-the-medieval/, accessed Jan. 15, 2022.

[36] François-Olivier Touati, *Maladie et Société au Moyen Age: La lèpre, les lépreux et les léproseries dans la province ecclésiastique de Sens jusqu'au milieu du XIVe siècle* (Bruxelles: De Boeck & Larcier, 1998) 19; Adam J. Davis, *The Medieval Economy of Salvation: Charity, Commerce, and the Rise of the Hospital* (Ithaca, NY: Cornell University Press, 2019), 22-27 et passim.

the Middle Ages."[37] Frequently, the Middle Ages occupy a paradoxical dual role in popular media, both that of the simpler past that is desired, and the barbarism and chaos from which modernity must escape, or which must be transcended in order that modernity may emerge.[38] Another constructed duality is one that David Matthews has defined as that of the gothic or grotesque Middle Ages vs. that of the romantic Middle Ages.[39] We can see in these options the legacies of Walter Scott, progenitor of many of the European medievalisms that persist to this day; while emphases and trends in ways of imagining the Middle Ages may come and go, the options for the imagined medieval set in the nineteenth century enjoy enduring influence.[40]

The contributors to this volume, using a variety of methods, examine the vibrancy and diversity of medievalism across multiple media. In doing so, they aim to contribute to what Geraldine Heng has called "a re-education of desire" for the medieval.[41] The goal of such a re-education of the imagination is not merely exporting the discipline of scholarly accuracy to contexts beyond the academy, but a liberation of the imagination to conceptualize a Middle Ages not limited by the clichés and prejudices of post-medieval tropes, however created. As Heng has observed, both public and academic desire shape the Middle Ages we see and seek in our interactions with the past.[42] Coming from different disciplines and different lived experiences, the scholars contributing to this volume present multiple visions of medieval medicine. In doing so,

[37] Eco, "Dreaming the Middle Ages," 61.

[38] Laurie A. Finke and Martin B. Shichtman, "Apocalyptic Medievalism: Rape and Disease as Figures of Social Anomie," in: *Cinematic Illuminations: The Middle Ages on Film* (Baltimore, MD: Johns Hopkins University Press, 2007), 288-334.

[39] Matthews, *Medievalism: A Critical History,* 15.

[40] On the influence of nineteenth-century medievalism, particularly in the Anglophone world, see Bull, *Thinking Medieval,* 7-41. On the legacy of Walter Scott, see James Watt, "Sir Walter Scott and the Medievalist Novel," in *The Oxford Handbook of Victorian Medievalism*, ed. Joanne Parker and Corinna Wagner (Oxford: Oxford University Press, 2020), 162-74.

[41] Geraldine Heng, "Medievalists and the Education of Desire," in *Whose Middle Ages? Teachable Moments for an Ill-Used Past,* ed. Andrew Albin et al. (New York: Fordham University Press, 2019), 276.

[42] Heng, "Medievalists and the Education of Desire," 275-90.

we are seeking not primarily to "rehabilitate" medieval medicine, nor to assess the authenticity of particular instances of medical medievalism.[43]

This book is aimed not simply at correcting misconceptions about the history of medieval medicine (by continuing the "battle between real history and fictional history" at play in 1990s Shrewsbury), although we do hope readers come away with a better understanding of how medieval healers and physicians actually worked. Rather, our contributors explore the elaboration and persistence of approaches to the history of medieval medicine that go far beyond the stereotypically Eurocentric medieval world of Cadfael. Echoes of medieval diseases and medieval medicine are found in the television sitcom *Seinfeld*, in the songs of U2, in many other novels besides the Cadfael Chronicles, in numerous video games, as well as in genres such as museum exhibitions and documentaries that purport to present the historical reality of medieval medical practice and practitioners. Each of these genres embraces and promotes its own versions of medievalism and of medical medievalism.

The Cadfael Chronicles give modern audiences a relatively positive portrait of medieval medicine. Yet many modern depictions of medieval medicine focus instead on only the most absurd and repulsive elements that existed – or have been imagined as existing – within medieval remedy books and healing practices. Such an approach to medieval medicine actively rejects the complexity, diversity, and rationality of premodern medical traditions, instead reducing medieval medicine to a few choice examples meant to shock and disgust. This approach occurs not only in fictional genres, such as novels, movies, and videos games, but even in recent historical texts intended for popular audiences. In most cases, the authors of these books aim to paint a sympathetic and historically accurate picture of medieval medicine, but their titles and covers tell a different story, one that aims to confirm many readers' assumptions about medieval medicine as closer to fantasy potions than to modern therapeutics. Such works include *Dragon's Blood and Willow Bark*, *Medicine in the Middle Ages: Surviving the Times*, and *Revolting Remedies from the Middle Ages*. While the first two of these books were published by

[43] Cf. Anne van Arsdall, "Rehabilitating Medieval Medicine," 135-41; April Harper, "Misdiagnosing Medieval Medicine: 'Magical' Muslims, Metanarrative and the Modern Media," in *The Middle Ages in Modern Culture: History and Authenticity in Contemporary Medievalism*, ed. Karl C. Alvestad and Robert Houghton (London: Bloomsbury, 2021), 58-73.

non-academics for presses that specialize in local and popular history for a British audience (Amberley Publishing and Pen and Sword Books), the last (*Revolting Remedies*) was edited by Dr. Daniel Wakelin, a medieval paleography scholar at the University of Oxford, and published by Oxford's Bodleian Library.

A closer look at Toni Mount's book *Dragon's Blood and Willow Bark* enables us to analyze how the tension between cover and text plays out in a popular book on medieval medicine. Mount's book is an entertaining survey of medieval medical traditions with the obligatory references to Hippocrates and Galen and their enduring influence but based primarily in later medieval England, the setting of Mount's other books, the Sebastian Foxley murder mysteries. While Mount does explain that "dragon's blood" is in fact the medicinal resin of the Socotra dragon blood tree (*Dracaena cinnabari*) and thus does not indicate medieval belief in mythological dragons, the title is nonetheless used to draw in readers looking for and expecting the grotesque and marvelous from a book on medieval medicine. In this spirit, the book's blurb promises a medieval medicine practiced by "butchers and executioners" prescribing "roasted cats" to a later medieval populace that is frequently "showered in poo". The connections between genuine medieval medicine and fantasy worlds are emphasized by a mock disclaimer on the back of the book: "N.B. No animals, large, furry or mythological, were harmed during the research for this book." Apparently either Mount or the press was uncomfortable with the original title of the book, because in its second printing in 2016, they republished it as *Medieval Medicine: Its Mysteries and Science.* Gone is the fantastic allure of "dragon's blood," replaced with a new focus on the "science" behind medieval medicine. Even though the text within the book did not change (nor did the blurb and mock warning on the back cover), the new title dramatically shifts its apparent purpose, from entertaining the reader with the backwardness of medieval medicine to educating the reader about its supposed validity in the context of modern biomedicine. Both approaches are far from atypical and both participate in a widespread othering of medieval medicine.

Going "beyond Cadfael" means examining diverse works across multiple genres to understand medical medievalism. It means stretching the boundaries of the field of medieval medicine geographically and chronologically, beyond just England and Northern France and beyond just the High Middle Ages. It even means leaving Europe entirely in our study of medieval medicine and medical medievalisms, to understand the important similarities and profound differences among the various medical traditions of the world. It is not enough to acknowledge the Eurocentrism of most medieval medicine and medical medievalisms. It is particularly incumbent upon professional medievalists to interrogate that Eurocentrism and explore the dangerous and constructive tensions created when we compare the premodern medical traditions of different cultures. "Medieval medicine" was not just European medicine. It belonged to a complex network of medical ideas and medical substances stretching across the whole of Afro-Eurasia. This new narrative of premodern medicine is only now being crafted and promoted by medical historians like Ronit Yoeli-Tlalim, who calls on medievalists to "ReOrient" our histories of medicine and to examine the intellectual and trade networks that connected medical practices from Europe to East Asia.[44]

The geographies of medical medievalisms tend to reflect the historically Eurocentric geography of medieval studies, focusing on Western Europe, and within that region focusing even more on just England, Scotland, Wales, and Ireland. Historians and popular writers frequently try to shoehorn the whole of "medieval medicine" into their preferred location or time period. Such is the case with a recent survey of medieval medicine, *Medicine in the Middle Ages: Surviving the Times*, by an author who has written primarily Tudor historical romances. Sure enough, many of the specific examples of "medieval" medicine come not from the Middle Ages from the biographies of King Henry VIII and Lady Margaret Beaufort.[45] But the Middle Ages, as imagined in the blurb for this book, are defined as a time when "people were subject to an array of not only deadly diseases but deplorable living conditions... [and] when cures for sickness were often worse than the illness itself."[46] This is a medieval world chosen to appeal primarily to an Anglophone readership, not only in the United Kingdom, but also in the United States, Canada, and Australia, where medievalism has often been linked to narratives

---

44 Ronit Yoeli-Tlalim, *ReOrienting Histories of Medicine: Encounters Along the Silk Roads* (London: Bloomsbury, 2021).

45 Juliana Cummings, *Medicine in the Middle Ages: Surviving the Times* (London: Pen and Sword, 2021).

46 The National Archives, London, https://shop.nationalarchives.gov.uk/products/medicine-in-the-middle-ages-surviving-the-times, accessed May 16, 2022.

"about white European possession of the land."[47] Many of the most popular medieval fictions take place in a recognizably "historic" Britain (the Brother Cadfael mysteries, Connie Willis's *Doomsday Book*, Mel Gibson's *Braveheart* [1995], and Kazuo Ishiguro's *The Buried Giant* [2015]) or in a fictional landscape clearly inspired by the geography of medieval Europe: George R. R. Martin's map of Westeros is essentially an inverted map of Ireland and Britain.[48] In her study of medieval crime fiction, Anne McKendry observes an unsettling nostalgia in the popularity of stories set in a fictionalized medieval "Britain" within non-European settler colonial states, a nostalgia that reflects a "deep (and often problematic) attachment to the fantasy of a medieval past by postcolonial societies."[49] One of the things this volume aims to do is to examine how the medieval past is fantasized as simultaneously diseased and curable, the locus of both grotesque illness and miraculous remedy.

Beyond Cadfael: Contents and Approaches

The medical medievalisms studied in this volume represent a significant branch of the "contemporary medieval", described by Clare Lees and Gillian Overing as "an emerging environment for interdisciplinary work within the creative humanities." [50] Medical medievalism specifically, however, remains under-studied and undertheorized. In contributing to a series on medievalism, this volume aims to showcase and stimulate such interdisciplinary work. Moreover, this volume found its genesis in academic conferences that promote the value of exploring, among many facets of medieval studies, the backgrounds and contexts of the contemporary medieval. These included the session, "Beyond Cadfael: Medieval Medicine in Popular Culture," organized and chaired by Lucy

[47] Young and Mudan Finn, *Global Medievalism*, 4-5, quoted at 4.

[48] "Game of Thrones' Westeros Is Really Just Britain and An Inverted Ireland," *Brilliant Maps*, March 7, 2015. https://brilliantmaps.com/westeros/, accessed June 11, 2022. George R.R. Martin admitted as much at the 2014 San Diego Comic Con in a "Rulers of the Realm" panel moderated by Ali T. Kokmen: www.youtube.com/watch?v=lUCz3c6-akU&t=930s, accessed June 11, 2022. On the Eurocentrism of Westeros, see Young and Mudan Finn, *Global Medievalism*, 26-31, 38-40.

[49] Anne McKendry, *Medieval Crime Fiction: A Critical Overview* (Jefferson, NC: McFarland & Co., 2019), 6.

[50] Clare A. Lees and Gillian R. Overing, "Doing It Differently: Medieval and Contemporary," in: *The Contemporary Medieval in Practice* (London: UCL Press, 2019), 5.

Barnhouse for the 54th International Congress on Medieval Studies (2019) at Western Michigan University (a conference well known among medievalists simply as "Kalamazoo"). More voices were added to this continuing discussion of medical medievalism in two conference sessions organized by Winston Black and chaired by both editors of this volume, "Mud, Blood...and Medicine? Modern Medical Medievalism", for *Medievalism Today*, the 36th Annual International Conference on Medievalism (2021), sponsored by the International Society for the Study of Medievalism and held at Delta College in Michigan.

The papers on medical medievalism presented in these two conferences, and the resulting essays in this collection, explore continuities between ancient and medieval medicine, between early and later medieval medicine, and between European and Asian medical traditions, as well as correspondences and contrasts between the medieval and the modern.[51] Moreover, they examine a range of historical medievalisms, from nineteenth-century imaginings of Ibn Sīnā to representations of medieval surgery in recent television, and from detective fiction to echoes of Victorian medievalism in contemporary music and other media. The following essays showcase both the Eurocentrism of much medievalism, and the richly varied realities of medieval cultures and responses to them around the globe. As they collectively demonstrate, while medical medievalism has hitherto been comparatively neglected in the field of medievalism, it provides fruitful material for study. Medieval medicine is the one subfield shared by all contributors to this volume. Severally, they have training in anthropology and history, archaeology and religious studies, with experience in lab and field work, as well as in the classroom. Collectively, they examine a range of ways in which medieval and modern medical knowledge, and narratives about that knowledge, enter into dialogue with each other. Whether through examining the imagined Middle Ages of the nineteenth century, parallels between medieval merchants and the herbalists of high fantasy, or medieval and modern uses of breastmilk, these essays bring multiple medievalisms into conversation. In so doing, they recognize

51 For this as a desideratum, see Horden, "What's Wrong with Early Medieval Medicine?", 5.

history as an endeavor of contact, of "resurrection," and of enabling and enacting transhistorical communities.[52]

This volume represents what we hope is only the first of many forays into the field of medical medievalism. So how should the contributions to this volume, the first on this subject, be arranged; what sort of principles and topics should guide inquiry into this field? When presented with the history of medicine, scholars and popular audiences alike tend to focus on the perceived differences between modern and premodern medical traditions. Most examples of medical medievalism, as described in this volume's essays, highlight the gulf, whether real or imagined, between the stereotypes of effective and clean modern medicine and barbarous and filthy medieval medicine. This focus on changes over time in the history of medicine only makes sense, as we can see all around us today the benefits of new systems of disease etiology, microbiology, and genetics, as well as a range of effective antiseptics, analgesics, and sedatives. Yet if we step back to look at the basic elements and participants of medical practice, whether in the eleventh or twenty-first century, in England or in Korea, we can see that little has changed: nearly every interaction that falls under the overarching concept of "medicine", whether medieval or modern, involves an essential triad of disease or complaint, a medical practitioner, and a treatment.

For this reason, the editors have organized the ten contributions to *Beyond Cadfael* into three thematic sections according to these three participants in a typical medical interaction: Section I, on "Disease, Medicine, and the Imagined Medieval," examines modern representations of "medieval" diseases (real and imagined) and medical interactions (literary and real) that can fruitfully be read through the lens of medical medievalism. Section II, "Doctors at Work in Medieval Worlds," looks at the practitioners themselves—surgeons, physicians, and herbalists, among others—as they appear in novels and movies, video games, and other popular representations. Finally, the three chapters of Section III, "Women's Medicine, Medieval and Modern," explore premodern medical treatments (herbs, fumigations, charms, and more) and their persistence in contemporary culture. This third section differs from the others in focusing not only on women's medicine, as distinguished from generic medieval medical ideas based on an assumed

52 Carolyn Dinshaw, *Getting Medieval: Sexualities and Communities, Pre- and Postmodern* (Durham, NC: Duke University Press, 1999), 46.

male body, but also on the medical traditions of East Asia, as a reminder that the study of "medical medievalism" should not be confined to the Western European borders of traditional medieval studies.

The contributors to Section I explore questions concerning modern representations of disease in the Middle Ages. Because almost every discussion of disease in the Middle Ages focuses unsurprisingly on plague, it is useful here to shift the discussion to other less-discussed diseases, some well-situated in the popular medieval imaginary (leprosy), others associated less with the Middle Ages but still possessing a significant medieval context (lupus), along with fictional diseases that are clearly based on elements of plague or leprosy, such as greyscale in *The Game of Thrones* novel and television series.

According to Luke Demaitre, in his contribution "'Is it Lupus?' — The Wolf in a Disease, from Metaphor to Medicine," synoptic histories of lupus leave gaps between the roots of this disease in vernacular metaphor and its analysis in modern medicine. A strictly scientific perspective leads some authors to disregard the historical context of lupus, to underestimate the significance of popular beliefs about the disease, and to oversimplify the genesis of a complex nosological entity. Demaitre offers a review of the provenance and vagaries of "lupus" (the "wolf") as a disease category, the interactions between learned discourse and lay imagination, the search for a rational classification of the disease, and the persistence of popular responses. The elusiveness of a definition for lupus, together with its continued appeal to imagination, echoes through pop culture in television shows such as *Seinfeld* and *House*.

Similar patterns of popular engagement can be seen in representations of leprosy (understood in medieval contexts as both Hansen's Disease and other skin conditions subsumed under that term) in modern media. Courtney Krolikoski explains in her chapter, "'Have you Come Here to Play Jesus?': The Use and Misuse of Medieval Leprosy in Modern Media," that even though the historiography of leprosy in the Middle Ages has evolved dramatically over the last three decades, modern perceptions of the disease have yet to follow. As such, the use of the terms "leper" and "leprosy" continue to follow popular ideas that have been firmly fixed for many centuries in Western culture, resulting in media images of disfigured individuals shunned by "healthy" society. Indeed, this longstanding image of the ulcerated, begging leper with clapper in hand persists in mainstream media, ranging from lyrics like

U2's *One*, "have you come here to play Jesus / to the lepers in your head?" to articles in magazines like *The Economist* which sensationalize the term through taglines like "Loneliness is the leprosy of the 21st century."[53] Krolikoski confronts this persistent narrative of leprosy, focusing on expulsion and exclusion, by disentangling modern usages of the disease from its historical actors. With over 200,000 new cases of Hansen's Disease each year worldwide, those affected by leprosy are haunted by nineteenth-century physicians' interpretations of medieval sources, read against the backdrop of colonialism.[54] By examining medieval medical texts, like the *Practica* of Bartholomaeus of Salerno, Krolikoski helps dismantle modern narratives of misunderstanding and exclusion by presenting how medieval physicians understood and treated the disease of leprosy. It is important to challenge the exclusion narrative of this disease by examining the historical reality of leprosy in the Middle Ages and to understand the legacy left by decades of research that emphasized exclusion and isolation.

Whereas lupus and leprosy were diseases that genuinely existed in the medieval world, traceable through textual and bioarchaeological evidence, and that continue to afflict people to this day, the disease of "greyscale" is wholly imaginary yet fully situated within an "Imagined Medieval". In her essay, "The Fantasy of Medieval Medicine: Poultices, Dusty Tomes, and the Spice Trade in the Medieval Mediterranean," Robin S. Reich guides us through the complex semiotics of how diseases and treatments are coded as "medieval" within modern fantasy literature, movies, and television series. One of her key examples is the fictional disease known as "greyscale" in George R.R. Martin's *Song of Ice and Fire* novels and their HBO adaptation, *Game of Thrones*. Reich also explores how diseases are diagnosed and treated by fantasy authors like J.R.R. Tolkien in *The Lord of the Rings* and J.K. Rowling in her *Harry Potter* books. These and other fantasy authors frequently situate their medical medievalisms on a binary of "wild wisdom" and "esoteric knowledge,"

---

[53] Maggie Fergusson, "How does it really feel to be lonely?" *The Economist: 1843 Magazine*, 22 Jan 2018, https://www.economist.com/1843/2018/01/22/how-does-it-really-feel-to-be-lonely, accessed June 1 2022.

[54] See Kathleen Vongsathorn and Magnes Vollset, "'Our Loathsome Ancestors': Reinventing Medieval Leprosy for the Modern Word, 1850-1950," in: *Leprosy and Identity in the Middle Ages: From England to the Mediterranean*, edited by Elma Brenner and François-Olivier Touati (Manchester: Manchester University Press, 2021), 347-82.

reproducing in their stories popularly held ideas about the nature of medieval learning as either overly pastoral or overly bookish.

In the final contribution to Section I, "Drinking the Word of God: Qur'anic Healing and Modern Science in Contemporary Egypt," Ana Vinea brings the tools of both medievalism and anthropology to the streets of modern Cairo. Her chapter focuses on a long-standing practice in the Islamic tradition: imbuing water with the Qur'an and drinking it, for prophylactic, therapeutic, and devotional purposes. She analyzes its articulations in contemporary Egypt, particularly in Qur'anic healing, a revivalist form of exorcism and counter-sorcery that in the context of the Islamic revival has gained increased visibility, stirring debates across the religious-secular divide. Through an anthropological analysis of both the pragmatic aspects of drinking the Qur'an and of the discursive space created around it, Vinea shows that Qur'anic healers have reconfigured this popular therapeutic technique, and Islamic healing more broadly, in ways that privilege a normative scientization of healing. Two intersecting threads comprise this reshaping process: a persistent emphasis on the normative, orthodox form of treatment has been fused with attempts to standardize and theorize therapeutic practices by deploying arguments, and notions framed as rooted in science. Qur'anic healers insist that only certain narrow forms of imbuing water with the Qur'an are permitted and argue that modern science demonstrates the effects of reciting the Qur'an over water. Through these processes, Qur'anic healers aim to create a modern science of orthodox healing that is simultaneously rooted in the "correct" Islamic tradition developed in the Middle Ages and aligned with modern, scientific knowledge.

The essays of Section II introduce us to medieval healers themselves—doctors, surgeons, herbalists, and medical teachers, among others—as they have understood and misunderstood in modern media. The first contribution to Section II takes the reader back to the healers and medical practices of the Early Middle Ages. In her chapter, "Early Medieval Surgery: Challenging Popular Stereotypes with Archaeological Evidence," Claire Burridge evaluates and challenges the portrayal in popular culture of medieval surgery, which has long been stereotyped as frightfully primitive. Images of unhygienic conditions, senseless bloodletting, and unrefined barber surgeons tend to come to mind. While research into Islamic medicine, highlighting sophisticated surgical writings and complex diagrams, has begun to influence popular understandings of medieval medicine and overturn these stereotypes, many negative preconceptions remain firmly entrenched in the popular imagination—would anyone have survived 'going under the knife'? Regarding the early medieval West, a period traditionally associated with the stagnation, if not retrogression, of medicine, the near total absence of textual evidence for surgery paints an even bleaker picture: was knowledge of surgery entirely lost during this period?

The archaeological record, and specifically the evidence presented by skeletal remains, offers a different – and less bleak – perspective. Markers of surgical intervention, including significant, invasive procedures like trepanations (the removal of sections of the skull), reveal that, despite a major lacuna in the written record, surgery certainly continued during this time. Furthermore, evidence of healing and long-term care, such as signs of healed infections or the incredible discovery of a lower leg and foot prosthesis, speak to the sophistication and success of some surgical treatments. This chapter will review archaeological evidence for surgery in the early Middle Ages, considering skeletal remains from both insular and continental contexts, to shed light on an area traditionally overlooked by the scholarship given the lack of textual sources. The integration of archaeological evidence offers a much-needed corrective to long-standing stereotypes, challenging popular portrayals of medieval medicine.

In the next chapter, "Avicenna, Prince of Physicians, in Modern Popular Culture," Winston Black shifts the geographical focus of the volume from Europe to Islamicate Asia and the subject matter to modern depictions of a single medieval physician. Black explores the nineteenth- and twentieth-century legacy of the Persian physician and philosopher Ibn Sīnā (ca. 980-1037 CE, known as "Avicenna" in the West). Avicenna's *Canon of Medicine* shaped medical thought and practice in Asia, Europe, and even the Americas for much of the last millennium. Thanks to his overwhelming influence on medical education, Avicenna has been lauded as a founder or "father" of intellectual fields as diverse as chemistry, nephrology, geology, and psychiatry, and is always presented as a clinical physician before his time. With the rise of both modern medicine and the history of medicine, Avicenna also earned a place among the ranks of pop culture icons and nationalist heroes. Black charts the shifting representations of Avicenna in popular culture from the later nineteenth century to the present day. He explores three different, yet overlapping, trends in the portrayal of Avicenna: the efforts of Western physicians like Sir William Osler, who praised Avicenna as a "founder" of medicine, to rebuild Avicenna's tomb in Persia; the adoption of Avicenna as a national Iranian hero by the Pahlavi dynasty (1925-1979) and their construction of the Avicenna Mausoleum and Library to replace his older tomb; and the nationalist adoption of Avicenna by other nations (such as Syria, Tajikistan, Uzbekistan) as witnessed especially by his depiction on their postage stamps. In doing so, Black demonstrates that Avicenna and his medical legacy serve as potent symbols for the validation of modern Islamic states as world leaders in the postcolonial era.

In the final essay of Section II, "Mysteries and Medicine: Medieval Medical Practitioners in Crime Fiction," Lucy Barnhouse provides a systematic and quantitative analysis of medicine in medieval crime fiction, from the descriptions of sickness and disability in the novels, to the depictions of medical practitioners and their materials and knowledge. In popular reviews and scholarship alike, such fiction has often been assessed as featuring anachronistically modern detectives against a realistic medieval background. This image, however, is not borne out by nearly half a century of crime novels featuring medieval medical practitioners as detectives. Rather, medieval Europe is exoticized as a place of dirt, danger, and sickness, where sleuths must solve the (imagined) difficulties of medieval society itself, as well as the crimes with which they are confronted. Modern crime fiction also presents one of the most striking examples of persistent modern ideas about medieval medicine, as the knowledge and skills of fictional medical practitioners (like Brother Cadfael) are often framed in terms of herbal knowledge: their ability to rapidly identify, gather, and apply various mysterious herbs for the treatment of disease and the solving of crimes.

The essays of Section III explore important and contentious areas of medicine and medical medievalism: the treatment of women, the representation of their bodies in medical literature, and the complicated question of continuity between medieval remedies and modern folk or popular medicine. All three of these essays, whether based in the medical traditions of premodern England, Korea, or China, provide examples of the continued use of medieval remedies in contemporary homes, saunas, websites, and birth chambers. Each author also demonstrates how contemporary, virulent debates over women's bodies, abortion, birth control, breastfeeding, infant formula, and sexuality can cloud popular and academic understandings of women's medicine in the Middle Ages.

In her essay, "Global Use of Mugwort in Popular Culture: Its Fumigation Treatment in the *Trotula* and Korean Modern Culture," Minji Lee examines cross-cultural usages of mugwort (understood as several species in the *artemisia* family) fumitory treatments for women's health. She uses mugwort as the focus of a comparison in how different cultures—medieval Europe and modern Korea—shaped the nature of a woman's body and how women wanted to solve their reproductive issues. For example, mugwort is recommended several times in the *Trotula*, a twelfth-century medical collection written in Latin Europe for women's diseases and treatments. According to the *Trotula*, artemisia can be used for treating menstruation retention. Western medieval medicine introduces fumitory treatments with mugwort to regulate the female cycle, but (perhaps surreptitiously) it could also be used as an abortifacient. The herb thus gave women power over conception, but nonetheless reinforced the supremacy of the biological when understanding woman, her power, and her societal possibilities. Mugwort fumitory practice is still present in Korean popular culture. Highly influenced by ancient Chinese medicine, modern Korean folk medicine understands mugwort to be beneficial to women's reproductive organs in general. It is not difficult to find mugwort fumigation in Korean saunas, which advertise that the herb can cure any disorder related to the reproductive body, including infertility or "coldness" from the womb. Looking to the past, we find evidence in the East and the West that suggests that the female body is deficient and needs to be activated from its "cold," "wet," passive state – to be called into the social, as it were, where a woman is only useful if she is a reproductive vessel.

Kristin Uscinski takes a similar approach in her chapter "For to Cause a Woman to Have Milk: Recipes to Promote Lactation for Medieval and Modern Women". Like Lee, Uscinski explores the use of specific plants (such as lettuce and fennel) in both medieval and modern medicine as galactagogues, that is, to increase breastmilk production. Uscinski draws her evidence from an extensive database of recipes drawn from medical texts and recipe collections produced or available in medieval England: the Medieval English Recipes for Women's Healthcare database (MERWH). Formal medical treatises from the Middle Ages, simpler medieval recipes, and popular breastfeeding websites recommend many of the same plants to promote lactation or maternal health in general, but, as Uscinski demonstrates, each is intended for a different sort of audience and provides a different logic behind the herbal pharmacy. A comparison of medieval and modern lactation remedies counters many of the widespread modern negative attitudes—the very same remedies are used today and promoted, if not by professional physicians, then by popular and prominent paramedical associations. It is the medieval recipes in particular, she argues, that provide some of our best evidence for the elusive subject of women's involvement in the supply and practice of medical care in medieval England.

Wee Siang Margaret Ng, in her essay "The Art of Giving Birth in China," examines how households prepared for the birth of a child in Middle Period China. Childbirth was a ubiquitous experience for women and their families and yet it was also described as a leading cause for death for many women. Childbirth took place at home and was handled by women, often with guidance from older women in the family or from midwives. However, most of what we know about childbirth was recorded by men for most of Chinese history. Ng examines how women and their families prepared for the arrival of a new family member, starting with the authoritative work of Chen Ziming's *Furen daquan liangfang* (*All Inclusive Good Prescriptions for Women*, ca. 1271), which contains a list of things a family should prepare a month before childbirth. Some items on this list include seven types of medicinal *san* (powdered formulae), four types of *wan* (pills), several types of roots commonly used in medicinal formulae, alcohol, vinegar, the urine of a young boy, kitchen implements, containers, soap, candles, and a stool. A study of these items will shed light on continuity and change in the material culture associated with childbirth and women's healing practices in medieval and modern Chinese medicine.

Attaining a thorough understanding of medical medievalism, an effort in which this volume can serve as a preliminary step, necessarily embraces not just the history of medicine and the study of medievalism, but also art history, media studies, medical anthropology, transnational and nationalism studies, and a variety of other approaches and disciplines. The three sections and ten contributions of this volume demonstrate that medical medievalism can be approached in many ways, whether through the examination of real and fictional diseases, herbal remedies and surgical procedures, specific doctors or types of healers, and different genres of medical writing and authority (recipes, textbooks, practical manuals, websites). Moreover, like other forms of medievalism, medical medievalism can also be defined by modern popular media. Fictional genres such as novels, comic books, video games, television shows and movies, and genres presented as factual, such as health websites, postage stamps, and medical journals, are thus also important sources for analysis and exploration. In bringing together critical studies of diverse medical medievalisms, this volume aims to provide an impetus for further study, even as it builds on previous work in the long art of scholarship.

SECTION I

Disease, Medicine, and the Imagined Medieval

"IS IT LUPUS?" – THE WOLF IN A DISEASE, FROM METAPHOR TO MEDICINE

LUKE DEMAITRE*

Most television comedies may be superficial and forgettable, but some shows remain vivid in memory, and a few add perspective to the past. This is the case for two popular sitcoms because of particular moments which enlivened the writing of this paper and, in addition, bear directly on the subject of medical medievalism. On a broad spectrum, both sitcoms highlight three simple yet pertinent verities: first, that the crab is not the only animal whose Latin name (*cancer*) has forever triggered dread; second, that the label "leprosy" is not the only one with an emotional impact sharpened by a lack of knowledge; and, third, that supposedly lowbrow and momentary humor can offer food for serious reflection. For thirty years, *Seinfeld* has drawn laughter with the cry, "Lupus, is it lupus?," when a hypochondriac George Costanza is panicking over an apparent cardiac incident.[1] More than a dozen years after the airing of *House,* guffaws still greet the gruff declaration, "It's never lupus!," when a grumpy Dr. Gregory House repeatedly dismisses the guesses of his staff about a patient's symptoms.[2] If, as is likely, this levity about a grave

* Independent scholar.

[1] *Seinfeld,* season 2, episode 8, "The Heart Attack," directed by Tom Cherones, aired April 25, 1991, on NBC.

[2] *House.* 2007. Season 4, Episode 8, "You Don't Want to Know," directed by Lesli Linka Glatter. November 20, 2007, on Fox.

disease is perceived as hurtful, it is helpful to keep in mind that the humor targets the ignorant rather than the affected.

The comical impetus of both sitcom memes flows ultimately from the mysteriousness of the disease's manifestations and processes. Paradoxically, and on parallel tracks, this mysteriousness is also a primary source of keen anxiety among the populace, while the elusiveness of diagnosis and identification has frustrated medical understanding for centuries. Both memes are of broader interest, as echoes of the closeness *and* the distance between common opinion and scientific induction (recent strife has made us more conscious of this distance). The bedside scenes, with their loosely clinical setting, hint at the divergences between everyday parlance and standardized nomenclature, between the given name and actual nature of a disease, and even between viewpoints within medicine. The broad and lasting appeal of both scenes suggests that the themes strike a common chord across viewers and years. This constancy, however, is not synonymous with continuity: the erratic itinerary of lupus disproves the linear view of history which prevails in surveys of the disease. It is worth emphasizing at the outset that medieval *lupus* has little in common with the nominal counterparts in immunology or dermatology, except for the generic references to ulceration and redness. There are multiple gaps and radical differences between the first mention of "the disease called *lupus*" and the current pathology of, to be precise, Systemic Lupus Erythematosus (SLE) and Discoid Lupus Erythematosus (DLE—aka Lupus vulgaris, or Tuberculosis luposa).[3] The differences should, in turn, make us cautious about drawing retrospective diagnoses from early or, worse, sketchy reports.

The association of a disease with the wolf, *lupus* in Latin, occurs first in medieval records. It appears that lupus is the longest extant medical category or concept with roots in popular lore rather than in the classical legacy of Hippocrates, Galen, and Celsus or, at least, that it is the oldest disease label with origins in German or French conversation rather than in the Greek or Latin vocabulary. The absence of the label among ancient disease names is surprising in view of the primeval presence of the wolf in the Mediterranean world. The association is first recorded in a Christian miracle story which dates back about a thousand years, and

[3] The distance is covered concisely yet with care by M. Rampudda, P. Marson, and G. Pasero, "Le principali tappe nella storia del lupus eritematoso sistemico – The main stages in the history of systemic lupus erythematosus," *Reumatismo*, 61 (2009), 145-152.

which is often cited, but arguably misinterpreted, in the current literature. The authors largely ignore the subsequent and probably independent development of lupus in medicine as a disease category. I hope to set the record straight by revisiting the early story and tracing the centuries-long course of medical teaching. My hope is tempered by a full awareness that, as a leading expert admitted in 2014, "We will probably never completely know the exact, true origins of the term 'lupus.'"[4]

The intellectual humility of this admission stands in direct contrast with the certitude of the brief histories which, while widely available, are in dire need of a revision. My search for the source and first uses of the label found an additional stimulus in the prevalence of inaccurate summaries in advertising posts and encyclopedia entries, as might be expected, but even in professional literature. Largely defective assertions have become stereotypical, reiterated without correction, and disseminated ever more widely over the internet. A simplistic synopsis is easily adopted as reliable, especially when it is created by a specialist for open access, as in the case of this garbled and misleading paragraph by a doctor of medicine:

> *A biography of St. Martin* gives us the first example of when the term lupus was used. St. Martin lived in the 4th century and *treated* the Bishop of Liège. The description of the disease is *consistent with lupus…* The history of lupus goes back even further than the 4th century. The *first known documented case of lupus* was recorded by Hippocrates in the year 400 BC.[5]

If the specific distortions do not immediately stand out in these lines, notwithstanding the italics, they will become obvious in the light of the evidence. The most deceptive misrepresentations lurk in historical sketches when these introduce seemingly knowledgeable discussions. This is particularly true for scientific articles, as in this instance from a medical journal:

---

[4] Donald E. Thomas, Jr., *The Lupus Encyclopedia. A Comprehensive Guide for Patients and Families* (Baltimore: Johns Hopkins University Press, 2014), 5.

[5] Robert A. Norman, "The History of Lupus Erythematosus and Discoid Lupus: From Hippocrates to the Present," *Lupus Open Access* 1:1 (2016), www.longdom.org/open-access/the-history-of-lupus-erythematosus-and-discoid-lupus-fromhippocrates-to-the-present-Lupus-1000102.pdf (emphases mine). Accessed March 15, 2022.

> The earliest usage of the term lupus in the *English* literature is in the *10th century biography of St. Martin*, written *in 963 AD*. Rogerius Frugardi (*1230 AD*) used the term lupus to describe erosive *facial* lesions. In t*he superstitious Middle Ages*, the *grotesque* appearance of some lupus sufferers brought the myth of *werewolves* to the minds of people.[6]

The highlighted misstatements and clichés in this quotation set markers for our review of, respectively, the time and place, cultural setting, anatomical assignment, and conceptual course of the original association.

Few authors have yet attempted to pinpoint the time and place at which a bodily condition was first associated with the wolf.[7] Anthropologists may be able to shed light on a potential context of surging awareness of the wolf in certain areas or eras. For our inquiry, it suffices to realize that no one has methodically pursued the documentary trail which was opened by a German pioneer in historical as well as scientific research almost 150 years ago. The "father of modern pathology," Rudolf Virchow, pointed to writings which he attributed to the School of Salerno and to the thirteenth century, but he did not consider this a conclusive estimate. He mused, "the history of lupus very likely goes back farther, to Constantine and the Arabs; at this time, however, I leave it to the research of others to find the original source."[8] He was right in pointing beyond the thirteenth and twelfth centuries, as we have learned since. With Constantinus Africanus and the Arabs, on the other hand, Virchow chose the wrong direction because the source may, ironically, have lain much closer to his own homeland.

---

[6] Ravi K. Mallavarapu and Edwin W. Grimsley, "The History of Lupus Erythematosus," *Southern Medical Journal*, 100.9 (2007), 896 (emphases mine). Even a detailed historical essay may transmit a far-fetched misrepresentation, such as, "dermatological descriptions of SLE were made by Herbernus of Tours in 916 and was termed herpes esthiomenos," Satoshi Hayakawa [M.D.] et al., "Rembrandt's Maria Bockenolle has a butterfly rash and digital deformities: Overlapping syndrome of rheumatoid arthritis and systemic lupus erythematosus," *Medical Hypotheses*, 68 (2007), 908.

[7] One of the few is the rheumatologist Donald Thomas, MD (see note 2 above), whose earnest interest in history was an appreciated source of encouragement and inspiration for my inquiry.

[8] Rudolf Virchow, "Historische Notizen über Lupus," *Archiv für pathologische Anatomie und Physiologie und für klinische Medizin* 32 (1865), 139-43, at 142.

The first person to enter history as a "lupus" patient was a tenth-century native of Saxony and close confidant of the German Emperor Otto I. The bishop of Liège from 959 to 971, Eraclius (*aka* Heraclius, Everaclus, Ebrachar, or Eracle), was reportedly cured at the tomb of St Martin (d. 397) in Tours. He had been a student in Cologne, master of students and then provost at the cathedral of Bonn, before he became abbot of the Benedictine abbey of Lobbes, which was a prize fief of the bishop of Liège. The city of Liège (presently the economic and cultural center of Wallonia, in Belgium) lay on the crossroads between the eastern and western realms that emerged from the division of the Carolingian Empire and which ultimately coalesced into the countries of Germany and France. Although it is now thoroughly francophone (with denizens who, some say, speak "the purest French"), Liège grew out of a foundation by Germanic Franks (*Vicus Leudicus* or "People's Settlement" in a record of 558 CE) and for centuries it was more closely aligned with the Rhine than with the Seine. The Germanic background and milieu of Eraclius will prove relevant to our inquiry, although they are easily overlooked because his cure was staged in the heart of West Francia, and the miracle story flowed from the original Latin versions into the French tradition.

The most captivating way to introduce the story, which evolved early in two directions, is to have it told in the first person. In this version, Eraclius himself recounts a visit to the tomb of Saint Martin in the 960s, after "hearing about the powerful miracles which happened incessantly there." The autobiographical style of the account immediately captures the reader's attention:

> When I was gravely stricken and nearly killed by the disease which is called "the wolf," I traveled to Tours in the hope of recovering my health. I stayed in the church of the illustrious saint day and night, with tears and sighs, vigils and fasts, and prayers. The seventh night, when from exhaustion I had fallen into a sort of ecstasy, Blessed Martin appeared to me.

The saint, who had been bishop of Tours six centuries earlier (371-397), "touched the affected place with the end of his staff," pronounced complete recovery, and "disappeared from my sight." The retinue of clergy and knights with their servants were summoned, and they arrived together with "the entire venerable college of Canons." They were unable to "find the place of the ailment which I had suffered in the buttocks, although a thin reddish line was left as a visible scar." The clergy celebrated this "bright and glorious miracle, and the devout people raised their voices to heaven with praise."[9]

The remainder of the purported testimony has Eraclius declare that, shortly after his return to Liège, he built a church "in honor of my healer," endowed it "most lavishly," and gave it a permanent chapter or *collegium* of thirty canons who followed "the custom of Tours." The use of this first-person account as an affidavit for certifying a foundation favors the doubts of skeptics. Such doubts are understandably reinforced by the concluding deference to the chapter of Tours – and by the chapter's assertive appropriation of the alliance.[10] Some of the skeptics not only dismiss "cette narration ridicule et certainement apocryphe" ("this ridiculous and certainly apocryphal story") but even insist that it originated outside Liège.[11] These dismissals have drawn passionate responses, as well as the sensible compromise proposition that, in spite of serious problems and inconsistencies, "au fond cette relation est véridique" ("at its root this story is truthful").[12] It is indeed too one-sided and misleading to reject the entire account as "ridiculous" and, even more categorically, as utterly worthless testimony. Neither the most exhaustive criticism of the account, nor the most cogent reasoning that it was forged in Tours, precludes the possibility – or even the likelihood – that an anecdote first told in Liège provided the nucleus for this and other accounts of Eraclius's affliction and healing. Furthermore, an anecdote usually has some basis, however trivial or tenuous, in someone's experience or impression. Similarly, even the most fantastic miracle story contains echoes, however faint, of an actual event, situation, or perception. What could have been the reason why Eraclius was reported to have been cured from a particular affliction that has no counterpart in

[9] Aubertus Miraeus [Albert le Mire], *Opera diplomatica et historica...: Codex donationum piarum*, second edition (Brussels: Francis Foppens, 1723), 1: 653. In this and subsequent quotations, translations into English are my own.

[10] See, for example, the versions of the charter reproduced in Jean Berthollet, *Histoire de l'institution de la Fête-Dieu avec la vie des bienheureuses Julienne et Eve, toutes deux originaires de Liège* (Liège: Jacques-Antoine Gerlach, 1781), 71-77 and xxi-xxxviii.

[11] Albert Poncelet, "Bulletin des publications hagiographiques," *Analecta Bollandiana* Tomus 23 (1904), 331.

[12] Edouard Maréchal, *Éracle et la fondation de la collégiale Saint Martin à Liége* (Liège: Dessain, 1894), 25.

other miracle stories? Ultimately, however, our inquiry aims neither to determine whether Eraclius wrote the testimony nor to verify that he actually incurred a disease called lupus.

Neither a debate about the authenticity of the affidavit nor skepticism about miraculous healing should blur our focus on the questions of when, where, whence, and how the wolf entered into the narrative – and how *lupus* wandered through the development of a medical category. If tentative answers forego Eraclius's authorship and his tenure in the See of Liège, they should allow for the likely agency of his successor Notger (972-1008), which extends the time frame, confirms the Liège setting, and continues the coexistence of Germanic and Gallic ties. Notger ostensibly favored the patron saint of Tours, who was venerated on both sides of the Rhine. His devotion to Saint Martin is a salient strand in his bonds with both the Capetian king Robert II and the wife of Emperor Otto I, Adelaide.[13] The most persuasive suggestion that Notger played a role in the development of the so-called affidavit is that he was the bishop who actually instituted the revenues for thirty canons to make the church of St Martin in Liège "collegial." In fact, he further managed to have Otto III convert a grant (*precarium*) to Eraclius into a donation to the same church.[14] It is clear that Notger would have been eminently motivated to legitimize the foundation with a compelling account of indebtedness to Saint Martin, to promote the story of a miracle which linked Liège and Tours, and to seize on a memorable incident in his predecessor's life.

The continuity between Eraclius and Notger sets the stage for the evolution of a rumor into a tale which was formulated for buttressing an ecclesiastical foundation. For our inquiry, the story introduces a popular tradition which associated wolf and disease. A fundamental factor in the continuity was the Germanic culture and language in which Eraclius and Notger were steeped as scions of, respectively, Saxon and Swabian aristocracy. Throughout their lives, they were regularly involved in the politics, court affairs, and family matters of the Ottonian dynasty. The involvement culminated in the ascent of Notger to the rank of prince-bishop with the imperial grant of a county. Both bishops traveled

[13] Jean-Louis Kupper, *Notger de Liège (972-1008)* (Brussels: Académie Royale de Belgique, 2015), 66-67 and 79-80. It is worth adding that, by virtue of her provenance, Empress Adelaide of Burgundy personified the cultural overlaps – as well as the territorial tensions – between the eastern and western realms.

[14] Kupper, *Notger de Liège*, 31n4 and 66n6.

extensively with the self-styled "Holy Roman Emperors," particularly to Italy on political missions, in military campaigns, and for ambitious coronations. The bishops' energetic travels occasionally sharpened their tensions with the papal claimants to the Roman legacy, as well as with dynastic kin in Francia. Notwithstanding such frictions, Eraclius and Notger cultivated relations with the See of Saint Peter as well as with their Gallicized neighbors. These elements of commonality expand the background for reconstructing the genesis of the "must read" (*legendum*) account of Eraclius's affliction and miraculous recovery. In addition, the continuity – together with their shared Germanic heritage – will shed light on the reason why the wolf appeared here, and even on the vagaries of *lupus* as a medical category.

If the "affidavit" of Eraclius is dismissed as a forgery, it nevertheless proves the existence of a story. What is more, it appears to represent one direction (even a stage, perhaps) in the development of the narrative, from a seminal anecdote to a full-grown legend. Before comparing this text with varying versions, we should note that neither an eleventh-century chronicle of Liège bishops nor a late-twelfth-century biography of Eraclius mentions the miracle.[15] This silence has served as a pivotal argument against the authenticity of the first-person account, but it does not prove that the story itself was complete fiction. Furthermore, in a search for the earliest association of an ailment with "lupus," the challenges to alleged authorship do not invalidate the proposition of Eraclius's and Notger's tenures as time frame. More important, these challenges should not raise doubts about contemporaneous Germanic – or, more precisely, Liégeois – familiarity with the wolf.

It is probably not by sheer accidental coincidence that, in the very same milieu, a teacher at bishop Notger's school featured the voracious animal prominently in a reader for his students. *Magister* Egbert of Liège poignantly played on the community's constant anxiety about the "swiftly roaming wolf" (*discurrens obiter lupus*) in his reader. In one little story, which "countryfolk (*pagenses*) know how to tell," he introduced a girl in "a dress woven of red wool." Running out of the house, "footloose and forgetting all danger," the girl is captured by a wolf who brings her

[15] Renier de Saint-Laurent (d. 1188), *Vita Evraclii*, in *Monumenta Germaniae Historica* 20 (1868), 561-565. Hubert Silvestre, "Notes sur la 'Vita Evracli' de Renier de Saint-Laurent. Contribution à l'histoire littéraire du XIIe siècle Liégeois," *Revue d'histoire ecclésiastique* 44 (1949), 29-86.

to his forest lair to be eaten by his cubs – but these, "dropping their wildness and unable to harm (*lacerare*) her," stroke her head.[16] Historians view Egbert's verses as the earliest Indo-European precursor to the tale of Little Red Riding Hood. The tale has broad relevance to our questions about the long, complicated, and mysterious development of a disease label, with parallel exchanges between oral and written transmissions, lay and learned interpretations, and between vernacular and Latin formulations – in fact, even between French and German versions.

The stories about Eraclius included a more directly pertinent coincidence between local "lupine" mythology, about which more below, and they retained their theatrical character for centuries. When the bishop returned to Liège from his arduous journeys on horseback, his retainers presented colorful travelogues which ended, in superb irony, at the "buttocks (*natibus*)" of the venerable bishop. An alert student of history cannot ignore the twofold likelihood that officials chose the most evocative label for the ailment healed in a consequential miracle, and that there was a layer of less dignified memories which endured – even if they were neither eternalized nor broadcast. Would rebellious vassals not have sneered at their lord's humbling weakness, or ribald *vilains* not have snickered about their prelate's inflamed behind? Be that as it may, the formal narrative preserved the earliest recorded mention of a widely known ailment. It is worth emphasizing that the story introduced neither a new medical label nor the first mention of the disease which is still called lupus. Hence, the challenge here is to learn where or how the label entered the medical nomenclature and, most important, what health-related category (or entities) it covered before the emergence of current definitions.

The colloquial origin of lupus as the name of an ailment, while self-evident in the Liège chronicle, was underscored when the medical authors adopted the phrase, "qui Lupus vulgo dicitur." The phrase "vulgo dicitur" covers a wide semantic range, with the latitude and looseness of premodern taxonomies, from "in vernacular parlance" or

[16] Egbert von Lüttich, *Fecunda Ratis*, Part II, verses 472-485, ed. Ernst Voigt (Halle: Max Niemeyer 1889), 232-233. English translation of the entire poem, by Robert Gray Babcock, *The Well-Laden Ship. Egbert of Liège.* Dumbarton Oaks Medieval Library, Book 25 (Cambridge, MA: Harvard University Press, 2013). See Jan Ziolkowski, "A Fairy Tale from before Fairy Tales: Egbert of Liège's 'De puella a lupellis seruata' and the Medieval Background of 'Little Red Riding Hood'," *Speculum* 67 (1992), 549-575.

"named by lay people" to the broader "commonly called." Physicians and surgeons suggested a distance between colloquial usage and their methodical approach or, eventually, between the general application and more narrowly focused discussions among teachers. The common factor, in the range of significations as well as in the overlap between the notarial and medical mentions, is the voracity for which the wolf was notorious. The vernacular association between the bishop's ailment "called *lupus*" and the "eating" or corrosive process is central to the Liège miracle story. This association foreshadowed two constants in the early and erratic attempts to classify lupus. First, corrosion as an essentially external process kept the disease outside the range of systemic malfunctions or, in less anachronistic terms, at the margin of the framework of humors and complexions – even as this framework guided a gradual but haphazard expansion of the combination, "corrosive and biting humors."[17] Second, the notion of eating continued to define lupus, not only in German and other vernacular mentions but also in the evolving taxonomy of diseases until at least the dawn of dermatology, as we shall see.

The facts summarized above indicate that the term "wolf" entered medicine from popular idiom, that German usage was common in Liège around 1000 CE, and that an affliction by that name became eternalized in memories of Bishop Eraclius. If we accept this as a threefold premise, with due reservations, the fate of the story itself presents a map for our further exploration. As primary (though not prime) evidence and evolving testimony, the narrative survives in a group of versions which, when compared with the first-person account, reveal the divergence – and even, I believe, the transition – between a commonplace saying and a medical category. It is impossible to certify a textual dependence or chronological sequence because there are no extant manuscripts to document direct or even intermittent transmission of the story. In the absence of successive copying, we depend on transcriptions which were printed after 1600. This dependence adds a shade of caution to inferences from a comparison of editions which were so far removed from the original sources. Nevertheless, certain variants stand out as shared by the third-person accounts and absent from the affidavit, and there is no

[17] See, for example, Gilbert of England (below, at n. 24). Later, in the surgical encyclopedia (1363) of Guy de Chauliac: *Guigonis de Cauliaco (Guy de Chauliac) Inventarium sive Chirurgia magna*, ed. Michael R McVaugh, Volume One: Text (Leiden: E.J. Brill, 1987), 215. Further, Ingrassia (see below, at n. 43).

reason to doubt that these variants took shape between 1000 and 1300. This assumption is sound enough for correlating the Liège tradition with other sources of that time, and for exploring the broader context of the convergence between wolf and disease.

Divergences in one particular alternate version of the Eraclius story demonstrate the range of imagination among copyists (and readers), as would be expected. More pertinently, they also indicate a degree of medicalization, an emerging distance between folklore and scientific discussion, and even a whiff of tension between physicians and surgeons. By means of textual collation, it is possible to strain out the earliest and arguably original version of the account as embedded in "The Miracles of Blessed Martin" which are attributed to an author now referred to as "pseudo-Hebernus" and dated (speculatively) to the late tenth century. In the early thirteenth century, Gilles (Egidius) of Orval adopted an apparently expanded version from an intermediate source which I am unable to identify. The Cistercian monk continued a chronicle which had covered the Liège bishops up to 1048 but which, as I noted earlier, was silent on the miracle.[18] Here again, silence does not prove absence, although it suggests that the memories congealed only after 1048 into an event worth chronicling.

It is safe to assume that Gilles drew on an established record for reporting, as a historical fact, that Eraclius suffered from a "disease which is commonly called 'the wolf'" (*morbo qui Lupus vulgo dicitur*). The narrator elaborated,

> The illness, which struck his buttocks, attacked his flesh so violently that it consumed, corroded and devoured it in a wolfish fashion (*lupino more*). The only relief was to apply two plucked and eviscerated chickens every morning and evening against this wolfish rage (*lupine rabiei*). With physicians despairing (*desperantibus medicis*) and with every treatment (*cura*) exhausted to no avail, the bishop was entirely deprived of human health as if about to die.

[18] The chronicle which Gilles continued was written by Heriger of Lobbes (d. 1007) and Anselm of Liège (d. 1056). See notes 15 above and 19 below.

The chronicler added graphic details, for example, that "great discomfort forced [the bishop] to remain prone" day and night. He was equally precise on the immediate reactions to the stunning recovery.

> The bishop, now awake, checked the place of the wound with his hand. But his servants, fearing that he would irritate the itch, stopped him. He said, "Fear not, Saint Martin has returned me to health." They suspected that he might be talking in his sleep, but he said, "Light the torches, come, and see the place where the disease was." They lit the torches and rushed after him into the chapter of the church.

The miracle story ended in a theatrical climax, with the servants removing the bishop's dressings and retrieving, "intact, the chickens which they had applied to the disease as if to an insatiable monster."[19]

The droll closing vignette should not distract us from the inference that the chronicle diverged from the first-person account by including the words *vulgo*, *medici*, and *cura.* Less striking variants suggest or presage several subtle yet meaningful developments in meaning. The difference between Eraclius as being "stricken" (*attritus*) and as having "suffered" (*patiebar*) echoes the shift in emphasis from acute to chronic. The added observation, that the affliction fed on the outside but "consumed internal matter even more intensely," presages a conceptual expansion of the simple popular idiom.[20] The digressions and variants become significant in the perspective of the twelfth century, which historians of the Middle Ages single out as fertile in a wide range of areas, including medical learning. One of many notable representatives of the spectrum was Peter of Blois who, after studying liberal arts in Tours, law in Bologna, and theology in Paris, served as diplomat in Angevin Sicily and in Henry II's England, from where he set out on the Third Crusade with Richard I Lionheart.

Peter's vast correspondence demonstrates a certain familiarity with medicine, for example in a letter to his brother around 1170.[21] He

---

[19] "Miraculum auctore Aegidio Aureaevallensi," *Gesta Episcoporum Leodiensium* II.48, in *Monumenta Germaniae Historica Scriptores* 25 (1880), 54.

[20] *Miraculum auctore Aegidio Aureaevallensi*, 25: 54.

[21] See Urban T. Holmes Jr. and Frederick R. Weedon, "Peter of Blois as a Physician", *Speculum*, 37 (1962), 252-256; François-Olivier Touati, "Maladies et pratiques médicales,

reported that Stephen, the archbishop-elect of Palermo, had died in Jerusalem after joining a crusading venture in order to escape seditious Sicily.

> The lord chancellor fell victim to fate when herpes estiomenus, which is commonly (*vulgo*) called "the wolf," severely afflicted his thigh, and all the tools of the medical men failed. In the ends, he expired in the Holy City of God, in the king's arms and in the midst of weeping princes. From the trustworthy report of travelers I have now also learned that, to avenge Lord Stephen, the city of Catania has been struck and knocked down by an earthquake.[22]

Our perspective on the wanderings of "the wolf" gains precision from a comparison between the accounts of Stephen's and Eraclius's predicaments. The narratives shared the tropes of tearful sighs, failing physicians, and deadly danger. The actualization of this danger, from the condition of Eraclius "as if about to die" to the tragic end of Stephen, subtly implies that *lupus* had acquired a more lethal character.

The date, together with the aside on Sicily, makes Peter's letter a key to a chronological and geographical context that is quite revealing. The lively twelfth-century flow between North and South accelerated the dissemination of the wolf idiom across linguistic borders, including between vernaculars and Latin, and, most significant, it promoted the medical adoption of "lupus." It is likely, though perhaps surprising, that this adoption took place south of the Alps. The same region and period also produced a landmark manual on surgery, written by Roger Frugardi, who was once known as "Salernitanus," although he was a Lombard. Although the designation of lupus by Roger is nearly contemporaneous with that of Peter, there are noticeable differences. On the basis of his educated knowledge of medicine, Peter presented lupus as a "commonly" (*vulgo*) used label, which he correlated with "herpes estiomenus," the classically established term for a creeping (Greek *herpes*, Latin *serpens*) corrosion. For Roger, herpes estiomenus was the principal

---

IXe-XIVe siècle. Pierre de Blois. La transmission d'un dossier médical à un confrère", in *Sources d histoire médiévale*, eds. Ghislain Brunel and Elisabeth Lalou (Paris: Larousse, 1992), 786-788.

[22] Jacques-Paul Migne, *Patrologiae Latinae cursus completus*, 207 (Paris: Garnier, 1855), col. 293.

entity which "is called 'eating itself' and, by another name, is called 'lupus.'" His statement may suggest that the appellation had moved from the "common" usage noted by Peter of Blois to the equivalence of "another name" in the learned vocabulary. The equation was subject to disagreement between those who wanted greater precision and others who preferred the simplicity of straightforward equivalence. Roger's *Cyrurgia* was still quite new when Lombard commentators specified that lupus was a type of cancer which affected the lower body, in distinction with *cingulus* and *noli me tangere*, which struck, respectively, the middle and the face. In contrast, when Guido d'Arezzo the Younger edited the same *Cyrurgia*, he seized on the equation for chiding the *medici* for making matters more complicated "in order to be seen doing *something*."[23]

The near-contemporaneous mentions of lupus by the Liège chronicler Gilles in the Holy Roman Empire, the French-Italian-English Peter of Blois, the Lombard surgeon Roger Frugardi, and the Tuscan Master of Arts Guido d'Arezzo, attest to European interactions – around the Mediterranean, through the Italian peninsula, and across the Alps, from Sicily to England. Such interactions were also evident in the entire career of Eraclius, particularly when he accompanied Emperor Otto I on his Calabrian campaign in 968. His entire life makes it tempting to conjecture that thoughts of the wolf for his affliction sprang spontaneously from the maelstrom of Gallic, Teutonic, and north-Italian mythology. It is equally tempting to assume that the category had roots in the medical learning which was beginning to thrive in southern Italy, especially in Salerno. Rather than confirming this assumption, however, my exploration of the writings which many still call "Salernitan" has not yet returned a mention of lupus by any of a half dozen or so associated "masters" (Archimatteus, Bartholomeus, Copho, Gariopontus, Johannes Platearius, Johannes de Sancto Paulo, and Petrocellus) even if they devoted considerable attention to skin diseases.[24]

This apparent silence may suggest the limited interest of *physica* in external afflictions as primarily the concern of *chirurgia*. Moreover, the

---

[23] *Rogerii, Cancellarii studii montispessulani, summa, sive Rogerina major, minor et media*, Paris, Bibliothèque Nationale de France, MS lat. 7065, fols. 58 and 59.

[24] Salvatore de Renzi et al., eds., *Collectio Salernitana*, 5 vols. (Naples: Filiatre-Sebezio, 1852-1859). Most typical: Gariopontus, *Passionarius*, Book V, in London, Wellcome Library, MS MSL 133 (late 12th century), fols. 89r-127v, available online at https://wellcome collection.org/works/z9xqdeax.

category was probably too new for the so-called Salernitan authors, who adhered to a traditional and rather basic classification of skin conditions. In contrast, the category drew the attention of thirteenth-century Lombard surgeons, although these, in turn, preferred tradition over some innovative classifications by physicians who taught in the new faculties of medicine. Thus, Bruno da Longoburgo set aside the classification of lupus by the *magistri* as a type of cancer, and he rejected their differentiation "according to complexional quality, as they say that lupus and cancer result from a red bile which is more fiery than the one which causes noli me tangere." For emphasis, he added, "I, Bruno da Longoburgo, do not see any truth in this [humoral] differentiation, for the simple reason that I do not find a trace of it in the books of the ancients."[25]

The place of lupus in the taxonomy of diseases proved unclear for mid-thirteenth-century writers. Around the time when Bruno was rejecting the physicians' differentiations, the encyclopedist Bartholomew the Englishman (cited more conventionally as Bartholomeus Anglicus) ranked lupus, among the corrosive *apostemata*, as more corrosive than "nolimetangere" and cancer, but less aggressive than "herisipila." However, Bartholomew did not clarify the ranking of lupus, and he fused "herisipila" with "estiomenus," as well as with sacred fire.[26] His contemporary and compatriot Gilbert the Englishman (Gilbertus Anglicus), on the other hand, adhered to the equation of lupus with herpes estiomenus and to the explanation by "yellow bile that is burned and thick," but he attempted to combine various qualitative and symptomatic criteria with the humoral differentiation.

> If unnatural [yellow] bile ascends and is burned, the result is erysipelas, that is, sacred fire. If it is greatly condensed, the result is lupus. If the bile is thin and liquid, it produces blisters resembling millet seeds [this was called *herpes miliaris*]. Lupus differs from erysipelas because the place blackens and the corrosion is greater; it differs from cancer because it corrodes more, deeper, and fast, and there is a strong foul

[25] Bruno da Longoburgo, *Chirurgia magna*, in *Cyrurgia Guidonis de cauliaco. Et Cyrugia Bruni, Theodorici, Rogerij, Bertipalie, Lanfranci* (Venice: Bonetus Locatelli, 1498), fol. 90ra.

[26] Bartholomeus Anglicus, *De proprietatibus rerum*, Paris, Bibliothèque Nationale de France, MS lat. 17817, fol. 78v.

> odor at the onset, with prickliness and burning. Advanced lupus is known from the hardness, blackening and in-depth corrosion of the part, and sometimes also from the consumption of the part.[27]

The distinctions lost much of their relevance, however, when Gilbert asserted that "all the things which cure cancer cure lupus and inversely."[28] This assertion was repeated in the therapeutic sections of many compendia, even though it often ran counter to the theoretical differentiations between *apostemata* due to bile, such as lupus or herpes estiomenus, and disorders due to black bile, most notably cancer.

The taxonomy of *apostemata* (which covered far more than the abscesses, ulcers, and tumors of the usual English translations) remained fluid and inconsistent for centuries, and yet there were threads of continuity. Shortly after Gilbert, Teodorico de' Borgognoni promoted the three-way equation of lupus, herpes estiomenus, and cancer. In the most authoritative of several textbooks known as *Magna chirurgia*, Teodorico devoted a relatively short chapter of his section on *apostemata* to "Herpestiomenus, or lupus" (III.9, between III.8, "De formice sive noli me tangere," and III.10, "De cancrenis").[29] He stated that herpes estiomenus "is called lupus by another name" and, even though he dismissed the assertion "by newcomers" (*a modernis*) that lupus was a type of cancer, he implied that the three were interchangeable in practice, since "in sum, the treatment of herpes estiomenus is the treatment of cancer." We are left to wonder whether he also treated cancer and lupus with the caustic and regenerative medications which, as he claimed, he had always applied to herpes estiomenus with good results, "Ego autem semper curavi sic, et bene."[30]

In 1275, Guglielmo da Saliceto maintained the three-way equation in the chapter on cancer in his textbook of surgery, *Cyrurgia*; it is worth noting that he did not mention lupus in his medical compendium titled

---

[27] Gilbertus Anglicus, *Compendium medicine* (Lyon: Portonaris, 1510), fol. CCCXXXIIv.
[28] Gilbertus Anglicus, *Compendium*, fol. CCCXXXIII.
[29] Teodorico, in *Cyrurgia Guidonis*, fol. 127va. It may be noted that Teodorico associates the facial *noli me tangere* with bites of the ant, *formix* (*formica* in conventional Latin). For the signal role of Teodorico, see Francesca Roversi Monaco, ed., *Teoria e pratica medica nel basso Medioevo. Teodorico Borgognoni vescovo, chirurgo, ippiatra* (Firenze: SISMEL - Edizioni del Galluzzo, 2019).
[30] Teodorico, in *Cyrurgia Guidonis*, fols. 126va and 127vb.

Summa conservationis et curationis, most likely because he considered it a surgical concern. The reader of the *Summa* could infer that lupus shared with other corrosive diseases not only the aggressive behavior but also a vernacular origin of the label and the elusiveness to classification. These three points are evident when Guglielmo speculates that *herpes estiomenus* continues:

> unceasingly to gnaw (*corrodere*) the body part, and to wander while gnawing, until it destroys and kills the body part unless it is restrained by medicinal or divine means. On account of the way it gnaws and wanders, it is called she-wolf (*lupa*) or erisipila by laypeople (*laicis*), although erysipelas differs from herpes estiomenus because erysipelas does not wander and it affects only the skin.[31]

Guglielmo's student, the surgeon Lanfranco of Milan, found that some of his "rustic" colleagues (*rudales chirurgici*) settled for the imprecision of laypeople; yet he, too, seemed rather nonchalant about the terminology for herpes estiomenus.

> Some call this disease cancer, some lupus, some – as in France – Our Lady's Evil; some Lombards call it Saint Antony's Fire, and some eating erysipelas. You should not worry about the different names, however.[32]

In a paradox that is at least as old as Galen, insouciant dismissals of name variants often came in one breath with insistent calls for differential nomenclature.

Henri de Mondeville, who studied with Teodorico and Guglielmo, stated that "herpes is generally (*communiter*) called lupus or cancer or eating erysipelas," and that the same *apostema* "goes by different names in

---

[31] *Liber Guilielmi Placentini de Saliceto in scientia medicinali qui Summa conservationis et curationis appellatur Cyrugia* (Venice, printer unknown, 1489), fol. 154. On the fortunes of the label "erysipilas" (modern spelling "erysipelas") until the mid-sixteenth century, see Angela Foscati, "Un'analisi semantica del termine erysipelas. Le Centuriae di Amato Lusitano nella tradizione dei testi dall'Antichità al Rinascimento," in Miguel Ángel González Manjarrés, ed., Praxi theoremata coniungamus. *Amato Lusitano y la medicina de su tiempo* (Madrid: Guillermo Escobar, 2019), 125-143.

[32] Lanfranc, *Practica seu ars completa totius cyrurgie* (Venice: Bonetus Locatelli, 1498), fol. 185ra.

various regions" – including "Saint Laurent's evil" in his native Normandy. Henri's acceptance of common equivalences was consistent with his position that, since the same treatment could address different conditions, "we surgeons, who are more practical, do not inquire in depth" into distinctions about which "physicians disagree among themselves."[33] By this time, physicians as well as surgeons were treating lupus as fully synonymous with herpes estiomenus, which became the dominant term – perhaps because they preferred a category with a classical pedigree over a label with unlearned roots. Nevertheless, the label endured on its own, and the precipitous voracity of the wolf was never eclipsed by the serpentine advance of herpes. In any event, both names perpetuated the notion of progressive corrosion or "eating."

Some medical authors dismissed literal interpretations of "eating" for lupus, while others extended the wolf metaphor to other diseases. Guy de Chauliac, in 1363, even declared that leprosy, *lepra*, "is named for the wolf, because it devours all the members like a cancerous wolf."[34] Whereas medical authors conventionally associated leprosy with the advancing "breakdown (*corruptio*)" of the entire body, they generally saw the epitome of voraciousness in cancer, which in their discussions often came close to being the same as lupus.[35] This closeness becomes explicit in Guy's report that many practitioners, when treating ulcerated cancer,

> mitigate the malignity and wolfishness (*lupacitatem*) with a scarlet cloth and with the application of the meat of hens: this is why people say that it is called "the wolf," because it eats one hen a day and if it did not have one, it would eat the person. Whatever may be the case, such things are rather harmless.[36]

---

[33] *Die Chirurgie des Heinrich von Mondeville (Hermondaville)*, ed Julius Pagel (Berlin: Hirschwald, 1892), 481 and 484 (with regard to cancer).

[34] *Guigonis de Cauliaco*, I.282 (with a strange attribution to Haly Abbas). The provincial surgeon Pierre Bocellin adopted the awkward attempt at etymology, almost two centuries after Guy, in *Practique sur la matiere de la contagieuse et infective maladie de lepre* (Lyon: n.p 1540), fol. 3.

[35] The nexus became more complex when authors combined both notions in their elaborations of Avicenna's teaching that *lepra* is "a cancer of the whole body."

[36] *Guigonis de Cauliaco*, I.283 and I.226. Folklorists have recorded, across Europe and far into the twentieth century, popular remedies of treating the voracious "animal cancer"

The alleged treatment by empirics and interpretations by the populace bring us right back to the Liège miracle story and the folksy vignette about the daily application of chicken meat. Guy's *Inventarium* may be the first medical work to incorporate this allegation. In a world where having poultry snatched by wolves was still relatively common, the experience may have fueled pervasive fears of wolfish rapacity. It is fair to speculate further that these fears, in turn, reinforced perennial legends about werewolves (French, *loups-garous*).[37] There is no evidence, however, of an inverse process whereby werewolf myths would have affected the medieval development of lupus as a medical category. Guy de Chauliac summarized the *actual* development of the category, although, surprisingly, he did not confirm the equation which had become commonplace. He emphasized that estiomenus kills a body part with putrefaction and softening,

> in contrast with lupus and cancer which destroy the part with gnawing and hardening. Therefore, they are not identical as Teodorico, Lanfranco and Henri said. Estiomenus is popularly called (*vulgariter dicitur*) the Fire of Saint Antony or of Saint Marcial.[38]

As for cancer, Guy reiterated Roger Frugardi's triple differentiation by affected place, with the third, lupus, occurring "on the fundament (*in coxis*)."[39] The word *coxa* designates the hip or thigh in the strict sense but,

with fresh meat. For background, see Alanna Skuse," Wombs, Worms and Wolves: Constructing Cancer in Early Modern England," *Social History of Medicine*, 27 (2014): 632-648. For a different application, see Erik A. Heinrichs, "The Live Chicken Treatment for Buboes: Trying a Plague Cure in Medieval and Early Modern Europe," *Bulletin of the History of Medicine* 91:2 (2017), 210-232.

[37] One "revival" of the legends in David Shyovitz, "Christians and Jews in the Twelfth-Century Werewolf Renaissance," *Journal of the History of Ideas,* 75 (2014): 521-43. One wonders about the semantic links in French, in view of (a) definitions such as "Le terme lupus est issu du latin 'loup', en référence à l'éruption rouge en forme de masque sur le visage, caractéristique de la maladie," www.sante-sur-le-net.com/maladies/maladies-auto-immunes/lupus/, (b) the evident popularity of the "masque loup" in France, and (c) the wide availability of the "masque loup garou."

[38] *Guigonis de Cauliaco*, I.75. The elucidation of this passage by the editor, Michael McVaugh, merits reading in full: *Guigonis de Cauliaco*, II.72. Concerning Teodorico, see above in notes 29-30.

[39] *Guigonis de Cauliaco*, I.224.

by extension, also the "sit bone." The context of imprecise anatomy, in addition to the degree of vagueness in everyday language, allows for the translation "on the fundament," which brings Guy's identification of lupus in line with the report that Bishop Eraclius was stricken *in natibus*. More significantly, the linguistic vagueness extended beyond daily usage, far enough to frame an effort by Guy to correct the claim of Bruno and Teodorico that the nomenclature and classification of lupus were new. Guy's effort was apparently disregarded, for in 1519 the surgeon Giovanni Vigo still insisted that the "modern and younger doctors" named the disease according to the affected location, and that he did not find "this modern distinction mentioned in the writings of the old." [40] Vigo considered it imperative to know the newly differential nomenclature.

The need for up-to-date nomenclature was emphasized by Vigo's contemporary and compatriot, the physician Giovanni Manardo, who wrote a long letter to a surgeon with the intention to "remove the confusion of names" by explaining them for each disease on the surface of the body. He argued, "Every day, big and numerous errors happen to common physicians from ignorance of such names, as they think that the same name in different authors always designates the same problem (*affectum*)." Before closing his *Epistola*, Manardo remembered:

> I have read many names of diseases occurring on the surface, which appear in the books of more recent physicians and which are not found with the old. One could rightly doubt about these whether, as they are new names, they also identify new diseases unknown to the older physicians.[41]

In this concluding thought, Manardo managed to sum up three hallmarks of Renaissance writing that affected the medical discussion of lupus. He and his sixteenth-century peers wrote during the height of a movement, which the Humanists had spearheaded, to sharpen the depth-

[40] Giovanni Vigo, *Prima pars practice in chirurgia: Practica in arte chirurgica copiosa Ioannis de Vigo* (Lyon: Vincent de Portonariis, 1519), fol. 34v. For authors after 1500, last names are used, in contrast with the customary use of first names for authors before 1500.

[41] Giovanni Manardo, *Epistolae medicinales diversorum authorum, nempe, Ioannis Manardi…* (Lyon, 1557), Liber Septimus, Epistola II "ad Michaelem Sanctannam Chirurgum de nominibus morborum in exterioribus corporis partibus evenientium," 43 and 52.

perception of the past, to correlate language and reality, and to accentuate the degrees of distance from their own literacy.[42]

The Renaissance hallmarks were voiced most eloquently by Giovanni Ingrassia, a student of Andreas Vesalius. In his compilation *De tumoribus praeter naturam* (which was based on Galen's treatise known by the same title), Ingrassia traced the appellations of 205 "tumors" back to Greek, Roman, and Arabic sources. He aimed consistently for documentary completeness and historical sequence, up to "the latest" (*recentiores*) authors and, in a sense, his "young" (*neoterici*) colleagues. His sense of "recent" was sharper than that of his predecessors who, at least as early as Teodorico, had cited the *moderni*. With obvious linguistic flair, Ingrassia interwove denomination, etymology, and taxonomy with etiology and therapeutics. This approach is strikingly illustrated in the coverage of "Tumor 118," that is, noli me tangere and related conditions.

> Some have presented these as kinds of cancer, but others distinguished them from cancer. Nevertheless, these are in agreement because what is a kind of cancer when taken in a generic sense (*generatim*) will differ specifically (*speciatim*) from the cancer of the Greeks and Romans."

The semantic problem was broader and older, and already Teodorico had considered cancer an equivocal name because previous authors understood cancer as covering phagedena (from Greek *phagein*, to eat). While resigning to the ambiguity of the relation between lupus and cancer, Ingrassia incorporated the conventional congruity between noli me tangere and lupus as both being caused by "overcooked bile." Lupus, he elaborated, was due to more completely burned bile, "so that it is eroding and advancing (*obambulans*) faster, as well as [occurring] lower down on account of the humor's heaviness."[43]

Different explanations, definitions, and even names of "eating diseases" were usually followed by correspondingly different treatments. Ingrassia did not cover therapeutics in *De tumoribus*, with the exception of cures linked with a name and explanation in a notorious tradition that

---

42 For an early stage, Luke Demaitre, "'Vita brevis, Ars autem prolixa': forging a medical language," in Monica Berté, Vincenzo Fera, Tiziana Pesenti, eds., *Petrarca e la medicina. Atti del Convegno di Capo d Orlando 27-28 giugno 2003* (Biblioteca umanistica 8) (Messina: Centro interdipartmentale di studi umanistici, 2006), 123-143.

43 Giovanni Filippo Ingrassia, *De tumoribus praeter naturam Tomus primus*, [Naples, 1562], 374.

gave him the opportunity to spotlight the distance between medical learning and lay lore. He singled out "certain common (*gregarii*, from Latin *grex*, herd) surgeons" when he cited Guy's report that "many (*multi*)" practitioners applied a scarlet cloth to mitigate the wolfishness of cancer. Then, for the tradition about lupus, Ingrassia applied a subtle substitution by replacing the *populus* of Guy's attribution with *vulgus*.

> Common people suppose that "lupus" is so named because it eats one hen a day and if it did not have one, it would eat the entire leg and then the entire person. This folly (*fatuitas*) continues until the present day with the common people, who think that this ulcer is fed by the meat of a hen and hold this for most proven.[44]

A few decades after Ingrassia, the French physician Laurent Joubert underscored Guy's rejection with the remark that, if the popular etymology made sense, "the disease should rather be called 'the fox,' and the applied meat should be mutton."[45] The tradition persisted nevertheless, and occasionally even in a more extreme form. In the early eighteenth century, a woman told an English physician that, at the display of "a piece of raw flesh at a distance from the sore, the Wolf peept out, discovering his Head, and gaping to receive it. *Tam facile decipitur Vulgus.*"[46]

The "deception," which blurred the line between the metaphorical and literal senses of eating, probably accounted for the reluctance of some medical authors to discuss lupus. It is surprising, for example, that neither the "first physiologist" Jean Fernel, nor the celebrated royal surgeon Ambroise Paré mentioned it in their comprehensive tomes. An additional reason for their inattention may have been the classification with diseases that were considered incurable and "reject the practitioner's efforts" (*medicantis opem respuunt*).[47] By the same token, the reputation of incurability encouraged a recourse to non-scientific attempts. Incurability

---

[44] Ingrassia, *De tumoribus*, 373.

[45] *Annotations de M. Laur. Joubert, sur toute la chirurgie de M. Gui de Chauliac* (Lyon: Estienne Micheand, 1585), 331.

[46] Daniel Turner, *De morbis cutaneis: a treatise of diseases incident to the skin.* The third edition Revised and very much Enlarged (London: R. and J. Bonwicke, [1726]), 114.

[47] Levinus Lemnius, *De habitu et constitutione corporis* (Antwerp: Guilielmus Simonis, 1561), 126.

made the miraculous healing of Bishop Eraclius more momentous, and it enhanced the memorability of his "wolfish" affliction. The historical momentum sparkles, as if preserved in amber, in a 19th-century commemoration of the ecclesiastical ties between Liège and Tours for which, as we have seen, Eraclius was the key figure on account of his healing by Saint Martin. The supporting documents stated that Eraclius recovered miraculously "from the incurable disease which is called lupus." In 1781, the "Preuves & Pièces Justificatives" emphasized the wondrousness of the miracle with the detail that Eraclius "was eaten up by a miserable disease, namely sacred fire [*sic*], which consumed two chickens in the morning and two in the evening."[48] It is puzzling that these lines were absent from the earlier and virtually identical publication of the book in 1746.[49] Whether they were taken from a newly discovered source or simply re-inserted, the lines attest to the stubborn longevity of popular notions in defiance of scientific understanding.

Many authors refuted literal associations between lupus and the devouring of chickens, but few tackled both the etymology *and* the practice as disparagingly as Samuel Hafenreffer in the *Nosodochium*, which is considered the first textbook of dermatology (1660).[50] In the chapter on cancer, he mentioned quite casually that "some" call a cancer lupus if it reaches the lower body and "erosion turns it into a horrible sight." He gave equal weight but less credit to the alternative explanation: "or, [the disease] has acquired the name of the wolf from the wrongheaded belief of some who applied the meat of hens or goats." It should be noted that Hafenreffer connected the appellation twice to "some," *quibusdam* and *quorundam*, in contrast with the conventional references to *vulgus*. This means that he left the field of common usage open (at least implicitly) for a different term which, serendipitously, he applied to an entry with possibly significant ramifications for our inquiry. In the chapter on excoriation, he described a condition caused by "riding a skinny, consumptive, and emaciated horse, with an ill-fitting caparison, or also by the hard run of a horse." This condition was known in medicine as intertrigo, and it retains the name *Hautwolf* in German. Hafenreffer

[48] Bertholet, *Histoire de l'institution de la Fête-Dieu*, xxj-xxij.

[49] Bertholet, *Histoire de l'institution de la Fête-Dieu*, xxxviij.

[50] For the 16th-17th-century context, see Hannah Murphy, "Skin and Disease in Early Modern Medicine: Jan Jessen's De cute, et cutaneis affectibus (1601)," *Bulletin of the History of Medicine*, 94 (2020): 179-234.

applied greater precision, however, when he noted, "commonly, it is called 'the wolf' or 'has ridden a wolf' (*vulgo dicitur wolff: oder hat ein wolff geritten*)." [51] His explicit distinction between medical and colloquial parlance, underscored by the bold Gothic font in the midst of the Latin text, suggests that he saw "der Wolff" as the default vernacular term for intertrigo caused by horseback riding.

Both the vernacular origin of the wolf idiom and the focus on horseback riding bring us back, full circle as it were, to Liège and Eraclius, who spent an extraordinary time in the saddle. More precisely, the image of saddle sores matches a poignant detail in the miracle story, namely, that the bishop was stricken "in the buttocks (*in natibus*)." Many an aristocratic churchman must have suffered the consequences of obesity for their extensive travels. After all, "royal illnesses follow royal dishes, including lupus and gout, which do not readily plague lean and industrious people," according to a sixteenth-century preacher.[52] In sum, Eraclius would have been a reasonable candidate for an ailment that was "commonly called the wolf" but did not fit the pattern of the disease which is called lupus in modern medicine. Furthermore, a cautious historian should keep an open mind for the possibility that the pious narrators endeavored to upgrade – or embellish, if this were the proper term – the bishop's condition to a miracle-level affliction. Their aim, after all, was to anchor a historic foundation in a miraculous recovery, not to enter a new medical category into history. Neither the use of the wolf label nor the depiction of the ailment is evidence that Eraclius was the first to be identified as a patient of a disease which is now categorized as lupus. The narrators in Liège and Tours took advantage of a popular label which, beyond designating intertrigo, had an inherent mystical power of suggestion. It makes sense to think of labels such as "leprosy" and a few others which, through history, have outrun reality and reason in their impact on imagination and emotion. This kind of label from common usage, *vulgo*, or a vague notion rather than a known condition, was the object of George Costanza's groan, "Lupus? Is it lupus?"

---

[51] Samuel Hafenreffer, *Nosodochium: in quo cutis, eique adhaerentium partium, affectus omnes, singulari methodo, et cognoscendi et curandi fidelissime traduntur* (Ulm: Balthasar Kuehnen, 1660), 155.

[52] Michel Ménot (d. 1518), *Sermones quadragesimales*, fol. 185v, cited in Charles Du Cange et al., eds., *Glossarium mediae et infimae Latinitatis* (Niort: L. Favre, 1883–1887), V155b http://ducange.enc.sorbonne.fr/LUPUS1.

Even medical discussions attested, for at least six centuries, to a substantial gap between lupus as a label and lupus as a defined disease. The gap typifies the lack of specificity which marks medical discussion before the nineteenth century as most fundamentally different from its later counterpart. When attempts were made to formulate a definition, lupus was usually equated with another generic disease concept, namely, herpes estiomenus. This equation was based more on written transmission than on clinical cases, more on casual impressions than on methodical observation, and more on the scheme of humors than on an understanding of physiology. There is irony in the fact that humoral explanations, although developed erratically, pointed towards the later change from external to internal treatment, and that the humoral implication of flow or flux, *rheuma*, is echoed in the eventual assignment of lupus to rheumatology.

The hold of humoral etiology was still evident in 1689, when Johann Dolaeus, in his surgical encyclopedia, attributed erysipelas, herpes estiomenus and, by extension, lupus to a disorder in "the littoral movement of the blood and fluids."[53] Dolaeus further associated lupus with "ulcerated" cancer when he summarized *apostemata* terminology. Paradoxically, his summary came right after the claim that he had little interest in "the diversity of meanings which we should better leave to philologists and lexicographers."[54] He would have agreed that the medical meaning of the term "wolf" was caught in semantic ambiguities between mythology and observation, between metaphorical and literal, between characterization and definition, or between generic and specific. The disease itself remained relegated to surgery, to the lower body, and to the shadow of herpes estiomenus.

The precise condition and process of LSE could not be identified without knowledge of cell defense and immunity; Lupus vulgaris – not to be confused with the disease "qui vulgo lupus dicitur" – could not find a place without the full understanding of tuberculosis. Even then, lupus continued to challenge bedside identification as well as unified explanation and consistent classification. It has, with the elusiveness of the wolf, defied the grasp of doctors and historians alike. The original aim of this inquiry was to review the early history of lupus, but the result

---

53 Johannes Dolaeus, *Encyclopaedia chirurgica rationalis: in qua omnes affectus externi corpus humanum unquam invasisse observati … pertractantur* (Frankfurt: Knoch, 1689), 1103.

54 Dolaeus, *Encyclopaedia chirurgica*, 1151.

is an early history of the label or, in way, a prehistory of the disease. The review neither confirms nor denies the pre-nineteenth-century incidence of lupus as it is currently defined. It does add up to a caveat about retrospective diagnosis. When we are tempted to identify a case from the mention of the label (or, for that matter, of "herpes estiomenus"), from partial descriptions, or from medical discussions, we might hear the gruff verdict of Dr House, "It's never lupus."

"HAVE YOU COME HERE TO PLAY JESUS?": THE USE AND THE MISUSE OF MEDIEVAL LEPROSY IN MODERN MEDIA

COURTNEY A. KROLIKOSKI*

> Have you come here for forgiveness?
> Have you come to raise the dead?
> Have you come here to play Jesus,
> To the lepers in your head?[1]

The archetype of the "medieval leper" has a long, troublesome history that can be traced from the Middle Ages to today.[2] While the historiography of leprosy has evolved over the last few decades, turning what we thought we understood about leprosy in the European Middle Ages on its head, modern society has held tenaciously to the figure of the medieval "leper" as society's ultimate exile. The implications of this are important both for understanding the place of leprosy in the medieval landscape and for addressing the stigma facing modern sufferers of Hansen's Disease (the preferred name of the disease in modern discourse).[3] Though the term "leper" is today considered by those with

* Department of History, Jacksonville University.

1 U2, "One," track 3 on *Achtung Baby,* Island Records, 1992, digital.

2 I would like to thank Dr. Lucy Barnhouse and Dr. Winston Black for their careful and insightful comments on this chapter during its evolution from conference presentation to the form it takes today.

3 A note: The terms "leper" and "leprosy" are still, as this paper shows, tied to a unique stigma that historians of medicine and advocates have fought to eliminate for decades. However, their use when discussing the medieval context reflects the sources and

Hansen's Disease to be a slur, in medieval Europe it was a label that could afford those diagnosed with the disease a measure of protection and support from their communities.[4] This could come in the form of alms for sustenance, membership in a *leprosarium* (hospital for those with leprosy), or the privileged status of a spiritual intercessor.[5] Despite this, contemporary interpretations of the "medieval leper" – especially those in popular culture – continue to perpetuate a centuries-old narrative of difference, disgust, and exclusion. In the AIDS charity benefit song "One," released by the Irish rock band U2 in 1992, the lead singer Bono asks if "you," his listener, have come to play Jesus to "the lepers in your head?" In another example, in George R.R. Martin's *A Dance with Dragons*, Tyrion Lannister bristles at the discussion his fellow passengers on the ship the *Shy Maid* are having about the Shrouded Lord, a legendary

---

attitudes of the time. Today the disease is commonly referred to as Hansen's Disease in an effort to alleviate the stigma for those who have been infected, especially in countries where the disease remains tied to social classes and accessibility to services. For a lengthier discussion on this, see: Carole Rawcliffe, *Leprosy in Medieval England* (Woodbridge: The Boydell Press, 2006), 11-12; Charlotte Roberts, "Reflections on the bioarchaeology of leprosy and identity, past and present," in *Leprosy and Identity in the Middle Ages: From England to the Mediterranean,* eds. Elma Brenner and François-Olivier Touati (Manchester: Manchester University Press, 2021), 21-44; Kathleen Vongasthorn and Magnus Vollset, "'Our loathsome ancestors': reinventing medieval leprosy for the modern world," in *Leprosy and Identity in the Middle Ages,* 347-82.

[4] Leprosy in the Islamicate world remains understudied. The classic work is Michael W. Dols, "The Leper in Medieval Islamic Society," *Speculum* 58 (1983), 891-916. Kristina L. Richardson, *Difference and Disability in the Medieval Islamic World: Blighted Bodies* (Edinburgh: Edinburgh University Press, 2012), 11-12, 45-47, 111-113, 118-119 discusses leprosy as a disability. On leprosy in Byzantium, see Timothy S. Miller and John W. Nesbitt, *Walking Corpses: Leprosy in Byzantium and the Medieval West* (Ithaca, NY: Cornell University Press, 2014), 27-95.

[5] A note for clarity: medieval leprosy is not necessarily identical to what is today known as Hansen's Disease. However, thanks to advances in modern bio-archaeological studies, we know there was considerable overlap with what was diagnosed as leprosy and the bacterium responsible for Hansen's Disease, to try and conflate the two for the medieval period is engaging in retrospective diagnosis and unnecessary. What matters, historically, is what happened to a person once diagnosed – whether or not they had the disease according to modern standards. For more on the concept of "leprosy/leper" as a meaningful identity in the Middle Ages, see Elma Brenner, *Leprosy and Charity in Medieval Rouen* (Woodbridge: The Boydell Press, 2015), esp. 38-57; Julie Orlemanski, "How to kiss a leper," *postmedieval: a journal of medieval cultural* studies 3 (2012), 142-57; Luke Demaitre, *Leprosy in Premodern Medicine: A Malady of the Whole Body* (Baltimore: The Johns Hopkins University Press, 2007), esp. 75-102.

figure who was believed to spread the fictional disease "greyscale" with his kiss.[6] We are told that the "thought made his flesh crawl. Death had lost its terror for Tyrion Lannister, but greyscale was another matter."[7] In the world of Westeros, greyscale is a severely contagious disease that bears a striking resemblance to leprosy and carries the same stigmas once thought to be associated with medieval leprosy: horror, shame, and exile.[8] These examples, among many others, highlight the use and misuse of the image of the medieval leper and the disease of leprosy in modern media, a practice that holds serious implications for changing the narrative – both the medieval and the modern.

In print and on screen, the universes of Tolkien's *Lord of the Rings* and *The Hobbit*, the tales of King Arthur in the movies of Guy Ritchie and Antoine Fuqua, and *Game of Thrones* have come to dominate modern imagination, with today's society showing an intense interest in fantasies of the medieval. Though these worlds may appear to be modeled on the medieval, they are in fact adapted from a "constellation of imagined medieval societies."[9] Yet the popular understanding of the "medieval" is one that was initially shaped by early modern thinkers attempting to distance their world from a past they saw as irrational and backwards, a so-called Dark Ages.[10] This image has persisted in multiple iterations to

---

[6] For a different analysis of Martin's use of "greyscale," see Robin S. Reich's chapter in this volume, "The Fantasy of Medieval Medicine: Poultices, Dusty Tomes, and the Spice Trade in the Mediterranean."

[7] George R.R. Martin, *A Dance with Dragons* (New York: Bantam Books, 2011), 116.

[8] It is important to recognize here that the tropes discussed in this paper are rooted in the medieval European Western tradition and are based on the Christocentric theology of the time. The use of the figure of the 'leper' as a trope, however, extends beyond both European and Christian boundaries. For a few examples, see: Susan L. Burns, "The Geography of Exclusion: Rai in Premodern Japan," in *Kingdom of the Sick: A History of Leprosy and Japan* (Honolulu: University of Hawai'i Press, 2019), 19-46; François-Olivier Touati, "Lepers and leprosy: connections between East and West in the Middle Ages," in *Leprosy and Identity in the Middle Ages*, 45-66; Miller and Nesbitt, *Walking Corpses*, 27-47.

[9] Carolyn Larrington, "Mediating Medieval(ized) Emotion in *Game of Thrones*," in *Studies in Medievalism XXVII: Authenticity, Medievalism, Music,* ed. Karl Fugelso (Cambridge: D.S. Brewer 2018), 35. For more on the imagined medieval world(s), see: Geraldine Heng, *Empire of Magic Medieval Romance and the Politics of Cultural Fantasy* (New York: Columbia University Press, 2003); Umberto Eco, "Dreaming of the Middle Ages," in *Travels in Hyperreality*, trans. William J. Weaver (New York: Harcourt Brace, 1986), 61-85.

[10] Many have pointed to Petrarch's writing in the 1300s as the first usage of the metaphor of "darkness" for the Middle Ages as a contrast with the "light" that came from the

the present day through art, entertainment, cultural beliefs, literature, scholarship, and more.[11] One early modern example comes from *The Rime of the Ancient Mariner*, wherein Samuel Taylor Coleridge draws from the fear of the disease to describe the chance nature of the Mariner's fate. The relationship between the skeleton ship with "the fleshless man" of Death and "Life-in-Death," whose skin is "as white as leprosy" highlights the fear of infection as divine retribution.[12] The disease was used more and more as a metaphor as "scientific" publications from this period described the symptoms and prognoses of leprosy, thus fanning the flames of the perceived social dangers of the disease.[13] In this way, the "Middle Ages was *never* simply a chronological concept, never simply a past time firmly fixed in the past," unhindered by interpretation.[14] Rather, the "medieval" can be both an ideological state worth returning to and one worth leaving behind. This is the essence of *medievalism,* a relationship between the present and the past wherein modern actors reinterpret, manipulate, and use the Middle Ages to tell compelling and exotic stories. As Leslie J. Workman defined the term at the foundation of the journal *Studies in Medievalism*, medievalism is "the continuing process of creating the Middle Ages."[15] Indeed, a continual creation and recreation of the Middle Ages often reflects more on the world that their creator(s) live in than the actual events, places, and ideals of the Middle Ages. In the places and ways where the medieval enters modern works of art, fiction, music, and more we can feel the creator's "sense of discontentment with the present," their desire to draw on collective memory, and/or their need to comment on contemporary issues.[16]

The "medieval leper" is undoubtedly one of the most easily identifiable tropes for creators to work with, either directly through the

intellectual and social rebirth of the Renaissance. Theodore E. Mommsen, "Petrarch's Conception of the 'Dark Ages'" *Speculum* 17, no. 2 (1942), 226-242.

[11] For more on the history of the term "Dark Ages," see Janet L. Nelson, "The Dark Ages," *History Workshop Journal* 63, no. 1 (2007): 191-201.

[12] Samuel Taylor Coleridge, *The Rime of the Ancient Mariner* (London: Sampson Low, Son & Co., 1857), 22.

[13] Rawcliffe, *Leprosy in Medieval England*, 34.

[14] David Matthews, *Medievalism: A Critical History* (Cambridge: D.S. Brewer, 2015), 46.

[15] Leslie J. Workman, definition cited from "A Brief History," *The International Society for the Study of Medievalism,* www.medievalisms.org/about, last accessed 3 December 2021.

[16] Tison Pugh and Angela Jane Weisl, *Medievalisms: Making the Past in the Present* (London: Routledge, 2013), 2.

inclusion of the disease itself or indirectly through the creation of a comparable disease in fantasy realms. However, the leprosy molded out of their imagination is not a product of the actual Middle Ages, but instead one that was crafted during colonial encounters of the nineteenth century into a narrative of exclusion and continuities be used and manipulated. These colonial contacts created the "historiographical myth" of leprosy: a monolithic understanding of a disease that was "emblematic of the dark Middle Ages" wherein the disease was seen as a scourge that wreaked havoc on a primitive and backwards society.[17] This imagined leprosy came predominantly from a misinterpretation of the Old Testament understandings of *tzāra'ath* (a generic Hebrew term for skin disorders) found in the thirteenth and fourteenth books of Leviticus.[18] These chapters describe in detail the process of diagnosing *tzāra'ath,* naming who was responsible for the examination, the symptoms to look for, and the resulting actions to be taken should the person be determined to have the disease. As Mosaic Law is primarily concerned with issues of pollution, the prescriptions of Leviticus also provided the process for a person's ceremonial exclusion from the community if diagnosed and their path for purification and ceremonial re-admittance to the community. Saint Jerome's translation of *tzāra'ath* to *lepra* thus also translated a variety of skin disorders that one could recover from to the singular leprosy which was instead a permanent state.[19] Victorian authors were able to construct a narrative using medieval sources that supported their "negative, one-dimensional view"

---

[17] François-Olivier Touati, "Contagion and Leprosy: Myth, Ideas, and Evolution in Medieval Minds and Societies," in *Contagion: Perspectives from Pre-Modern Societies,* ed. Lawrence I. Conrad and Dominik Wujastyk (Aldershot: Ashgate, 2000), 180.

[18] Demaitre, *Leprosy in Premodern Medicine*, 83.

[19] Though this chapter focuses primarily on uses of the figure of the "medieval leper" from a Christian basis, the history of leprosy in Judaism is vast and presents an interesting point of comparison. For more on leprosy in Jewish history and law, see: Ephraim Shoham-Steiner, *On the Margins of a Minority: Leprosy, Madness, and Disability Among the Jews of Medieval Europe* (Detroit: Wayne State University Press, 2014); Irven M. Resnick, "The Jews and Leprosy," in *Marks of Distinction: Christian Perceptions of Jews in the High Middle Ages* (Washington D.C.: Catholic University of America Press, 2012), 93-143; Ephraim Shoham-Steiner, "Pharaoh's Bloodbath: Medieval European Jewish Thoughts About Leprosy," in *Jewish Blood: Reality and Metaphor in History, Religion, and* Culture, ed. Mitchell B. Hart (London: Routledge, 2009), 99-115; Hyam Maccoby, *Ritual and Morality: The Ritual Purity System and Its Place in Judaism* (Cambridge: Cambridge University Press, 1999), esp. 118-40.

of their modern contact with the disease.[20] The resulting myth of leprosy was so strong that the historiography of the disease in the Middle Ages bred scholarship well into the 1990s (and in some cases beyond) that overwhelmingly supported a narrative that leprosy sufferers were purposely and forcefully excluded from mainstream society, avoided at all costs, and the anguishing effects of their disease were used as a warning to healthy society against sin and deviance.[21] Academic works and popular understandings of leprosy both perpetuated this narrative, asserting that those affected by the disease in the medieval West were excluded, ostracized, and despised.[22] In this view, they were truly the social and medical outcasts that needed to be sent "outside the camp so they will not defile" their community.[23]

This historiographic orthodoxy persisted almost unchallenged until the later twentieth century, when interdisciplinary research into the disease and its history brought both reevaluation of this narrative and a renewed interest in the field. It was only in the 1990s that leprosy was revisited in a way that detangled the historical reality of the disease from its longstanding myth. The publication of foundational works by scholars including Luke Demaitre, Carole Rawcliffe, and Francois-Olivier Touati jettisoned the exclusion narrative of leprosy in favor of a narrative that emphasized society's inclusion of and compassion towards the sick.[24] We now understand that leprosy was overwhelmingly viewed in the Middle

[20] Rawcliffe, "Isolating the Medieval Leper," 230.

[21] For examples of this "exclusion narrative," see: Saul Brody, *The Disease of the Soul: Leprosy in Medieval Literature* (Ithaca, NY: Cornell University Press, 1974); R.I. Moore, *The Formation of a Persecuting Society: Authority and Deviance in Western Europe 950-1250,* 2nd edition (Oxford: Blackwell Publishing, 2007), esp. 42-56; Susan Zimmerman, "Leprosy in the Medieval Imaginary," *Journal of Medieval and Early Modern Studies* 38 (2008): 559-63; Miller and Nesbitt, *Walking Corpses: Leprosy in Byzantium and the Medieval West* (Ithaca, NY: Cornell University Press, 2014).

[22] We see this myth perpetuated even today in articles like Maggie Ferguson's "How Does it Really Feel to Be Lonely?" wherein she describes loneliness as the "leprosy of the 21st century." Maggie Ferguson *The Economist. 1843: Stories of an Extraordinary World.* February/March 2018. www.1843magazine.com/features/in-solitude-what-happiness.

[23] Numbers 5:3

[24] See Luke Demaitre's chapter in this volume, "Lupus, From Wolf to Butterfly: Vagaries of a Disease;" Demaitre, *Leprosy in Premodern Medicine,* passim; Rawcliffe, *Leprosy in Medieval England*; François-Olivier Touati, *Maladie et société au Moyen Âge: la lèpre, les lépreux et les léproseries dans la province ecclésiastique de Sens jusqu'au milieu du XIVe siécle* (Bruxelles: De Boeck Université, 1998).

Ages as a deeply personal tragedy for an individual and, after the turn of the twelfth century, society came to see those who suffered from the disease as privileged intercessors between this world and God.[25] This period also saw a renewed focus on the importance of redemptive almsgiving, wherein donations, gifts, and service to the needy were believed to generate spiritual rewards. Hospitals, *leprosaria,* and other charitable institutions thus benefitted greatly from this development in lay piety and religious devotion and, as a result, found themselves receiving broad support from many sectors of society, including ecclesiastics, aristocrats, merchants, military orders, municipalities, and townspeople.[26] While not fully integrated into everyday life, those with leprosy were in fact interconnected with their communities socially, spiritually, and physically. It is, as Rawcliffe has noted, that the development and longevity of the myth of medieval leprosy is one that was "less a matter of selection than invention – or at least serious distortion.[27] Indeed, though none of the information presented in the pre-1990s historiography was falsified, it was greatly distorted, misquoted, or given undue emphasis, while information that contradicted the exclusion narrative was ignored or discounted. Despite the evolution of the historiography of leprosy in the Middle Ages over the last three decades, modern society's perception of the disease's place

---

[25] André Vauchez, "Assistance et Charité en Occident, XIIIe -XVe Siècles," in *Domanda e consumi. Livelli e strutture (nei secoli XII-XVII),* ed. Vera Barbagli Bagnoli (Florence: L.S. Olschki, 1978), 152.

[26] For more on the study of the growth in donations to assistive institutions in the Middle Ages, see: Richard C. Trexler, "Charity and the Defense of Urban Elite in the Italian Communes," in *The Rich, the Well Born, and the Powerful: Elites and Upper Classes in History,* ed. Frederic Cople Jaher (Urbana: University of Illinois Press, 1973), 56-109; Michael Mollat, *Les Pauvres au Moyen Âge: étude sociale* (Paris: Hachette, 1978); Sharon Farmer, *Surviving Poverty in Medieval Paris: Gender, Ideology, and the Daily Lives of the Poor* (Ithaca: Cornell University Press, 2002); Mark R. Cohen, *Poverty and Charity in the Jewish Community of Medieval Egypt* (Princeton: Princeton University Press, 2005); James Brodman, *Charity and Religion in Medieval Europe* (Washington D.C.: Catholic University of America Press, 2009); Anne M. Scott (ed.), *Experiences of Charity, 1250-1650* (Farnham: Ashgate, 2015); Sharon Farmer (ed.), *Approaches to Poverty in Medieval Europe: Complexities, Contradictions, Transformations, c. 1100-1500* (Turnhout: Brepols, 2016).

[27] Rawcliffe, *Leprosy in Medieval Medicine*, 39.

in medieval society has yet to follow.[28] As such, the use of the terms "leper" or "leprosy," especially in relation to something medieval or perceived as medieval, is frequently linked to images of disfigured individuals shunned by "healthy" society.

As will be shown, leprosy is often used as a catch-all descriptor for any diseased, excluded, or marginalized individual or population. Almost always when someone or something is said to be "like a leper" we are meant to picture an unclean, unwanted individual who has no place in polite society; the imagined medieval leper of today is to be shunned. However, on occasion, some uses of medieval leprosy pull from a separate, but equally prominent, Biblical story of leprosy – and one that casts the "medieval leper" as worthy of compassion despite their situation. Consider the lyrics of "One" by U2 quoted at the start of this chapter. This verse of the song recalls a story from the Synoptic Gospels of the New Testament where Jesus heals people from leprosy – something seen as both a miracle and an act of compassion. In the Gospel of Matthew, for example, a person suffering from leprosy approached Jesus in the street, emerging from a crowd moments after the "Sermon on the Mount." The man said to Jesus, "Lord, if you are willing, you are able to cleanse me."[29] Jesus reached out a hand, touched the man, and he was instantly healed. So, when Bono asks if you have "come here to play Jesus to the lepers in your head," he is insinuating that we all have the power to heal ourselves of something terrible but, perhaps, worthy of compassion and healing. It is worth noting that "One" was released as a benefit single to raise money for AIDS research at the height of the AIDS epidemic. As AIDS has often been referred to as the iconic disease of the late twentieth century, so leprosy is often referred to as emblematic of the Middle Ages.[30] The juxtaposition of the song's lyrics with its social impact for another largely misunderstood

28 Recent works that similarly challenge modern misconceptions of medieval leprosy include Elma Brenner and François-Olivier Touati (eds.), *Leprosy and Identity in the Middle Ages* and Elma Brenner, *Leprosy and Charity in Medieval Rouen.*

29 Matthew 8:2. A transcription and analysis of the place of healing episodes in the Synoptic Gospels can be found in Will Eggers, "Selected Episodes on Healing and Disability from the Vulgate Bible - Matthew, Mark, Luke, and John," in *Medieval Disability Sourcebook: Western Europe,* ed. Cameron Hunt McNabb (New York: punctum books, 2020), 113-37.

30 "Pour bien des esprits, le Moyen Âge, c'est la lèpre," Touati, *Maladie et société au Moyen Âge*, 19; see also Rawcliffe, *Leprosy in Medieval England,* 17.

disease further highlights the ways in which perception of a disease can be shaped and reshaped over time.[31]

U2's more positive use of the medieval leper contrasts with Christopher Moore's use of it in his national-bestselling satirical novel entitled *Lamb: The Gospel According to Biff, Christ's Childhood Pal,* published in 2002. The book chronicles what might have happened during the 30-year gap between Jesus's (called Joshua in the story) birth and adulthood – as told by his best friend, the wise-cracking Biff. Though set in the first century CE, *Lamb* perpetuates the nineteenth-century myth of medieval leprosy, including descriptions of people with leprosy being required to call out "unclean" to alert others of their presence, as vagrants who live far removed from society, and as people who lived lives dictated by Mosaic Law.[32] In one instance, Biff and Joshua are approached by a group of leprosy sufferers who implore Joshua to heal them, echoing the New Testament story discussed above. When Joshua calls the group to him so he can "put his hands on the lepers," Biff describes them as "three piles of rags" who "ooz[e] over" to the savior.[33] Once healed, the group "threw off their rags and praised Joshua," prompting Biff to remark that they "looked like perfectly normal people who just happened to be all wrapped up in tattered rags."[34] While Joshua's compassion towards those with leprosy reflects the savior of the Gospels, Biff's repulsion towards those with the disease instead reflects the enduring legacy of the 'medieval leper' as unclean, disgusting, and meant to be avoided. Indeed, though the Biblical tradition provides no description of the disease, Biff's comment "no matter how many healings I saw, lepers always gave me what we Hebrews call the willies" reflected how today's society expected premodern persons to react to its presence.[35] This is also reminiscent, in

---

[31] It is worth noting that the revival of scholarship on medieval leprosy in the 1980s and 1990s occurred at the same time of the AIDS epidemic and, perhaps, can account for the parallels drawn between the two by historians of the time, including Rawcliffe, *Leprosy in Medieval England*, 17-19, 90; Demaitre, *Leprosy in Premodern Medicine,* 278-9.

[32] These depictions of leprosy come from the often-cited book thirteen of Leviticus wherein it is said that "whosoever shall be defiled with leprosy" shall be separated from the community, forced to wear loose clothing and "cry out that he is defiled and unclean…he shall dwell alone without the camp." Leviticus 13: 44-46.

[33] Christopher Moore, *Lamb: The Gospel According to Biff, Christ's Childhood Pal* (New York: William Morrow, 2004), 342.

[34] Moore, *Lamb*, 342.

[35] Moore, *Lamb*, 341.

many ways, of the mid-thirteenth century *vitae* of Saint Francis of Assisi who is said to have initially felt "terrified and revolted" by persons with leprosy, but ultimately accepted and cared for them.[36] Though Francis is projected in his *vitae* as a Christ-like figure, his actions only emulate Jesus's meetings with persons with leprosy. Instead of healing the leprous, however, Francis overcomes his revulsion in order to provide them with alms, care, and compassion.[37] Though we are meant to aspire to Joshua and Francis's humility and compassion, the tone of the novel assumes that the audience likely still reacts to leprosy and those who suffered from it with repulsion, or what Biff calls "the willies."

Where *Lamb* reimagines a lived past wherein those with leprosy were shunned, more fanciful interpretations of leprosy are also formed by, and perpetuate, the stigma of the "medieval leper." The *Game of Thrones* television show and George R. R. Martin's *A Song of Fire and Ice* novels on which the show is based is perhaps the most recent popular franchise to perpetuate the image of the abhorred and isolated person suffering from a leprosy-like disease. Martin has asserted that his fantasy world of Westeros is "more realistic," both "historically and sociologically, than other neomedieval fantasy."[38] Indeed, *Game of Thrones* reimagines the power struggles of medieval Europe, especially the many wars of succession. However, while Westeros may draw more directly from the lived medieval than other works in its genre, it still relies on and sustains many tropes of the medieval that are not based in historical fact. Like other neomedieval works of science fiction and fantasy, *Game of Thrones* accesses and manipulates the medieval though "a medievalist intermediary."[39] Even with Martin's desire to better represent the medieval than his peers, as a work of fantasy *A Song of Fire and Ice* cannot

---

[36] *Vita secunda,* translated in Regis J. Armstrong, J. A. Wayne Hellmann, and William J. Short, ed., *Francis of Assisi: Early Documents – The Saint* (New York: New City Press, 1999), 248-9. For more on Saint Francis and his relationship to leprosy, see: Courtney A. Krolikoski, "Kissing Lepers: Saint Francis and the Treatment of Lepers in the Central Middle Ages," in *Leprosy and Identity in the Middle Ages*, eds. Elma Brenner and François-Olivier Touati, 269-93.

[37] *Vita secunda,* Armstrong, Hellmann, and Short, ed., *Francis of Assisi: Early Documents - The Founder*, 248.

[38] Shiloh Carroll, "Rewriting the Fantasy Archetype: George R. R. Martin, Neo-medievalist Fantasy, and the Quest for Realism," in *Fantasy and Science-Fiction Medievalisms: From Isaac Asimov to A Game of Thrones*, ed. Helen Young (Amherst: Cambria Press, 2015), 60.

[39] Amy Kaufman, "Medieval Unmoored," *Studies in Medievalism* 19 (2010), 4.

fully and accurately depict the medieval as it reimagines it through a modern, fictional lens. In this "more realistic" medieval world of Westeros a fatal disease called "greyscale" exists which greatly disfigures and torments (both mentally and physically) those who become infected.[40] Though audiences are shown that residents of Westeros feel sympathy for those suffering from greyscale, referred to as "Stone Men," they nevertheless remain excluded from society for fear of contagion.[41] Greyscale is conceptualized as a progressive and highly contagious disease that kills its host slowly and painfully. In its early stages, greyscale causes the skin to become discolored, thin, and cracked, with the color of the skin changing slowly from grey to black. As the disease advances, the skin hardens further causing the limbs to become increasingly stiff and hard to move. These progressive symptoms provide the impetus for the pejorative label of "Stone Men" to refer to all who are infected. Should a person live long enough, greyscale ultimately infects the brain, causing severe pain which often causes them to become excessively violent and unstable. Physically, greyscale's symptoms and progression parallel those of leprosy – changes in the skin's appearance and texture, the disfigurement, and the death and decay of the flesh. Socially, the fear of greyscale and the imperative need to isolate any cases of the disease is clearly reminiscent of the stigma of leprosy. However, unlike those with leprosy in medieval Europe, catching greyscale almost universally led to exile in the ruined cities of Essos, a landmass east of Westeros.[42]

Leprosy was widely considered by medieval authorities to be incurable, save through a miracle. This seems also to be the case with greyscale in *Game of Thrones:* those infected by the disease were considered almost certainly doomed. Yet some medieval physicians and medical writers nevertheless wrote recipes they thought might be capable of

[40] *Game of Thrones*, season 5, special feature, "Histories & Lore: Greyscale & The Stone Men," HBO, 2016, DVD.

[41] *Game of Thrones*, season 5, episode 3, "High Sparrow," directed by Mark Mylod, written by David Benioff and D.B. Weiss, aired 26 April 2015, in broadcast syndication, HBO, 2016, DVD; *Game of Thrones*, season 5, episode 5, "Kill the Boy," directed by Jeremy Podeswa, written by Bryan Cogman, aired 10 May 2015, in broadcast syndication, HBO, 2016, DVD.

[42] *Game of Thrones*, season 5, episode 4, "Sons of the Harpy," directed by Mark Mylod, written by Dave Hill, aired 3 May 2015, in broadcast syndication, HBO, 2016, DVD.

curing, or at least caring for, those with the disease.[43] There are likewise certain cases in the *Game of Thrones* franchise wherein someone who caught greyscale was able to survive the disease. In one striking example, Princess Shireen Baratheon had contracted greyscale as an infant after her father, Stannis Baratheon, gave her a doll that (unbeknownst to him) had been infected when it had come into contact with someone suffering from the disease. Subsequently, Stannis called on every healer, apothecary, and Maester (members of a respected and celebrated order of religious intellectuals) to heal her and his efforts prevailed. Though cured of the disease, Shireen's face remained visibly marked by the effects of the disease for the rest of her life.[44] The method of transmission of greyscale in this example, through an object that had come into contact with an infected person, parallels the medieval understanding of disease transmission by miasma (corrupted, diseased air).[45] However, we see in *Game of Thrones* the merging of the medieval narrative of leprosy with that of the Black Death – a profound event from the Later Middle Ages that has shaped narratives of disease ever since. The Black Death, in many ways, is "one of the most important medievalist tropes" of the present world as it ties into modern fears of the apocalypse, disease, and death.[46] By tying these two tropes of fantasy medievalism together, the writers are able to emphasize the severity of greyscale in the world of Westeros. In Martin's self-professed attempt to combat escapist, traditional fantasy, he emphasizes greyscale as a disease

[43] For a discussion of the medieval medical understanding of leprosy, see: Demaitre, *Leprosy in Premodern Medicine;* Rawcliffe, *Leprosy in Medieval England,* esp. 44-103; Touati, "Contagion"; Luke Demaitre "The Description and Diagnosis of Leprosy by Fourteenth-Century Physicians," *Bulletin of the History of Medicine* 59 (1985): 327-44. For a discussion of miraculous cures of medieval leprosy and their Biblical foundations, see: Rawcliffe, *Leprosy in Medieval England,* esp. 168-79.

[44] *Game of Thrones*, "Sons of the Harpy."

[45] For a more in-depth discussion of miasma theory, see: Vivian Nutton, "Did the Greeks Have a Word For It? Contagion and Contagion Theory in Classical Antiquity," in *Contagion: Perspectives from Pre-Modern Societies*, 137-62; Touati, "Contagion and Leprosy;" Carole Rawcliffe, *Urban Bodies*, esp.116-75; Richard Palmer, "In bad odour: smell and its significance in medicine from antiquity to the seventeenth century," in *Medicine and the Five Senses,* eds. William F. Bynum and Roy Porter (Cambridge: Cambridge University Press, 1993).

[46] Adam Whittaker, "A Plague of Medievalism upon You All: Medievalism, Music, and the Plague," *Studies in Medievalism XXVII: Authenticity, Medievalism, Music* (Woodbridge: D.S. Brewer, 2018), 201.

worthy of extreme oppression and exclusion. However, this ultimately plays into the medievalism that he ostensibly disdains – if greyscale, like leprosy, is meant to be feared, its legacy must also come from the nineteenth- and twentieth-century manipulations of medieval perceptions of the disease.

Like the medievalesque leprosy of Westeros, modern media continues to turn to the "medieval leper" in order to tell (and retell) stories from history, literature, and myth. While most of these works are said to be "based on a true story" or a modern adaptation of a medieval story, many fall back on longstanding stereotypes of the Middle Ages as dark, backwards, and primitive. The portrayal of leprosy in these works often, again, follows the narrative of exclusion. In the second season of the History Channel's *Knightfall*, the Order of Saint Lazarus, a military order founded by crusaders at the *leprosarium* of Jerusalem, is introduced. In the fourth episode of the season, the Knights Templar are warned by Gabriel, a leprous knight of the Order of Saint Lazarus, that Philip, King of France, is sending an army to kill them.[47] A small group of the Templars escort Gabriel, who had been injured by the French troops, back to the Church of Saint Lazarus, where they are invited to stay, pray, and dine with them. The Church of Saint Lazarus is located far beyond the boundaries of any city or civilization, standing alone in a barren field, echoing the portrayal of *leprosaria* as places of exclusion and isolation.[48] The knights of the Order of Saint Lazarus are depicted, through their movements, makeup, and dialogue, as experiencing diverse stages of the disease. They wear masks made of metal as well as chainmail and long-sleeved green tunics adorned with white crosses. This serves both to mark their status in the Order and to hide all visible signs of the disease. Moreover, while *Knightfall* is filmed in grey and earthen tones, the scenes with the knights of Saint Lazarus are presented largely in darkness.[49] The Church of Saint Lazarus is shown with the windows closed and the rooms are bathed in darkness, the only illumination coming from the candles the brothers carry. Their world is one shrouded in darkness and death, with their faith as their only source of light.

---

[47] *Knightfall,* season 2, episode 4, "Equal Before God," directed by David Wellington, written by Kristen SaBerre, released 15 April 2019, Netflix.
[48] *Knightfall,* "Equal Before God".
[49] *Knightfall,* "Equal Before God".

The Order of Saint Lazarus was indeed one of the crusading Orders of the Middle Ages. It was founded around the 1130s at Jerusalem's *leprosarium* (a hospital for those suffering from leprosy) and recognized as a hospital and military order in 1255 by Pope Alexander IV. The historic origins of the order, however, are "obscure and controversial," making it difficult to fully understand the relationship between the Order and the *leprosarium* of Jerusalem it was initially meant to serve.[50] The knights of the Order of Saint Lazarus were initially charged with caring for those affected by leprosy, but the brothers did not need to have the disease themselves in order to join. Indeed, initially it was only the master who was required to be leprous.[51] However, the composition of the Order shifted in the twelfth century with the legal code known as the *Livre au Roi* (c. 1198-1205). This document stated that a knight or sergeant with leprosy should join the Order of Saint Lazarus "where it is established that people with such an illness should be."[52] Moreover, the wife of the leprous knight should join a convent and all their remaining property should go to their heirs or their lord. Similarly, the *Règle du Temple* (The Rule of the Templars) stated that any brothers afflicted with the disease could, if they wanted, transfer to the Order of Saint Lazarus.[53] Those who elected to remain Templars continued to be cared for by the Order but were required to live apart from their brothers.

Though their temple is isolated from the world, the brothers of the Order of Lazarus in *Knightfall* can move freely about in the world and interact with other orders. The fact that Gabriel travelled safely and openly to the Chartres temple to warn his brothers in the Templars suggests that, while not a regular occurrence, this sort of movement was not unheard of. While Landry, the protagonist of *Knightfall*, and a few of his brothers were excited to see their friend from the Crusades and harbored no fear of his disease, one of the newly initiated Templars,

---

[50] David Marcombe, *Leper Knights: The Order of St Lazarus of Jerusalem in England, 1150-1544* (Woodbridge: The Boydell Press, 2003), 6.

[51] Marcombe, *Leper Knights*, 10.

[52] "Le Livre au Roi," in *Assises de la Haute Cour, Recueil des Historiens des Croisades, Lois: Assises de Jérusalem ou Recueil des ouvrages de Jurisprudence composés pendant le XIIIe siècle dans les Royaumes de Jérusalem et de Chypre* vol.1 (Paris: Imprimerie Royale, 1841), 636-7; Barber, "The Order of Saint Lazarus and the Crusades," 444.

[53] *La Règle du Temple,* ed. Henri de Curzon, *Société de l'Histoire de France* (Paris: Librarie Renouard, 1886), 239-40; Barber, "The Order of Saint Lazarus and the Crusades," 444.

Rhone, was clearly uncomfortable with the "leper knights."[54] Rhone's disgust for people with leprosy is revealed to be founded on a local myth of the disease and is, moreover, tied to a family tragedy. Before Gabriel arrives at the Chartres Temple, Rhone is having a conversation with some of his brothers about the causality of leprosy. One of the Templars states that they should give alms to the leprous because "lepers were anointed by God to suffer in Christ's name." Rhone disagrees, saying that "their curse is God's punishment for poisoning wells and murdering children – they bear the mark of Cain." He then tells his brothers how his "sister was killed by a leper when she was five years old." He explains that his father had sent her into the woods to collect berries but, later that night, "a leper returned her to our home, carrying her in his arms" and hours later "a fever took her and she died." His brothers respond that it was "hard to blame the leper" as it was a fever that killed her, not leprosy.[55] Rhone stays firm throughout this interaction in his belief that people infected by leprosy were monsters who took pleasure in watching the healthy suffer. In this way, Rhone showcases the paranoia and disgust that the makers of the show assumed medieval society felt about people who had developed leprosy.

Rhone and his brothers' assorted statements about the cause of leprosy and the nature of those with the disease play on numerous other tropes and legacies of medieval leprosy. The contrasting perceptions of leprosy discussed by the Templars in *Knightfall* – as both God's elect and the damned – coexisted in the Middle Ages and can be seen in the differing responses to the disease across this period in Europe.[56] Though an increasing effort went into supporting and caring for persons with leprosy over the course of the Middle Ages, the image of the unwanted "leper" in medieval hagiography was often used to highlight a potential saint's sanctity.[57] Further, the idea that people with leprosy sought out

---

[54] *Knightfall,* "Equal Before God".
[55] *Knightfall,* "Equal Before God".
[56] For examples of the divergent perceptions of leprosy in the Middle Ages, see Courtney A. Krolikoski, "Malady or Miracle? The Influence of St Francis on the Perception of Leprosy in the High Middle Ages," MA Thesis (Central European University, 2011).
[57] Lily Stewart, "Leprosy, Chastity, and Desire in Medieval Hagiography," *Magistra* 27, no. 1 (2021): 49-78; Courtney A. Krolikoski, "'No More Horrified by Them': Royal Holy Women and Lepers in Twelfth- and Thirteenth-Century Hagiography," in *Living on the Edge: Transgression, Exclusion and Persecution in the Middle Ages,* ed. Delfi Nieto and Laura Miquel Milian (Berlin: De Gruyter, 2022), 59-74; Krolikoski, "Malady or Miracle?"

ways to maliciously transmit their disease to healthy members of society likely stems from the infamous "lepers' plot" of 1321 in the Kingdom of France. This event, recorded in only one extant source, saw persons with leprosy accused of being recruited by Jews in a plot to poison wells and fountains and overthrow Christian rule.[58] This resulted in persons with leprosy being rounded up, questioned, and sentenced to death. Though often pointed to in the historiography of leprosy and the history of persecution as proof of the exclusion and persecution of leprosy sufferers, the events of 1321 were an isolated incident that did not have a significant impact on the perception of leprosy sufferers in the later Middle Ages.[59]

In a final example, Ridley Scott's 2005 film *Kingdom of Heaven* showcases another attempt to depict a more "historical" picture of leprosy in the Middle Ages. While the movie is often discussed by historians as an inherently problematic portrayal of the Middle Ages for a number of reasons, I would like to focus here on how writers and producers chose to tell the story of King Baldwin IV (d. 1185), the "leper king of Jerusalem." The Baldwin of *Kingdom of Heaven* is regularly adorned in beautiful silver and white regalia which, though projecting his status as king, allows him to cover every inch of his body and hide the state of his disease. For the same reason, his face is also covered with a metal mask (something which *Knightfall* likely took as inspiration for their Knights of the Order of Saint Lazarus). In the historical sources, we are told in the *Chronicon* of William of Tyre, Baldwin's tutor, that leprosy rendered Baldwin blind, disfigured, and disabled to the point that he had to be carried onto the battlefield on a litter.[60] William claims he was the first to notice and report the symptoms that would later be determined

[58] The "lepers' plot" was recorded only in the fourteenth century chronicle of Guillaume de Nangis. H. Géraud, ed., *Chronique Latine de Guillaume de Nangis de 1113 à 1300 avec les Continuations de cette chronique de 1300 à 1368,* vol. 2 (Paris: Société de l'Histoire de France, 1843). For a recent contextualization of this episode, see Tzafrir Barzilay, *Poisoned Wells: Accusations, Persecution, and Minorities in Medieval Europe, 1321-1422* (Philadelphia, PA: University of Pennsylvania Press, 2022), 38-70.

[59] For example, see Malcom Barber, "Lepers, Jews and Moslems: The Plot to Overthrow Christendom in 1321," *History* 66, no. 216 (1981), 1-17; David Nirenberg, *Communities of Violence: Persecution of Minorities in the Middle Ages,* Second Edition (Princeton: Princeton University Press, 2015); Steve Tibble, "Medieval Strategy? The Great "Leper Conspiracy" of 1321," *Yale University Press Blog,* 11 September 2020, https://yalebooks.yale.edu/2020/09/11/medieval-strategy-the-great-leper-conspiracy-of-1321.

[60] Bernard Hamilton, *The Leper King and His Heirs: Baldwin IV and the Crusader Kingdom of Jerusalem* (Cambridge: Cambridge University Press, 2000), 202.

to be leprosy in Baldwin to the King. Though these initial symptoms suggested that the young Baldwin might be developing leprosy, William stated that the disease became clear as he "began to approach the age of puberty." [61] As time passed, and as the physicians "made more comprehensive observations," they realized that "this was the beginning of an incurable disease."[62] Yet, even with his body ravaged by leprosy, "the hearts of his faithful men were touched by compassion when they looked at him."[63] Yet he was a cunning and courageous leader who was skilled on horseback and used those skills, even when his condition worsened, to defeat Saladin in 1177 at Mont Gisard after the sultan attacked his kingdom in Jerusalem and again at the battle of Le Forbelet.[64]

Despite the medieval image of Baldwin as a successful leader and compassionate king, the image of leprosy presented in *Kingdom of Heaven* is nevertheless one shaped by the long historical myth of the disease. While it has been argued that the high profile enjoyed by the historic Baldwin as a "noble leper" with "unimpeachable moral character" was an important factor in promoting a positive image of the disease in the twelfth century, this is not how he is depicted in the *Kingdom of Heaven.*[65] In the film, Baldwin's condition and the state of his body, rendered almost non-human by leprosy, is only revealed upon his death, a reveal that is meant to be a great surprise to both the characters in the film and the audience. In one part of the film, Baldwin reveals his condition to

---

[61] "...cum ad pubertatis annos cepit exsurgere morbo elephantioso visus est periculosissime laborare." William of Tyre, *Chronicon,* ed. R.B.C. Huygens, vol 2. (Turnhout: Brepols, 1986), 962. It is worth noting that we should avoid reading too much into William's discussion of Baldwin's leprosy as he was in many ways using his text to defend Baldwin and his disease from those who believed that he had been punished by God with the disease for his actions in Jerusalem. P.W. Edbury and J.G. Rowe, *William of Tyre: Historian of the Latin East* (Cambridge: Cambridge University Press, 1988), 45-6; Philip Handyside, *The Old French of William of Tyre* (Leiden: Brill, 2015), 5.

[62] "Erat enim, ut processu temporis ipso rerum experimento postea plenius cognovimus, amplioris et penitus incurabilis doloris initium quod premittebatur." William of Tyre, *Chronicon,* 962.

[63] "Quo per dies singulos ingravescente nimium, extremitatibus maxime lesis et facie, fidelium suorum corda, quotiens eum intuebantur, compassionis affectu molestabat." William of Tyre, *Chronicon,* 962.

[64] Marcombe, *Leper Knights,* 13; Hamilton, *The Leper King and His Heirs,* 132-58, 171-78, 241-42.

[65] Rawcliffe, *Leprosy in Medieval England,* 54.

Balian, a blacksmith turned Crusader who had caught the king's attention, stating simply "I am a leper."[66] This revelation was prompted by Balian having killed a Saracen who happened to be a close friend of the king. Baldwin explains that this was the man who had "noticed that [he] felt no pain" in his youth and had concluded that the young Baldwin had contracted leprosy.[67] By depicting King Baldwin in *Kingdom of Heaven* as reluctant to expose the state of his health to anyone beyond his closest supporters the film reinforces the narrative that people in the Middle Ages saw the disease as shameful and worthy of fear.

It is, as David Matthews has noted, the task of medievalism studies to "hunt [the] revenants" of medieval history in the modern world so that we may understand how our responses to, and uses of, the Middle Ages have been shaped.[68] As medievalism arguably comprises everything medieval that was crafted *after* the Middle Ages, the variety of works analyzed in this paper highlight how varied the modern uses and interpretations of medieval leprosy can be. With the nineteenth- and twentieth-century explications of medieval sources, modern authors formed their own medievalisms concerning leprosy and the image of the "medieval leper" that have remained influential in Anglophone popular culture to the present day. From U2 and Christopher Moore's use of the Biblical foundations of the conception of leprosy, to the re-imaginations of historical persons with leprosy in *Knightfall* and *Kingdom of Heaven*, and to the manipulation of the medieval disease of leprosy in George R.R. Martin's books and HBO's *Game of Thrones,* the leprosy of the Middle Ages has been interpreted as a disease that is morally and physically repulsive. The "medieval leper" in these examples is thus the perpetual "other" – excluded from normative society and yet, simultaneously, at society's mercy.[69]

Acknowledging the place(s) of the medieval leper in contemporary media allows us to further engage with how our perceptions of the past have been shaped and, in turn, allows us to question how we understand

---

[66] *Kingdom of Heaven*, directed by Ridley Scott (2005; Los Angeles: 20th Century Fox, 2005), DVD.

[67] Scott, *Kingdom of Heaven.*

[68] Matthews, *Medievalism: A Critical History*, 1.

[69] For further discussion of representations of leprosy in mystery novels, see Lucy Barnhouse's chapter in this volume, "Mysteries and Medicines: Medieval Medical Practitioners in Crime Fiction".

and interpret our present. In this way, the continued portrayal in modern media of persons suffering from leprosy in the European Middle Ages as outcasts says more about our present situation than it does our past. A growing number of scholars have argued that "genuine historical neutrality does not exist," meaning that historians cannot claim that their work on the past is entirely divorced from the present world and their own personal situation.[70] As Paul Strohm has shown, no matter how hard we may try to tell the truth of the past, we will never be able to "get it right."[71] Much the same can be said about how leprosy, both medieval and modern, is depicted in contemporary media. With over 200,000 new cases each year worldwide as reported by the World Health Organization,[72] people diagnosed with Hansen's Disease today continue to be affected by the nineteenth-century invented narrative of exclusion of leprosy sufferers in the Middle Ages. Today's scholarship, especially public-facing scholarship, on medieval leprosy has the power to shift the discourse in a way that can simultaneously emphasize the lived realities of those diagnosed with leprosy in the European Middle Ages and adjust modern perceptions of those living with Hansen's Disease today. This, in a sense, involves erasing – or at least qualifying – today's medievalisms concerning leprosy in favor of understanding that medieval society's approach to leprosy in the Middle Ages was one of inclusion, care, and support. Instead of forcefully excluding those who had contracted the disease, medieval society came together to support its most vulnerable members. Perhaps our modern world might benefit from learning how to be just a little more medieval.

---

[70] Celia Chazelle, Simon Doubleday, Felice Lifshitz, and Amy G. Remensnyder, eds., *Why the Middle Ages Matter: Medieval Light on Modern Injustice* (London: Routledge, 2012), 3.

[71] Paul Strohm, "Historicity without historicism?" *postmedieval* 1 (2010), 387.

[72] "Leprosy (Hansen's disease)," *World Health Organization,* last modified 10 May 2021, https://www.who.int/news-room/fact-sheets/detail/leprosy.

THE FANTASY OF MEDIEVAL MEDICINE: ORIENTALIZING EXPERIENTIAL AND TEXTUAL TRADITIONS IN THE IMAGINED MEDIEVAL PAST

ROBIN S. REICH*

Author Robert Jordan once described the setting of his popular book series, *The Wheel of Time,* as "not the medieval period, not a fantasy with knights in shining armor … imagine it as the late 17th century without gunpowder."[1] Jordan used this setting to construct a fantasy world defined by an absence of technology and even of scientific knowledge. This absence is made conspicuous throughout the series, especially as characters with knowledge of an earlier, more technologically-advanced age lament the loss of their civilization.[2] Although Jordan explicitly distanced his temporal setting from the Middle Ages, he chose to set the technology of this world farther in the past to make it seem regressive from a modern-coded earlier period in this fantasy world.[3] This technological medievalism challenges the characters to overcome the

* Center for Medieval Studies, Fordham University.

1 "Robert Jordan: The Name Behind the Wheel," *Locus Magazine*, March 2000, http://www.locusmag.com/2000/Issues/03/Jordan.html.

2 See, for example, Robert Jordan, *Lord of Chaos* (New York: Tor Books, 1994).

3 Hilary Jane Locke, "Beyond 'Tits and Dragons': Medievalism, Medieval History, and Perceptions in Game of Thrones," in *From Medievalism to Early-Modernism: Adapting the English Past*, ed. Marina Gerzić and Aidan Norrie (New York: Routledge, 2019), 172; Kelly DeVries, "Gunpowder Weaponry and the Rise of the Early Modern State," *War in History* 5, no. 2 (1998): 129; Elly Rachel Truitt, *Medieval Robots: Mechanism, Magic, Nature, and Art* (Philadelphia: University of Pennsylvania Press, 2015), 2.

limits of their knowledge. The character Nynaeve, for instance, builds her healing skills in two conflicting contexts: the orally transmitted herbal tradition within which she was raised and the text-based magical study to which she aspires. In Nynaeve's struggle, Jordan's technological medievalism becomes a balancing act between tradition and advancement. Not only in Jordan's work, fantasy literature and media often use pretextually medieval settings to explore the complexities of navigating competing medical systems and theories. These can be beneficial reflections, but they also have the potential to develop tropes that reinforce harmful biases, such as an Orientalist contrast between the "traditional" and the "Western."[4]

In this essay, I consider how medieval and medieval-coded fictional settings present medical knowledge, and how these fictional presentations can reflect on the study of medieval history and literature. While fantastical uses of medieval themes and settings typically are not directly informed by medievalist scholarship, this literature has the power to articulate and influence attitudes towards the medieval that can extend to new scholarship.[5] Fantasy literature, as the case of Nynaeve illustrates, frequently constructs two types of medical knowledge: one that is esoteric, obscure, even magical, and accessed only through specialized study; and one that is inherited through oral or experiential tradition, innate, and democratically available. As we will see, these types have cogent equivalents in the current scholarly understanding of medieval medicine, and in that sense the fictional exploration of them in fantasy settings can be an imaginative way to access the medieval past.[6] At the same time, these categories can easily map onto the Orientalist divide

[4] We can find some precedent for the articulation of this dichotomy in Edward Said, *Orientalism* (New York: Random House, 1978), as the notion that European and North American societies are driven by progress and development, while others are timeless and mired in the past. On the particulars of this theory and its subsequent development, see Bryan S. Turner, *Orientalism, Postmodernism and Globalism* (London: Routledge, 1994), 7–8; Wael B. Hallaq, Restating Orientalism: A Critique of Modern Knowledge (New York: Columbia University Press, 2018), 36–7; Mohammad R. Salama, Islam, Orientalism and Intellectual History*: Modernity and the Politics of Exclusion Since Ibn Khaldun*, Library of Middle East History (London: I.B. Tauris, 2011), 7–8, 12–14.

[5] Helen Young and Kavita Mudan Finn, *Global Medievalism: An Introduction* (Cambridge: Cambridge University Press, 2022), 7.

[6] Locke, "Beyond 'Tits and Dragons', 175–76.

between East and West, modern and premodern, and can thus reinforce harmful and unfounded distinctions.[7]

I begin by considering the relationship between fantasy fiction and medieval history. Based on some of the most popular works of fantasy – some of which have gained their widest appeal through video media – I identify depictions of medicine as the contrasting Orientalist tropes of scholarly and indigenous knowledge. I follow these categories through medieval traditions of herbal medicine, fictional Westeros, and the quick thinking of one brave hobbit. In my historical examples, I concentrate on the twelfth-century Mediterranean, the focus of much scholarship on medieval medicine. Finally, I pursue these themes through to a problematic result, examining how scholarship has often misinterpreted the report on Crusader medicine by Usama ibn Munqidh. I find that while it is easy to dismiss ahistorical depictions of medieval tropes as uninformed, these tropes are themselves grounded in outdated scholarship and thus still have the ability to encourage uncritical thinking about the Middle Ages in both popular media and current scholarship.

I. Fiction and Medicine

Fantasy fiction offers a lens for perceptions of technology and medicine in a way that illuminates modern attitudes towards both the present and the past. In contrast to science fiction, which often proposes speculative technologies, and can indeed inspire scientific innovation, fantasy is typically retrospective, reflecting more on progress already made.[8] As Marie Sachiko Cecire and Irina Ruppo Malone have each argued, fantasy can have a humanizing effect on the modern world, a Romantic overlay on the dreary, cold reality constructed by the objectivity of modern science.[9] Cecire argues that this function was established by C.S. Lewis

[7] See Note 5 above. For an overview of this concept in the premodern periods, see Ivan Kalmar, *Early Orientalism: Imagined Islam and the Notion of Sublime Power* (London: Routledge, 2012); Nikolaos G. Chrissis, Athina Kolia-Dermitzaki, and Angeliki Papageorgiou, eds., *Byzantium and the West: Perception and Reality (11th-15th C.)* (London: Routledge, 2019).

[8] Bill Pomidor and Alice K Pomidor, "Essay: 'With Great Power…' The Relevance of Science Fiction to the Practice and Progress of Medicine," *Medicine and Creativity* 368 (December 1, 2006), 13–14.

[9] Maria Sachiko Cecire, *Re-Enchanted: The Rise of Children's Fantasy Literature in the Twentieth Century* (Minneapolis: University of Minnesota Press, 2019), 2; Irina Ruppo Malone,

and J.R.R. Tolkien, fantasy authors who were also medievalist scholars and who found a more potent reality in a medieval past that stepped "outside of the relentless linear narratives of progress."[10]

Other scholars have seen this humanistic contrast between fantasy and science as instructive. For instance, Harvey B. Simon has argued that medical doctors should read well-crafted novels to humanize their practice, because they challenge the reader to evaluate complex and ambiguous information such as morality, emotion, and social relationships.[11] Jennifer J. Conn extends Simon's argument to fantasy literature specifically, arguing that J.K. Rowling's *Harry Potter* series and its offshoots provide both role models and useful conceptual approaches for clinicians.[12] Indeed, biomedical scientists have found surprisingly deep applications for fantastical literary metaphors, as in the 2020 paper by Garrido et al., titled "Lord of the NanoRings: Cyclodeztrins and the Battle against SARS-CoV-2," in which the authors extend Tolkien's ring of power to describe the microscopic structure of organic anti-viral devices.[13] Perhaps more superficially, however, others, such as the National Library of Medicine, have used the loose relationship between the representation of science in this literature and current STEM fields to encourage children to pursue futures in the biomedical sciences.[14]

Representations of medicine in fantasy literature thus have real power to influence our understanding of what medicine can do in the present or future, by making comparisons to what it has not been able to do in the past, or indeed, what the fantasy genre often relegates so far into the

---

"What's Wrong with Medievalism? Tolkien, the Strugatsky Brothers, and the Question of the Ideology of Fantasy," *Journal of the Fantastic in the Arts* 27 (2016), 212.

[10] Cecire, *Re-Enchanted: The Rise of Children's Fantasy Literature in the Twentieth Century*, 3.

[11] Harvey B. Simon, "Reading Fiction," *The American Journal of Medicine* 127, no. 4 (April 1, 2014): 357; David Comer Kidd and Castano Emanuele, "Reading Literary Fiction Improves Theory of Mind," *Science* 342, no. 6156 (October 18, 2013), 377–80.

[12] Jennifer J Conn, "What Can Clinical Teachers Learn from Harry Potter and the Philosopher's Stone?," *Medical Education* 36, no. 12 (December 1, 2002), 1176–81.

[13] Pablo F. Garrido et al., "The Lord of the NanoRings: Cyclodextrins and the Battle against SARS-CoV-2," *International Journal of Pharmaceutics* 588 (October 15, 2020), 119689. See also Kavita Mudan Finn, ed., *Game of Thrones*, Fan Phenomena (Bristol: Intellect Books, 2017), 179–90.

[14] The exhibit, titled *Renaissance Science, Magic, and Medicine in Harry Potter's World* included modules on potions, herbology, and immortality. It is permanently available, as of publication of this volume, on the library's website at www.nlm.nih.gov/exhibition /sciencemagicmedicine/index.html.

realm of impossibility that such medicine is only achieved through magic.[15] Fantasy literature itself seems to use descriptions of medicine and biomedical technologies as part of its worldbuilding, as in the quote from Robert Jordan above, to establish the rules and limitations of the setting that might become obstacles for the characters. Epic fantasy book series and their film adaptations [16] take different approaches to the medieval setting, often using features that are coded as medieval, such as castles, infectious skin diseases, and a lack of automation or electricity (the literal darkness of the "Dark Ages"), to signal medical regression from the real-world present.[17] Even in explicitly fantastical works, these aspects, including depictions of frameworks for medical knowledge, often read as historical.[18] We can see this interpretation most clearly in the numerous essays that have been published in the last decade that try to distinguish between the "real" and "fake" medieval history in HBO's *Game of Thrones,* based on the book series *A Song of Ice and Fire* by George R.R. Martin.[19] A similar work that parses the historical and mythological influences in *Wheel of Time* has recently appeared.[20] Indeed, aspects of the

---

[15] Truitt, *Medieval Robots: Mechanism, Magic, Nature, and Art*, 1–3. This is something of an inversion of Arthur C. Clarke's third law, "Any sufficiently advanced technology is indistinguishable from magic." Eugene P. Wigner, "Time and Effort Reports Defended," *Science* 159, no. 3812 (1968): 255–255, https://doi.org/10.1126 /science.159.3812.255.a; Arthur C. Clarke, *Profiles of the Future; an Inquiry into the Limits of the Possible*, [1st ed.] (New York: Harper & Row, [c1962]).

[16] I consider the adaptations of these works as part of their canon because it is through video media that these works have realized even more widespread and integrated cultural influence.

[17] See John M. Ganim, "Medieval Noir: Anatomy of a Metaphor," in *Medieval Film*, ed. Anke Bernau and Bettina Bildhauer (Manchester: Manchester University Press, 2009).

[18] Locke, "Beyond 'Tits and Dragons', 174.

[19] "The Real Medieval History Behind Of 'Game Of Thrones,'" accessed December 14, 2021, www.wbur.org/radioboston/2019/04/15/game-of-thrones; Richard Marsden, "Game of Thrones: Imagined World Combines Romantic and Grotesque Visions of Middle Ages," The Conversation, accessed December 14, 2021, http://theconver sation.com/game-of-thrones-imagined-world-combines-romantic-and-grotesque-visions-of-middle-ages-105141; "Game of Thrones Effect Seen in Medieval Studies Scholarship | Time," accessed December 14, 2021, https://time.com/ 4837351/game-of-thrones-real-medieval-history/. See also Kavita Mudan Finn, ed., *Game of Thrones.*

[20] Michael Livingston, *Origins of the Wheel of Time: The Legends and Mythologies that Inspired Robert Jordan* (New York: Tor Books, 2022).

depiction of medicine and medical knowledge in these works often are historical, but they are not necessarily medieval.[21]

II. Ways of Knowing in Medieval and Fantasy Medicine

Although fantasy literature invokes a sense of medievalness, its historical references are at times more medieval*ism* than medieval, and instead present modern readings of the medieval past. Recalling Cecire and Malone's understanding of Tolkien and Lewis as Romantics, even Luddites, in the face of the common characterization of particularly twentieth-century medical innovation as the steady march of upward progress, the medieval past is a foil, the Age of Uninformation against which progress is made.[22] Implicitly, then, the medieval past is valued as negative or perhaps impotent in this narrative. This contrast between progress and backwardness reflects a colonialist or Orientalist approach to knowledge in which the oral or experiential transmission of knowledge is framed in opposition – and made implicitly inferior – to systematized written transmission.[23]

On the one hand, fantastical depictions of medieval medicine can show knowledge of healing that is rooted in tradition, a connection to the inhabited land, and personal grit. This depiction maps onto the notion of the indigenous, traditions that are primarily transmitted orally or experientially, and tied to an intimate knowledge of the environment.[24] In Nynaeve's story from *The Wheel of Time,* above, Jordan characterizes Nynaeve's talent for healing as not only innate, but inherited: through the oral tradition by which she learned it; tied to her region of the Two Rivers, a landscape that functions as an essential identifier for Nynaeve and her companions throughout their story; and preserved in her travels by means of a frequently-remarked upon "stubbornness" that is also

[21] Young and Finn, *Global Medievalism,* 30-1.

[22] Charles E. Rosenberg, "Disease in History: Frames and Framers," *The Milbank Quarterly* 67, no. 1 (1989): 8; James Delbourgo, "The Knowing World: A New Global History of Science," *History of Science* 57 (September 1, 2019), 378–81

[23] See Young and Finn, *Global Medievalism,* 5.

[24] For more on indigenous medical traditions and their suppression by colonialism, see the National Library of Medicine exhibit "Native Voices" www.nlm.nih.gov/nativevoices/index.html.

understood as characteristic of her people.[25] On the other hand, fantasy often displays knowledge derived through book learning, limited to characters who are able to read in largely illiterate societies. This invokes the Orientalist, the archaeologist, even the historian, as the pursuit of someone struggling to uncover known truth in written records that has been lost or made inaccessible. One category relies on the other as a foil.[26] Again, in Nynaeve's story, upon her arrival at the White Tower, the institution where she is meant to formalize her medical knowledge, Nynaeve's stubbornness becomes an obstacle to her success, as she discovers that she can only access her magical healing powers when she is angry, a struggle that literalizes the conflict between her indigenous-coded tradition and the esoteric knowledge to which the White Tower allows her access.[27] Iona McCleery has argued that late-medieval adaptations of oral or experiential indigenous knowledge traditions similarly treated the information itself as useful, but found the unwritten system difficult to access.[28] Implicit in these relationships is the understanding that oral or experiential medical systems are less potent than written traditions because they are not formalized in writing, and that the process of uncovering them harnesses them more effectively. It is for this reason that the two kinds of knowledge exist as a pair in fantasy literature, creating a tension around the acquisition or use of medical knowledge that can drive the plot.

As the parent of the modern fantasy genre, *Lord of the Rings* set the precedent for this dichotomy of medical ways of knowing. In the first book of the series (and the first movie of the film adaptations), *The Fellowship of the Ring*, the characters require both kinds of knowledge to save the protagonist, Frodo, from certain death. Frodo has been stabbed by a deadly magical blade and needs exceptional medical attention. But the party is far away from any help. So, two of his companions, Aragorn, a Ranger, and Samwise Gamgee, a gardener, go off in search of an herb

---

[25] See, for example, Robert Jordan, *The Eye of the World* (New York: Tor Books, 1990); Robert Jordan, *The Shadow Rising* (New York: Tor Books, 1992); and Robert Jordan, *A Crown of Swords* (New York: Tor Books, 1996).

[26] Madhuri Sharma, *Indigenous and Western Medicine in Colonial India* (New Delhi: Foundation Books, 2012), 1–2.

[27] Jordan, *Lord of Chaos*, 310-27.

[28] Iona McCleery, "What Is 'Colonial' about Medieval Colonial Medicine? Iberian Health in Global Context," *Journal of Medieval Iberian Studies* 7, no. 2 (2015), 161.

called kingsfoil.[29] It is their wild wisdom – Aragorn's knowledge of the occult forces behind Frodo's stab wound (and, in the movie adaptation, Sam's ability to identify what he sees as a weed in the wild) – that keeps Frodo alive until he can be treated. But this knowledge only takes them so far. Frodo must be seen by the elves at Rivendell, who understand the plant's healing powers, to cure him of the malicious magic and the wound. The elves appear several times throughout the series and its prequel novel *The Hobbit* as custodians and mediators of an esoteric past: keepers of ancient knowledge and artifacts.[30] It is implied that the elves save Frodo in part because of the secretive and ancient knowledge they represent. In Tolkien's Romanticist vision of the medieval past, the wisdom of the elves is a textually recorded but rapidly fading source of knowledge. Sam and Aragorn's understanding of the land is a related but less potent form of medicine.

This framing of medical knowledge has become a trope in fantasy literature written over the last thirty years. Late in the *Game of Thrones* television adaptation, Samwell Tarly (a character heavily inspired by Samwise Gamgee) serves as a plot device through his esoteric knowledge.[31] In Season 7, while studying at the Citadel, seemingly the only educational institution in the world of *Game of Thrones*, Samwell steals a book from the library in order to learn the cure for a disease known as greyscale.[32] *Game of Thrones* depicts the inaccessibility of the knowledge in this library literally, showing the books chained to the shelf so that only those with permission and status may read them – a fantastical take on the chained libraries of the Middle Ages such as the one that survives at Hereford Cathedral.[33] Samwell's mentor has already warned him that the cure for greyscale is too dangerous even to attempt,

[29] J.R.R. Tolkien, *The Fellowship of the Ring* (London: Allen & Unwin, 1954).

[30] J.R.R. Tolkien, *The Hobbit* (London: George Allen & Unwin, 1937).

[31] In response to a reader's inquiry on this topic, author George R.R. Martin wrote in 2001: "There are a number of homages to LOTR [Lord of the Rings] in my book. I am a huge Tolkien fan." https://www.westeros.org/Citadel/SSM/Entry/1165.

[32] Dermatologists have considered the historical comparisons to greyscale, particularly leprosy. Jules B. Lipoff, "Greyscale – A Mystery Dermatologic Disease on HBO's Game of Thrones," *JAMA Dermatology* 152, no. 8 (August 1, 2016), 904, https://doi.org/10.1001/jamadermatol.2015.5793.

[33] See Burnett Hillman Streeter, *The Chained Library: A Survey of Four Centuries in the Evolution of the English Library* (London: Macmillan and Co., 1931); Joan Williams, *The Chained Library at Hereford Cathedral* (Hereford: Hereford Cathedral Enterprises, 1996).

and it is partially for this reason that the book has been locked away. In this episode, text-based knowledge is a complex maze of forbidden information. The disease of greyscale is famously incurable, and yet the truth that Samwell learns is that there is in fact a known cure, but the *knowledge* of it has been locked away. It is intentionally kept secret by a large and powerful institution because the members of that institution believe they are protecting society.

There is a way in which we can interpret Samwell's story as an allegory of modern medical anxieties, such as the inaccessibility of healthcare. The inaccessibility of medical treatment was the focal point of much public discourse in the US throughout the early years of the twenty-first century, punctuated by the release of documentaries highlighting the failures of the American healthcare system, such as Michael Moore's 2007 documentary, *Sicko*, as well as the landmark legislation of the Obama presidency, the Affordable Care Act, enacted in 2010. In this context, the central struggle was indeed a distance between medical knowledge and access to treatment, seemingly created by powerful institutions. It would be comforting, therefore, to understand barriers to healthcare access as relics of an unfree past society. Writers such as Martin and the adaptation's showrunners can find easy evidence for a superficial reading of their medieval European setting in the fact that the majority of medieval medical manuscripts were produced by or for either the wealthy or religious institutions such as monasteries upon which the Citadel appears to be based.[34]

However, we can also see this depiction of the inaccessibility of medical knowledge as a modern understanding of medieval medical texts *themselves* as inaccessible. A modern reader attempting to discern medical practice from medieval texts might be stymied by many aspects of the ways that these works recorded medicine, such as the fact that some of these writings were apparently not intended to be instructional. In Samwell's story, he can access instructions to a full medical procedure in

[34] Cornelius O'Boyle, *Thirteenth- and Fourteenth-Century Copies of the Ars Medicine* (Cambridge: Cambridge Wellcome Unit for the History of Medicine, 1998), xi–xv; Florence Eliza Glaze, "The Perforated Wall: The Ownership and Circulation of Medical Books in Medieval Europe, ca. 800-1200" (Doctoral Dissertation, Duke University, 1999), 12–18; Monica Green, "Medical Books," in *The European Book in the Twelfth Century*, ed. Erik Kwakkel and Rodney Thomson (Cambridge, UK: Cambridge University Press, 2018), 278–82.

a single text. There is not an exact medieval parallel to this, particularly for the later medieval setting that often serves as inspiration for these fantasy worlds.[35] Some types of later medieval medical works, such as the *Articella* collections, which served as the foundation for medical instruction starting in the twelfth century, focused more on theory than practice.[36] None of the works included in this collection instruct the reader on cures; instead, they theorize aspects of diagnostics and describe various diseases.[37] For instance, most *Articella* manuscripts from around the thirteenth century include the work *De urinis* of Theophilus Protospatharius, an influential treatise that theorizes in detail how the visual examination of urine can be used for diagnosis.[38] In this text, we see a more theoretical approach, as the method of uroscopy, the actual practice of examining urine, is not described.[39]

There were also more practical texts that did describe procedures, and these could have been used as guides to varying degrees. For instance, surgical texts, such as the highly influential work of Abū al-Qāsim Khalaf ibn al-ʻAbbās al-Zahrāwī al-Ansari, known in Latin as Albucasis or Abulcasis, described procedures in limited terms, giving more detail on specialized tools than specific actions.[40] Meanwhile, collections known

[35] For a discussion of the differences between surviving medieval surgical texts and the evidence from the skeletons themselves of medieval people, see Claire Burridge's chapter in this volume, "Early Medieval Surgery: Challenging Popular Stereotypes with Archaeological Evidence".

[36] Green, "Medical Books," 286; Danielle Jacquart, "Review: Thirteenth- and Fourteenth-Century Copies of the Ars Medicine: A Checklist and Contents Description of the Manuscripts by Cornelius O'Boyle; The Articella in the Early Press, c. 1476–1534 by Jon Arrizabalaga; Papers of the Articella Project Meeting: Cambridge, December 1995 by Roger French," *Isis* 94, no. 4 (2003), 717–18.

[37] O'Boyle, *Copies of Ars Medicine*, i–xvi.

[38] O'Boyle, *Copies of Ars Medicine*, v.

[39] Faith Wallis, "Signs and Senses: Diagnosis and Prognosis in Early Medieval Pulse and Urine Texts," *Social History of Medicine* 13, no. 2 (2000): 266–67; Laurence Moulinier-Brogi, *L'uroscopie Au Moyen Age – "Lire Dans Un Verre La Nature de l'homme"* (Paris: Champion, 2012).

[40] Emilie Savage-Smith, "The Practice of Surgery in Islamic Lands: Myth and Reality," *Social History of Medicine* 13, no. 2 (2000): 315; M.S. Spink and G.L. Lewis, eds., *Albucasis on Surgery and Instruments* (Berkeley: University of California Press, 1973). Nancy Siraisi also emphasizes that Latin surgical texts often segregated descriptions or explanations of practice to handbooks, keeping them separate from texts that addressed specific conditions. Nancy G. Siraisi, "How to Write a Latin Book on Surgery: Organizing

as *Practica,* which were organized systematically by body part and disease, often gave detailed instructions for treatment, as did *materia medica* texts.[41] Scholars like Linda Voigts have argued that in the early medieval period, medical handbooks were intentionally instructional, meant to record for the purposes of reproduction the steps required to undertake a cure.[42]

It is not always clear to a modern reader, though, that this was the case, as texts can at times give deceptively incomplete pictures of medieval medicine. For instance, one *materia medica* text of Salerno, *Circa Instans* of Matthaeus Platearius, composed between 1150 and 1170, offers the following imprecise recipe for bladder retention: "For resolving painful or difficult urination, a large quantity of cypress, once pounded, should be infused in a good quality oil, and, after having been strained, it should be applied as a poultice to the abdomen. It will then induce urine and should dissolve humors."[43] This recipe would be nearly impossible to produce from the written explanation alone, since it does not explain the quantities of the ingredients, how to choose ones of appropriate quality, how finely to crush the cypress, or how long to infuse the oil. Aspects of practice such as time, quantity, and quality are omitted from written instructions such as these, but likely would have been known to medical practitioners through the tacit, experiential, and oral aspects of their training.[44] While this is most evident in works attributed to the twelfth century, this distance between what is written regarding practice and what was able to be undertaken extended into the later Middle Ages and the early modern period, even as texts became more detailed in their

Principles and Authorial Devices in Guglielmo Da Saliceto and Dino Del Garbo," in *Practical Medicine from Salerno to the Black Death*, ed. Luis Garcia-Ballester et al. (Cambridge: Cambridge University Press, 1994), 93–94.

[41] For a summary of conventions of *Practica*, see Winston Black, "Review: *La* 'Practica' *de Plateario: Edición Crítica, Traducción y Estudio*," *Speculum* 93, no. 3 (2018), 895–97.

[42] Linda E. Voigts, "Anglo-Saxon Plant Remedies and the Anglo-Saxons," *Isis* 70, no. 2 (1979), 251–52.

[43] "Contra stranguriam et dissuriam in multa quantitate quassati aliquantulum ciperi in oleo decoquantur bene, post pectini et peritoneo cataplasmentur, provocant urinam et humores dissolvunt." Matthaeus Platearius, *Circa Instans. Text Und Kommentar*, ed. Hans Wölfel (Berlin, 1939), 37.

[44] See Pamela H. Smith, Amy R.W. Meyers, Harold J. Cook, eds., *Ways of Making and Knowing: The Material Culture of Empirical Knowledge* (Ann Arbor: Univ. of Michigan Press, 2014).

instructions.[45] Contemporary medical education similarly formalizes the instruction of practice through experiential modules rather than the teaching of medical procedures in writing.

Modern readers of these medieval medical texts will therefore find that a lot is missing, or that much seems to be hidden. Historians have often interpreted these gaps in the literature as a reflection of knowledge of medicine that was lost in Latin between the end of the Roman Empire and the twelfth century or so.[46] Although it is no longer how medievalist scholars understand medicine or knowledge more broadly, this notion of loss was essential to how writers of the Enlightenment envisioned themselves in comparison to a "dark" medieval past, articulating the Renaissance as the rediscovery of lost Classical knowledge. This understanding of loss is present throughout fantastical depictions of esoteric knowledge: in Martin's work it is in the waning of culture, perhaps metaphorically represented in the decreasing presence and power of dragons; in Jordan's work it is the literal loss of technology as the result of the apocalyptic event referred to as "the Breaking of the

[45] Pamela Smith and Pamela Long both address this distance between written and practical knowledge in the sciences related to artisanal crafts in the Early Modern period. Pamela H. Smith, *The Body of the Artisan: Art and Experience in the Scientific Revolution* (Chicago: University of Chicago Press, 2004), 6–8; Pamela O. Long, *Openness, Secrecy, Authorship: Technical Arts and the Culture of Knowledge from Antiquity to the Renaissance* (Baltimore: Johns Hopkins University Press, 2001), 1–2. For a specifically medical context, see Katharine Park, *Secrets of Women: Gender, Generation, and the Origins of Human Dissection* (New York: Zone Books, 2006), 13–14.

[46] This narrative was articulated for scientific texts generally by Charles Homer Haskins, *The Renaissance of the Twelfth Century* (Cambridge, MA: Harvard University Press, 1927). More recently, scholars such as Charles Burnett and Monica Green have extended and updated this claim to focus specifically on the translation of Arabic scientific texts in particular and the production of new medical texts in Latin based on them. Newer scholarship such as this has increasingly deemphasized the notion of loss, attempting to understand medieval science more in its own terms. Burnett; Monica Green, "Rethinking the Manuscript Basis of Salvatore de Renzi's Collectio Salernitana: The Corpus of Medical Writings in the 'Long' Twelfth Century," in *La Collectio Salernitana Di Salvatore de Renzi*, ed. Danielle Jacquart and Agostino Paravicino Bagliani (Florence: SISMEL, 2008), 17–18. On the earliest translations in this so-called movement, see Charles Burnett and Danielle Jacquart, eds., *Constantine the African and 'Alī Ibn Al-'Abbās Al-Magūsī: The Pantegni and Related Texts* (Leiden: Brill, 1995); Charles Burnett, "Manuscripts of Latin Translations of Scientific Texts from Arabic," in *Taxonomies of Knowledge: Information and Order in Medieval Manuscripts*, ed. Emily Steiner and Lynn Ransom (Philadelphia: University of Pennsylvania Press, 2015), 80–89.

World"; in Tolkien's work it is the dying age of the elves, who hold both institutional memory and sophisticated knowledge of the world; and even in J.K. Rowling's work this loss is understood through the lens of childhood, as the teenage protagonists must struggle with the adults in their lives keeping information from them, even to the point of restricting their access to certain books.

While fantasy characters can overcome inaccessible information through personal diligence – in Samwell's case, simply stealing the book he needs – medieval peoples have often been understood by historians as working through a more arduous process of uncovering old knowledge through translation. Indeed, to medievalist scholars of the late nineteenth and early twentieth centuries (such as Tolkien himself), this is how these texts appeared: novel reinvigorations in the later Middle Ages of Ancient knowledge.[47] Because Tolkien helped to establish many of the tropes of the modern fantasy genre, including its presentation of book learning, subsequent fantasy writers may have perpetuated this attitude even as the scholarship has updated its own. Historians no longer understand the Middle Ages broadly as a period of loss but must still grapple with the realities of knowledge lost from the medieval period to the *present*. Importantly, scholars who work with these texts perceive them to be incomplete, whether intentionally or incidentally. Iolanda Ventura has shown how modern scholars can only track a portion of the knowledge of how to make and use medicines in medieval southern Italy through the translation and transmission of medical texts; much of the medical practice implied in such works was likely conveyed entirely outside of writing.[48] This is ultimately a product, even a flaw, of our reliance on texts to convey information. But for medieval peoples, this was only one facet of their medical tradition, it was only one way in which they recorded medical knowledge. In the highly literate, highly textual societies of modern Britain and America, all information is expected to have a written component. But for medieval peoples, writing was a

[47] This narrative of loss and rediscovery was most influentially articulated by Charles Homer Haskins. See Charles Homer Haskins, "The Sicilian Translators of the Twelfth Century and the First Latin Version of Ptolemy's Almagest," *Harvard Studies in Classical Philology* 21 (1910), 75–102.

[48] Iolanda Ventura, "Medieval Pharmacy and Arabic Heritage: The Salernitan Collection *Circa Instans*," in *The Impact of Arabic Sciences in Europe and Asia*, Micrologus: Nature, Sciences and Medieval Societies, XXIV (Firenze: SISMEL, 2016), 339–401.

specialized skill, one that was, especially in Latin prior to the twelfth century, reserved mostly for religious activities.[49] In that sense, the depiction of hidden knowledge is more a reflection of our modern expectations of medieval sources than of the medieval use of medical texts.

The issue here is not the factual accuracy in fantasy depictions of medieval European settings – whether they present medieval medical knowledge and practice as it was or not – but the perspective informing how these depictions approach their subject matter. The image of the studious expert poring over dusty tomes is not the experience of the medieval medical scholar or practitioner, but of the medievalist. That this trope perhaps originates with Tolkien is not surprising, since Tolkien himself imbued his work with medievalist methodology. He presented medieval knowledge as he himself experienced it: through manuscripts and mythology.[50] Just as Tolkien established many of the tropes, structures, and elements of twentieth-century fantasy, he also established how subsequent fantasy narratives would depict medical knowledge. His genre successors, then, did not have to be medievalists to present the medieval world as he did.[51] This allowed medievalist scholarly readings of the early twentieth century to become encoded into fantasy literature as part of a metaphorical vocabulary for depicting the past.

We have already seen that medieval medicine was transmitted in ways more complex than a single text on its own could convey. Similarly, we can find a middle ground in the Orientalist dichotomy between oral and text-based learning, where literate individuals might not read medical texts or be trained in indigenous traditions, but they could still have common knowledge of practical medicine. Indeed, we can see this in Tolkien's story of how Samwise Gamgee helped to save his friend Frodo.

---

[49] Rosamond McKitterick, ed., *The Uses of Literacy in Early Medieval Europe* (Cambridge: Cambridge University Press, 1990), 1–10; M.T. Clanchy, "Parchment and Paper: Manuscript Culture 1100-1500," in *A Companion to the History of the Book*, ed. Simon Eliot and Jonathan Rose (Malden, MA: Blackwell, 2007), 194; M.T. Clanchy, *From Memory to Written Record* (Malden, MA: Blackwell, 1979), 226–34.

[50] On Tolkien's medievalism, see Malone, "What's Wrong with Medievalism? Tolkien, the Strugatsky Brothers, and the Question of the Ideology of Fantasy"; Chance, *Tolkien the Medievalist.*

[51] David Williams similarly argued that medieval content in movies is derived not from medieval sources but from nineteenth and twentieth century intermediaries. David Williams, "Medieval Movies," *The Yearbook of English Studies* 20 (1990), 1–32.

Sam is certainly literate, but not bookish. His skill in this episode comes from his acquired knowledge as a gardener, which affords him the ability to identify medicinal herbs in the wild. Unlike that of the elves, Sam's medicine is simple and provides merely a stopgap measure. The framework of indigenous medicine can become problematic in the dual implication that it is both less effective at providing medical treatment and limited to exceptional practitioners. But in Tolkien's portrayal, it is not just that Sam is an uneducated bystander that makes his help limited, but that he is not part of the culture that is capable of healing Frodo's wound. In the Middle Ages, as today, some types of medical knowledge were widely available to those without any form of medical training, whether institutional or tacit. And so, we can expand this literary trope beyond its Orientalist roots to appreciate a mundane kind of knowledge of medicine that might have been more widely available. A letter from two brothers recommending cumin to their sick mother shows how knowledge of medical substances gained without special skills or training could be applied.

In 1153, two brothers, Perahya and Moses Yiju, wrote a letter from Messina, Sicily to their father Joseph. Failing business had forced the brothers to leave home in the small trade hub of Mazara del Vallo, on Sicily's southwest coast, to find work in Messina, in the northeast corner. The trip proved disastrous for the family, as the brothers found little work and their parents each contracted increasingly dire illnesses. Their father explained in the subsequent letter, likely in 1156, that his own illness was indescribable, and his wife's failing health and her concern for the welfare of their sons had made her unable to eat.[52] Their sons, deeply concerned for their parents' wellbeing, instructed the following:

> Please accept my best wishes and greetings to my mother. Let me know how she is and whether you received the mail I sent you, and the lock. I wrote you what is suitable for her, namely a mithqal (4.2 grams) sagapenum every three days and a trace of cumin. Our orders are that you should not be negligent and that you should not burden yourselves with fasts, nor weep.[53]

[52] Cambridge, Cambridge University Library, Taylor-Schechter 16.288.
[53] Shlomo Simonsohn, *The Jews in Sicily*, vol. 1 (Leiden: Brill, 1997), 407.

According to their appearance in similar trade records, cumin and sagapenum were likely readily available throughout Sicily without trade. In fact, these two goods appear very rarely in trade documents, precisely because they were likely available through local gardening. It is not clear whether merchants would have grown these themselves or purchased them in the market. Sagapenum is not present in most medical treatises or *materia medica* texts of this time, but *Circa Instans* explains that cumin grows freely in the region that both that text and this letter were written. It recommends soaking it in wine to treat stomach illnesses, essentially as a laxative.[54] This is consistent with the father's description of the mother being unable to eat, as one interpretation could be that she is suffering from digestive issues, or perhaps melancholy. This recommendation therefore offers insight into what is essentially a common-knowledge cure.

III. Usama's Physicians and the East/West Dichotomy

We have seen so far that an Orientalist framing of medieval medical ways of knowing can be wrapped up in modern confusion over medieval sources and confounded by overly strict categories such as literacy. These problems exist in scholarship as well, particularly in the perceived divide between the sophistication of medical traditions in the so-called East and West. Since Enlightenment thinkers' invention of the Middle Ages, European historians have used the concept of the "Western" tradition to elevate European intellectual production, connect it to authorities that were not at the time considered explicitly European (such as Classical Greece), and exclude Asian and African contributions.[55] As the effects of this kind of Orientalist framing have been so strongly felt in the decades since decolonization, over the last twenty years or so historians of medicine have made a more concerted effort to emphasize the

[54] "Est autem semen herbe in multa quantitate nascentis. Non sophisticatur propter multam eius copiam per 5 annos servatur. Virtutem habet diureticam et inde subtiliandi furmositatem. Unde sumptum in cibo et potibus et salsamentis digestionem confortat. Vinum decoctum eius et feniculi seminist dolorem stomachi et intestinorum torcionem ex ventositate mitigat." Platearius, *Circa Instans. Text Und Kommentar*, 35.

[55] William J. Bulman, ed., "Literature and Violence," in *Anglican Enlightenment: Orientalism, Religion and Politics in England and Its Empire, 1648–1715*, Cambridge Studies in Early Modern British History (Cambridge: Cambridge University Press, 2015), 26–31, https://doi.org/10.1017/CBO9781139683609.004.

importance of the Islamicate intellectual sphere in particular to the development of what would become modern Western medicine. However, as we will see, such scholarship has often represented medieval Europe as a barbaric foil.[56] There, an East/West dichotomy emerges in a presentation of the Latin world as largely uneducated, even barbaric, in comparison to the literate and sophisticated Arabic scholars of the Middle East as well as Islamic Spain. This is a kind of positive Orientalism, one that elevates rather than denigrates the imagined "East," but still distorts historical realities. Both approaches hinge on the logical fallacy that the two cultures are separate and must be compared critically. Stereotypical understandings of the medieval world (and of its medicine in particular) have encouraged the frequent misuse of medieval sources to show "Western" medieval medicine as barbaric in comparison to a sophisticated Middle East.

We can return to the story of Samwell Tarley and his cure for greyscale. There, the slow torture of death from a necrotic skin disease is transformed into the acute agony of Samwell's treatment. The narrative of the HBO adaptation especially encourages the audience to see this treatment as gruesome in and of itself, not a mistake on Sam's part, after an increasingly gritty montage of Sam's life in the Citadel as well as depictions in earlier seasons of casual amputation as a necessary form of battlefield medicine. *Game of Thrones* presents these treatments as realistic interpretations in a fantasy setting of historical forms of medicine, reflecting the popular expectation that medieval "Western" medicine was necessarily harsh.

This understanding of medieval European medicine as barbaric is also perpetuated in medievalist scholarship. An oft-cited example is a story from the *Book of Contemplation* of Usama ibn Munqidh, a memoir written by a Muslim Syrian knight who lived during the Crusades and fought on both sides. In it, a Frankish (European) physician arrives in a Crusader settlement in the Levant to treat a sick woman and a knight with a leg abscess. The physician diagnoses the woman with demonic possession, first shaving her hair and then carving a cross into her head and rubbing

[56] Charles Issawi, "Europe, the Middle East and the Shift in Power: Reflections on a Theme by Marshall Hodgson," *Comparative Studies in Society and History* 22, no. 4 (1980), 487, 492–93. For a more general overview of this issue, see also Matthew Gabriele and David M. Perry, *The Bright Ages: A New History of Medieval Europe* (New York: Harper, 2021).

it with salt, killing her immediately. The knight is subjected to faulty amputation, which on the second try drains his bone marrow and kills him. But this example is not, in fact, meant to illustrate the barbarity of European medicine. Indeed, in the context of Usama's story, this anecdote is presented as the report of a Syrian physician employed by Usama's uncle, which the author immediately casts doubt on. He follows the physician's anecdote with one of his own, which he introduces by saying "Now I have observed in [the Franks'] medicine a case exactly the opposite of this."[57] He goes on to relate two more stories in which Frankish physicians administer effective treatments such as proper hygiene and simple ointments to cure festering wounds. This juxtaposition shows that the purpose of the first story is to caution Usama's contemporaries against believing all the tall tales they heard about the Franks, even though Usama himself often believed they were crude or uninformed.

Scholarship has often interpreted Usama's story exactly opposite to its intent by decontextualizing the anecdote of the Frankish physician.[58] Representations of this anecdote as an example of European barbarism (or the Middle Eastern perception of European barbarism) hinge on a further uncomplicated reading of the text, assuming that Usama's presentation of the "Franks" was wholly negative, rather than ambivalent. These readings often support arguments that hinge on strong divides within the medieval world.[59] One scholar, writing on the subject of Christian physicians in the medieval Islamicate world, says: "The author of the story, Usāma ibn Munqidh, includes this anecdote in a section of his memoirs wherein he demonstrates, with story after story, that the Frankish crusaders[sic] were primitive, uncivilized, backward people in comparison with the Arab Islamic civilization."[60] This reading essentially serves as a straw man to separate Eastern Christians of the Islamicate world from Latin Christians.

---

[57] Usama ibn Munqidh, *The Book of Contemplation: Islam and the Crusades*, trans. Paul M. Cobb (London: Penguin, 2008), 146.

[58] Paul M. Cobb, *Usama Ibn Munqidh: Warrior-Poet in the Age of Crusades* (Oxford: Oneworld, 2005), 108.

[59] On the depiction of such divides as a worldbuilding device in fantasy literature, see Young and Finn, *Global Medievalism*, 28-31.

[60] Jason R. Zabrowski, "Arab Christian Physicians as Interreligious Mediators: Abū Shākir as a Model Christian Expert," *Islam and Christian-Muslim Relations* 22, no. 2 (2011), 187.

Other uses of this anecdote are meant to support the notion that the Crusades themselves were brutal, both in the experience of warfare and as a reflection of an intolerant society. For instance, David Nicolle uses this anecdote as an example of "the crude efforts of [Middle Eastern 'field surgeons']'s Western European colleagues," editorializing that "the occasionally barbaric methods of the latter were also described by Usamah."[61] Instead, as Piers Mitchell has argued, our evidence from Crusaders themselves shows that their battlefield medicine was reasonable and appropriate.[62] This is an insidious, rather than malicious form of Orientalism that allows what a scholar "knows" to supersede what they see. Similarly, Avner Falk summarizes this story by saying: "[Crusader] medicine was hopelessly primitive, ignorant, and cruel. There were 'Frankish' patients whom Ibn Munqidh personally and successfully treated with simple, natural means, and whom the Frankish physicians then killed with their ignorant, superstitious, and brutal treatments."[63] This last version of Usama's story is likely based in the author not having read the text at all, but instead asserting an expected reading on the text based on the perception that the Crusades reflected a real difference between two competing societies. That such a reading is unflattering to the Latin Christians is still consistent with the dichotomy we have already seen in fantasy tropes; such an unflattering portrait is a necessary part of juxtaposing modern "Western" progress from an uninformed European past.

The message that medieval Europeans were brutal and careless toward human life, and unscientific in their approach to medicine, is more a popular cultural trope, a joke of the twentieth century, than an argument made by historians. In fact, one of the most nuanced interpretations of this trope is found in comedy, as in the famous "Theodoric of York" *Saturday Night Live* sketch performed by Steve Martin, which first aired in 1978.[64] In it, Martin appears as the

[61] David Nicolle, "Wounds, Military Surgery, and the Reality of Crusading Warfare; The Evidence of Usāmah's Memoires," in *Medieval Warfare, 1000-1300*, ed. John France (Burlington, VT: Ashgate, 2006), 607–8.

[62] Piers D. Mitchell, *Medicine in the Crusades: Warfare, Wounds, and the Medieval Surgeon* (New York: Cambridge University Press, 2004).

[63] Avner Falk, *Franks and Saracens: Reality and Fantasy in the Crusades* (Routledge, 2010), 141.

[64] The "Theodoric of York" skit is also discussed by Claire Burridge in her chapter in this volume, "Early Medieval Surgery: Challenging Popular Stereotypes with Archaeological Evidence".

stereotypical medieval barber, hacking away at trusting peasants and bleeding one poor girl to death. This sketch is, superficially, a criticism of a barbarous past, but it makes a subtle point about modern medical hubris. It ends with a monologue by Theodoric in which he pontificates about medical advancement and the ushering in of a new era of learning that, distinct from the rest of the sketch, sounds very much like a modern doctor expounding on recent medical advancements. Coming out of the mouth of a man smeared with dirt and blood, this monologue is obvious satire, but its sting comes from prevalent concerns during the 1970s, when doctors had, within recent memory, performed such dubious medicine as prescribing Thalidomide to pregnant patients to treat nausea, causing debilitating birth defects.[65] This sketch is thus directed not primarily at the barbarity of the medieval past, but at modern doctors who cannot see their own faults. And that is indeed the danger of simplifying our understanding of medieval medicine: allowing ourselves to be uncritical of our own medical shortcomings based on the notion that we are advanced in comparison to the past.

Currently, we are in the midst of another crisis of confidence in healthcare due in part to the rise of antibiotic-resistant bacteria, the overprescribing of painkillers that has addicted many people to opioids, and a global pandemic.[66] In response to these developments, more medical professionals and institutions, particularly in the United States, are looking for ways to integrate approaches previously dismissed as invalid, precisely because they are based on indigenous traditions.[67] Continuing to hold this medicine apart from the "West" prevents us from gaining the full benefit of both. The balanced integration of both

---

[65] James H. Kim and Anthony R. Scialli, "Thalidomide: The Tragedy of Birth Defects and the Effective Treatment of Disease," *Toxicological Sciences* 122, no. 1 (2011), 1–6.

[66] United States Senate Hearing of the Committee on Health, Education, Labor, and Pensions One Hundred Fifteenth Congress, Second Session, *The Opioid Crisis: The Role of Technology and Data in Preventing and Treating Addiction. February 27, 2018*, United States. Congress. Senate. S. Hrg.; 115-782 (Washington: U.S. Government Publishing Office, 2020).

[67] For instance, a Harvard University initiative in partnership with the Culinary Institute of America to integrate dietary practices with medical treatment. "Overview," *Healthy Kitchens, Healthy Lives* (blog), accessed October 27, 2021, www.healthykitchens.org/overview. There has also been an increased acceptance of indigenous medical systems such as Ayurveda and homeopathy both in India and abroad. Shinjini Das, *Vernacular Medicine in Colonial India: Family, Market, and Homeopathy* (Cambridge: Cambridge University Press, 2019), 2–3.

experiential and textual medicine is truly what characterized medieval medicine, both in Latin Europe and the Middle East.

DRINKING THE WORD OF GOD: MODERN SCIENCE AND RECONFIGURATIONS OF ISLAMIC HEALING IN CONTEMPORARY EGYPT

ANA VINEA*

I. Introduction

"Marwa, that's the name of the case we're going to see," Shaykh Khalil[1] clarifies, "has been having splitting headaches for some months now. She cannot read the Qur'an anymore, she says; as soon as she tries, her mind wanders. I recited over her last time and a jinni appeared, but he is still inside her. We have work to do today!" It is May 2012. I sit in the back of the shaykh's car, slightly concerned about his impulsive driving, but feeling lucky that Marwa has agreed I join the healing session at her sister's place in one of Cairo's satellite cities.

"Hamdulillah, we arrived!" Shaykh Khalil exclaims and quickly gets out of the car. A retired mechanical engineer in his early sixties, the shaykh is quite agile for his age, so I hurry to follow him. Knowing that I will accompany the Qur'anic healer, Marwa's sister Leila has prepared coffee and treats to welcome me. Shaykh Khalil, however, is impatient: "Let's start with the session, and then we chat!" He asks Leila if she had prepared the water over which the Qur'an has been recited *(mayya maqrū'a bi-l-qur'ān)*. She nods and gestures towards a one-liter plastic bottle, traces

* Department of Asian and Middle Eastern Studies, University of North Carolina at Chapel Hill.

[1] With the exception of published authors, all names used in this chapter are pseudonyms.

of a Pepsi label still visible, placed nearby on a side table. The shaykh begins to recite the *ruqya*, the Qur'anic verses healers use to exorcise the invisible spirits known as jinn.[2] Seated on the couch, Marwa keeps her eyes closed. She is still at first, then, slowly, her left leg starts trembling. Continuing the recitation, Shaykh Khalil grabs the bottle and starts sprinkling Marwa. She shivers, her facial expressions and light moans suggesting pain. By now her leg is shaking and jerking. Undisturbed the shaykh continues the Qur'anic recitation, periodically spraying water until gradually Mawra calms down. In about half an hour, the session is over. "The jinni is weakened, but he did not depart the body you need another session next week," the shaykh concludes and gives Marwa a list of Qur'anic verses for daily recitation. "And don't forget to drink the recited upon water twice per day." It is coffee time now.

On the way back to Shaykh Khalil's apartment, we start discussing the healing session, as we typically do after attending such home consultations. During my ethnographic research among Cairene Qur'anic healers,[3] I observed many times the employment of water over which the Qur'an has been recited, but up to this point it has never come up in my conversations with Shaykh Khalil. Hearing my question, the shaykh gets animated: "I am glad you asked about this! Of course, this is part of religion (*guz' min al-din*), there are hadiths that talk about it." He continues to tell me how Muslims have always used recited upon water in different forms, "some better than others," he adds. "But this is not all! There are also scientific experiments (*tagārib 'ilmiyya*) carried out by a Japanese scientist that prove the effect of the Qur'an over water. You see, modern science (*al-'ilm al-hadith*) has confirmed what we knew all along!"

Here, Shaykh Khalil introduces the practice of imbuing water with the Qur'an and drinking it for curative purposes as an ancient one with a double epistemic grounding, in Islam's revealed texts and in modern science, with the second corroborating the already established evidence

[2] In Arabic, *jinn* is a collective noun that refers to this category of invisible beings. The singular is *jinni* (masc.) and *jinniya* (fem.).

[3] The ethnographic research this chapter draws on was conducted over a total period of 20 months in Cairo, between 2006-2016. Besides Qur'anic healers, the research included mental health professionals, religious scholars, patients, and other Egyptians interested in jinn possession and Islamic healing. Unless otherwise specified, the quotes I include here are all from interviews I conducted with various Qur'anic healers and other interlocutors during this field research.

provided by the first. The shaykh's statement sums up the main way this technique with a long genealogy in Islamic spiritual therapies has been framed and explained in Qur'anic healing (*al-'ilaj bi-l-qur'an*), a form of jinn exorcism that has raised to prominence in Egypt and beyond in the last decades of the 20th century in the context of the Islamic revival.[4] Aided by the popularity of this therapy, the idea that water imbued with the Qur'an is twice authorized, from within the Islamic tradition and from without, by modern scientific experiments, has gained a foothold in today's Egypt. This idea was often repeated to me when Egyptians from all walks of life learned about my research. Yet, as I show, this perspective is not without its skeptics and detractors, with some Qur'anic healers and other observers raising questions about the potential damaging effects of using science to explain a tradition-bound practice.

This essay traces the articulations of Qur'anic infusion and ingestion in contemporary Egypt, focusing on the way it has been employed by Qur'anic healers and discussed in the public sphere. It intertwines thus a consideration of the pragmatic aspects of this therapeutic technique with the discursive space created around it, which has been central for this practice's uptake and understanding. Of course, Qur'anic healers do not have a monopoly over this practice in Egypt, nor are invocations of science in connection to it, be they supportive or critical, universally embraced. My aim here is not to provide an exhaustive overview of drinking the Word of God in today's Egypt, but to analyze one of the ways, a popular and publicly visible one, in which it has been taken up.

Through this anthropological analysis, I show how Qur'anic healers have reconfigured the long-standing use of recited upon water in ways that privilege I call a normative scientization of healing that combines an attention to religious permissibility with a recourse to modern science as an authoritative framework. Thus, as Shaykh Khalil does above, Qur'anic healers have argued that some forms of Qur'anic ingestion are preferable, and that modern science demonstrates the effects of Qur'anic recitations

[4] See Mikkel Bille, "Seeking Providence through Things: The Word of God versus Black Cumin," in *An Anthropology of Absence: Materializations of Transcendence and Loss*, ed. Mikkel Bille et al. (New York: Springer, 2010); Elizabeth Coker, "Claiming the Public Soul: Representations of Qur'anic Healing and Psychiatry in the Egyptian Print Media," *Transcultural Psychiatry* 46, no. 4 (2009), 672–94; Emilio Spadola, Emilio, *The Calls of Islam: Sufis, Islamists, and Mass Mediation in Urban Morocco* (Bloomington and Indiana: Indiana University Press, 2014).

over water. Through these processes, Qur'anic healers have not only reshaped specific therapeutic practices, like the recitation of the Qur'an over water on which I focus on in this essay, they have also aimed to create something akin to a modern orthodox science of Islamic healing. That such attempts have not gone unchallenged draws attention to how debates over health and cure serve as a lens into broader epistemic and ethical contestations over Islamic practice in the present. It also shows that the question of how religion and science relate, or should ideally relate, at the center of such debates is not fixed, but continuously up for (re)consideration. My concern in this essay is not with the veracity of Qur'anic healers claims to either orthodoxy or scientificity. The first has long been debated in the Islamic tradition and the second has its own complexities as detailed in science and technology studies. Instead, I trace both the shapes and the stakes of this science of orthodox healing as concretized in the practice of imbuing water with the Qur'an, as a window into modern epistemological transformations of Islamic healing.

This focus on the contemporary transformations of the tradition-bound practice of ingesting the Qur'an both challenges and extends existing scholarly approaches to this particular use of Islam's scripture and, more broadly, to the employment of the Qur'an in healing. A significant trend in this body of work has been to situate such therapeutic practices at Islam's periphery, be it a geographical periphery, in an imaginary that takes the Middle East as the center of Islam, or, more frequently, a religious periphery, as the domain of heterodox, superstitious practices, the realm of "popular Islam" allegedly separated from normative, textual traditions.[5] Framed in this way, the persistence of this and other related healing practices in the present has also been seen, explicitly or more often implicitly, as a symptom of Islam's stuckness in the past.

---

[5] E.g., Abdullahi El-Tom, "Drinking the Koran: The Meaning of Koranic Verses in Berti Erasure," *Africa: Journal of the International African Institute*, 55:4 (1985), 414-31; Edward Westermarck, *Ritual and Belief in Morocco* (New York: Routledge, 2014, first published 1926 by Macmillan (London); and James Robson, "Magic Cures in Popular Islam," *The Muslim World* 24:1 (1934), 33–43. For a similar point, see also Rudolph Ware, *The Walking Qur'an: Islamic Education, Embodied Knowledge, and History in West Africa* (Chapel Hill: The University of North Carolina Press, 2014), 58 and Travis Zadeh, "An Ingestible Scripture: Qur'ānic Erasure and the Limits of "Popular" Religion," in *Material Culture and Asian Religions: Text, Image, Object*, ed. Benjamin J. Fleming and Richard D. Mann (New York and London: Routledge, 2014), 98.

More recently, some scholars have moved away from such explicitly or implicitly normative assessments to provide instead an analysis of Qur'anic imbuement and ingestion. Using theoretical approaches ranging from speech act theory and semiotics to embodiment and materiality, they have provided conceptually sophisticated analyses of this practice and of the transformations at play within.[6] Such analyses have also, if only indirectly at times, re-centered the practice of ingesting the Qur'an as a widespread and normative use of the Word of God.[7] It is especially Travis Zadeh who has most extensively investigated the rich medieval and early modern range of Islamic discourses around this and related practices, convincingly demonstrating that far from being always already marginal and heterodox, forms of ingesting the scripture were normative employments of the Qur'an "grounded in the religious authority of law, theology, and prophetic tradition."[8]

Building on this latter body of work, in this chapter I approach the contemporary transformations of Qur'anic ingestion and the debates around them not by labelling them as forms of popular Islam, but by showing how they rework notions of normativity and orthodoxy into the present, especially in relation to modern science. The debates I focus on

---

[6] Michael Lambek, *Knowledge and Practice in Mayotte: Local Discourses of Islam, Sorcery, and Spirit Possession* (Toronto: University of Toronto Press, 1993), Webb Keane, "On Spirit Writing: Materialities of Language and the Religious Work of Transduction," *Journal of the Royal Anthropological Institute* 19, no. 1 (2013), 1-17; Finbarr Flood, "Bodies and Becoming: Mimesis, Mediation, and the Ingestion of the Sacred in Christianity and Islam," in *Sensational Religion: Sensory Culture in Material Practice*, ed. Sally Promey (New Haven: Yale University Press, 2014), 459–93; Ware, *The Walking Qur'an,* 57-64.

[7] Christiane Gruber, "The Arts of Protection and Healing in Islam: Water Infused with Blessing," *Ajam Media Collective*, May 6, 2021, The Arts of Protection and Healing in Islam: Water Infused with Blessing (Ajam Media Collective). See: https://ajammc.com/2021/04/30/water-infused-with-blessing/.

[8] See Travis Zadeh, "Touching and Ingesting: Early Debates over the Material Qur'an," *Journal of the American Oriental Society* 129, no. 3 (2009), 443–66 and Zadeh, "An Ingestible Scripture." As Zadeh shows, the fact that some religious figures have raised objections to Qur'anic ingestion shows not the practice's non-normativity, but how it was the focus of discourses and debates over what is normative and what not within the Islamic tradition (Zadeh, "An Ingestible Scripture," 116). Through this analysis, Zadeh not only questions the equation of Qur'anic ingestion with popular region, but more importantly questions the static distinction between two allegedly separate realms, that of "popular" versus "normative" Islam (Zadeh "An Ingestible Scripture," 99, 116). In fact, drinking the Word of God has been throughout Islamic history simultaneously a pervasive part of the lived experiences of Muslims and of Islamic law and theology.

here, unlike those analyzed by Zadeh, are not restricted to religious scholars, but encompass instead a wider group of actors in debate, including psychiatrists and lay Egyptians.

I begin this chapter by providing a short overview of the practice of Qur'anic ingestion and move then to introducing Qur'anic healing, the popular form of Islamic therapy whose employment of Qur'anic ingestion is at the center of my analysis. Then, I discuss the two main elements of Qur'anic healers' normative scientization of Qur'anic ingestion, briefly touching on their concern with delineating the most correct form of the practice and discussing in greater depth these practitioners' use of science to explain and give it authority.

II. Qur'anic Ingestion: Past and Present Trajectories

Conceptualized as God's verbatim speech, his eternal, uncreated words (*kalām allah*) as they were gradually revealed to Muhammad over more than 20 years, the Qur'an is central both in Islamic ritual and in Muslims' everyday devotions and lives. The Qur'an's first chapter (sura), *al-fātiḥa*, and other verses are recited during the five obligatory daily prayers. During Ramadan, the entirety of the Qur'an is recited over the course of the month as part of the *tarāwīḥ* supererogatory prayers that end each day's fast. In many Muslim majority countries, like Egypt, brief Qur'anic recitations also mark the beginning of many secular events, from the inauguration of a business to, as I witnessed during my research, the opening of a psychiatric conference. For pious Muslims, reciting, listening to, or just reading the Qur'an are central daily forms of devotion, integrated in the rhythms of everyday life. Quotes from the Qur'an mark buildings as well as the speech of many Muslims as commentary, advice, or admonition. Even in Cairo, the mega-city where I conducted my research, the sounds of Qur'anic recitation manage to penetrate through the usual cacophony.

Emphasizing the essentially oral character of the divine scripture, the term *al-qur'ān* refers to a recitation and is distinguished from the *muṣḥaf*, the physical codex. Yet, as a receptacle for the Word of God, the *muṣḥaf* and by extension anything that carries parts of the Qur'an cannot be treated like other objects, leading to debates in the early centuries of

Islam and the establishment of rules for its handling.[9] With the introduction of the print medium and more recently of digital technologies, such rules have been revisited and reformulated.[10] This special status of the material Qur'an transpired in countless mundane instances and daily gestures I observed in Cairo, from placing a *muṣḥaf* on top of the car's dashboard to the care given of not placing anything on top of it.

The centrality of the Qur'an in Muslim life, in both its recited and physical form, is also manifested in the practice, or family of practices, I focus on in this chapter. "Qur'anic ingestion" covers a wide variety of historical and contemporary practices ubiquitous throughout the Muslim world from sub-Saharan Africa to India to the Middle East.[11] At their core, these practices are forms of transferring and dispensing the Qur'an into another medium, typically water. Starting from this basic principle, the specific forms and processes have varied and included the direct recitation of the Qur'an over water or other substances, often accompanied by blowing or spitting; writing Qur'anic verses on paper and dissolving it in water; washing with water the wooden tablets used Qur'anic schools; or engraving drinking bowls with Qur'anic verses.[12]

Despite the pervasive historical and geographical presence of Qur'anic infusion and ingestion, these employments of the scripture never had a ritual role, nor have they been formalized during medieval and early modern times. Nevertheless, they have been used both in the mundane setting of traditional Islamic schooling, and in more specialized contexts of healing and protection. In this way, drinking the Qur'an is,

---

[9] Among these rules, the most important ones concern the prohibition of touching the *muṣḥaf* while in a state of ritual impurity (*najāsa*). See Zadeh, "Touching and Ingesting," 445-448.

[10] Natalia Suit, *Qur'anic Matters: Material Mediations and Religious Practice in Egypt* (London: Bloomsbury Academic, 2020).

[11] See, for example, Ware, *The Walking Qur'an*, 57-58, Joyce Flueckiger, *In Amma's Healing Room: Gender and Vernacular Islam in South India* (Bloomington: Indiana University Press, 2006), 68, Eleanor Doumato, *Getting God's Ear: Women, Islam, and Healing in Saudi Arabia and the Gulf* (New York: Columbia University Press, 2000), 138-146. While beyond the scope of this essay, forms of ingesting the sacred and of materializing scripture are not specific to Islam; they have been documented in both Christianity and Judaism (see Keane, "On Spirit Writing" and Flood, "Bodies and Becoming").

[12] E.g., John Bowen, *Muslims through Discourse: Religion and Ritual in Gayo Society* (Princeton, NJ: Princeton University Press, 1993), 149; Lambek, *Knowledge and Practice*, 142; Doumato, *Getting God's Ear*, 141; Ware, *The Walking Qur'an*, 57, Gruber, "The Arts of Protection."

on one hand, complexly connected with an understanding of the transmission of Islamic knowledge as an embodied process, of epistemology qua embodiment, an approach to knowledge that was dominant up until the modern period as historian Rudolf Ware has brilliantly demonstrated.[13] On the other hand, practices of infusion and ingestion of the Qur'an are part of and connected to a broader sphere of practices and discourses concerning the special qualities of the Qur'an (*faḍā'il al-qur'ān*) and its apotropaic and talismanic properties (*khawāṣṣ al-qur'ān*), Prophetic medicine (*al-ṭibb al-nabawī*), as well as forms of licit magic.[14]

Unifying these diverse practices and usage contexts is the idea that the Qur'an's charismatic powers, its *baraka*, as well as its curative powers, mentioned in the Qur'an itself,[15] are transferable. Thus, the Qur'an's beneficent powers are carried by sounds or script and are transferred into another substance, water typically, and, through its intermediary, into the human body. At the core of Qur'anic ingestion then are both processes of (re)materialization across different semiotic modalities and of embodiment that speak to the transformative power of divine words over the human body.[16] That, as Travis Zadeh has shown, some medieval religious scholars expressed ambivalence and concern with these processes that connect scripture and the human body only demonstrates the desire of religious authorities to establish the normative limits of this widespread engagement with the Word of God.[17]

Many of the forms of Qur'anic infusion and ingestion documented by historians and anthropologists continue to be practiced in today's Egypt. During my research, I observed two principal forms. The first consists of writing verses on a piece of paper, typically with saffron or

13 Ware, *The Walking Qur'an.*

14 Zadeh, "An Ingestible Scripture," 98.

15 There are several Qur'anic verses that associate the Qur'an with the word "cure," collectively known as the cure verses" (*āyāt al- shifā'*): *al-tawba*: 17, *yūnus*: 57, *al-naḥl*: 69, *al-isrā'*: 82, *al-shu'arā'*: 80, and *fuṣṣilat*: 44.

16 On these points, see Lambek, *Knowledge and Practice*, Keane, "On Spirit Writing," Flood, "Bodies and Becoming," and Ware, *The Walking Qur'an.*

17 These concerns have to do with early anxieties about the status of the Qur'an in material form, such as the potential that the Word of God might be corrupted inside the human body, and the possibility of using the material Qur'an in illicit forms of magic or of reducing it to a series of incantations (Zadeh, "An Ingestible Scripture" and Zadeh, "Touching and Ingesting," 461-466).

ink, and then submerging the paper in water so that the still wet substance carrying the words dissolves. The second involves the direct recitation of the Qur'an over water, then using it to drink, wash the body, and sprinkle the house. Occasionally, other substances are similarly infused, particularly olive oil, and either ingested or smeared over painful areas of the body. Both healers of various orientations and lay Egyptians use this practice, reflecting on the one hand its specialized use as a therapeutic technique, and, on the other hand, a more diffuse and quite widespread employment as a general prophylaxis, a way of getting closer to God, or of a means of achieving a state of well-being. This generalized usage and the centrality of the Qur'an itself in this practice explain why Qur'anic ingestion has not been criticized as unscientific and non-modern as other medieval medical practices that have been revived in the last decades.

The preoccupation with the proper uses and the kinds of transformations at play in Qur'anic ingestion manifested in the history of the practice have not disappeared in present-day Egypt. These issues have particularly interested Qur'anic healers, the practitioners at the center of this essay that I introduce more fully in the following section.

III. Qur'anic Healing and the Normative Scientization of Islamic Therapies

In 1990, an article entitled "A Heated Debate among Physicians, Religious Scholars, and Qur'anic Healers: The Treatment with the Qur'an Is Proven and Valid… and Yet!!" appeared in the magazine *Al-Majalis*.[18] The article recounted the proceedings of a seminar organized at the magazine's editorial office which brought together Qur'anic healers and psychiatrists to debate the reality of jinn possession, the healing capacity of the Qur'an, the correct diagnosis of patterns of behaviors and emotions, and the forms of knowledge and practice that can be employed to treat them.

Since then, many other articles touching on this therapy have appeared in the Egyptian press[19] and, with the satellite revolution of the

[18] Abu Al-Abbas Muhammad, "Munazara Sakhina bayna al-Atibba' wa-l-'Ulama' wa-l-Mu'alajin bi-l-Qur'an al-Karim. Al-'Ilaj bi-l-Qur'an al-Karim Thabit wa Sahih wa Lakin!", *Al-Majalis*, June 26, 1990.
[19] See Coker, "Claiming the Public Soul."

2000s,[20] they have been accompanied by televised debates. Such media representations point not simply to the rich discursive field formed around this therapy, but to the emergence of Qur'anic healing itself as a distinctive therapeutic orientation within a broader field of Islamic spiritual practices.

A therapy of jinn exorcism and counter-sorcery through Qur'anic recitations (hence its name in Egypt, *al-'ilaj bi-l-qur'an*, literally "treatment with the Qur'an"), Qur'anic healing has asserted itself in the existing therapeutic landscape not only through practitioners' savvy use of forms of mass mediation, but also through their double claims of therapeutic orthodoxy and similarity to biomedicine and psychiatry. Through these intertwined assertions, Qur'anic healers have proposed what I call a normative scientization of Islamic healing.

Thus, these practitioners have persistently attempted to delineate and construct a normative, orthodox treatment (*'ilaj shar'i*) for jinn afflictions,[21] claiming that only Qur'anic healing meets this normative threshold due to its rootedness in the Qur'an and the Prophet's practice (*sunna*) as recorded in the hadith corpus. Qur'anic healers have coupled this orthodox self-identification with a persistent critique of a host of other therapeutic forms, regrouped and relabeled as superstitious, ignorant, and un-Islamic, despite their distinctive genealogies and varying evaluations of their permissibility: amulets, Sufi-inflected therapies, and the *zār* ritual based on the appeasement, not the exorcism, of jinn.[22] These efforts to reconfigure the Egyptian landscape of Islamic spiritual cures have not been completely futile, even if the above-mentioned therapies have not disappeared. What they did achieve, aided also by Qur'anic healers' use of forms of mass media, was to create and sustain

---

[20] Marwan Kraidy and Joe Khalil, *Arab Television Industries* (London: Palgrave Macmillan, 2009).

[21] I use this term to encompass the two main afflictions Qur'anic healers claim expertise in treating, jinn possession (*mass*, *talabbus*, *labs*, *lamsa*, or more descriptively, *dukhūl al-jinn,* "the entering of the jinn") and sorcery/black mafic (*siḥr, 'amal*), because both are conceptualized by Qur'anic healers as forms of possession by the jinn or at least as the result of jinn's interference. Occasionally, Qur'anic healers themselves use this term as well: *amrāḍ al-jinn*.

[22] For more on the religious assessment of some of these therapies see Zadeh, "Touching and Ingesting" and "An Ingestible Scripture." On the *zār* ritual, Janice Boddy, *Wombs and Alien Spirits: Women, Men, and the Zār Cult in Northern Sudan* (Madison: University of Wisconsin Press, 1989).

a public discursive sphere around the permissibility of such therapies and a palpable, though uneven, concern with normativity among some patients that was evident during my research.

Furthermore, this normative thread in Qur'anic healing has been fused with attempts to scientize healing, by standardizing, classifying, and theorizing therapeutic practices based on healers' practical experience of healing (*tajriba*)[23] and by deploying arguments, notions, and practices framed as rooted in science, specifically in medical sciences (biomedicine and psychiatry). For example, healers have adopted a concept and language of symptoms and checklists of symptoms for different types of jinn afflictions that are reminiscent of, without being fully identical with, biomedical and psychiatric ones. Qur'anic healers have also claimed that their diagnostic techniques, their reliance on symptoms to diagnose types of possession, and their practices of experimentation to devise new therapies make their practice akin to biomedicine and psychiatry. "I work like a psychiatrist. I talk with the patient, see what the symptoms are and diagnose the illness," one of my interlocutors once told me. In this way, Qur'anic healers have attempted to carve out a space for themselves, as jinn afflictions specialists, alongside physicians and psychiatrists.

Through these dual processes of normativization and scientization, Qur'anic healers have aimed to create a modern science of orthodox Islamic healing they see as simultaneously rooted in the correct Islamic tradition and aligned to modern scientific knowledge, with the two facets mutually supporting each other. The mass dissemination of these authoritative assertions facilitated by healers' use of print and televised media has stirred anxieties and concerns across the religious/secular spectrum, attracting especially the critique of Egyptian psychiatrists.[24] Debates bringing together different actors and opinions, such as the one organized in the office of *Al-Majalis* in 1990, have continued, including on the television screen. In this way, Qur'anic healing has emerged as a

---

[23] For more on the use of practical experience in Qur'anic healing, on its role as both an evidentiary technique for developing therapies and for making authoritative claims see Ana Vinea, "What is your Evidence? A Salafi Therapy in Contemporary Egypt," *Comparative Studies of South Asia, Africa, and the Middle East*, 39:3 (2019).

[24] As my interviews with psychiatrists revealed, many mental health professionals claim that those diagnosed by Qur'anic healers as possessed suffer in fact from mental disorders (especially schizophrenia, bipolar disorder, or other disorders with psychotic features, as well as OCD or anxiety) or at least from subclinical psychological symptoms resulting from daily stresses.

node in wider societal debates over notions of affliction, causality, and cure, over what experts and knowledges should be given authority to treat, and over the "proper" relationship between science and religion in a modern society.

The kind of therapeutic rearticulation proposed by Qur'anic healers and the debates stirred by this therapy emerged in Egypt against the backdrop of the Islamic revival that since the 1970s has pushed the question of the role of religion in all aspects of life, including health and healing, into the public sphere.[25] Among the various, often contrasting, orientations that comprise the Islamic revival, Egyptian Qur'anic healers have been particularly close to the Salafi strand that foregrounds correct religious practices purified from innovations through an unmediated return to the Qur'an and *sunna*.[26] If this Salafi concern with correct practice and doctrine smoothly transfers into Qur'anic healers' attempts to demarcate a uniquely orthodox Islamic healing, their invocations of modern science sit at odds with widespread framings of Salafis as anti-modern and opposed to Western cultural formations.[27]

Yet, Qur'anic healers' employments and invocations of modern science are just a contemporary articulation of more than a century-long history of Muslim engagement with scientific disciplines. It was especially in the context of nineteenth- and early-twentieth-century colonialist and Orientalist attacks on Islam as anti-scientific and irrational that Muslim scholars became preoccupied with the question of the relationship between Islam and modern science. The most coherent response came from the representatives of the modern reformist movement who argued for the inherent compatibility of modern science and a properly understood Islamic faith.[28] Basing this interpretation on a positivist understanding of science as a universal, meaning not grounded in any

[25] E.g., Saba Mahmood, *Politics of Piety: The Islamic Revival and the Feminist Subject* (Princeton, N.J.: Princeton University Press, 2005) and Sherine Hamdy, *Our Bodies Belong to God: Organ Transplants, Islam, and the Struggle for Human Dignity in Egypt* (Berkeley: University of California Press, 2012).

[26] Roel Meijer, ed., *Global Salafism: Islam's New Religious Movement* (New York: Columbia University Press, 2009).

[27] For more on this point, see Vinea, "What is your Evidence?".

[28] Albert Hourani, *Arabic Thought in the Liberal Age, 1798–1939* (Oxford: Oxford University Press, 1970) and John Livingston, "Muḥammad 'Abduh on Science," *The Muslim World* 85:3/4 (1995), 215-234.

culture or society, and constantly evolving practice,[29] this view has become one of the most prevalent ways of approaching science in contemporary Egypt, one that is embraced by many Qur'anic healers as well.[30]

Later, with the advent of the Islamic revival, other problematics, rooted in previous debates, started to gain more prevalence, most notably the scientific exegesis of the Qur'an[31] and the "Islamization of science and knowledge" movement.[32] Moving in opposite directions, with the former asserting that modern scientific findings are foreshadowed in the Qur'an and the latter questioning the epistemological compatibility of modern science and Islam, these two approaches to questions of science and Islam have shaped Qur'anic healing, including the practice of reciting the Qur'an over water and its interpretations, as I show below.

Besides echoing previous engagements with modern science, Qur'anic healers' endeavors to scientize Islamic therapeutics should not be surprising in a society like Egypt where biomedicine has been adopted, though not uncritically,[33] for more than a century. The development of Western-inspired medicine in the country, beginning with the nineteenth century,[34] has reshaped the medical field, including through the creation

---

29 Ahmad Dallal, *Islam, Science, and the Challenge of History* (New Haven, CT: Yale University Press, 2010), 160–162.

30 Beyond Egypt, this framing of modern science can be encountered in other colonial and postcolonial contexts, especially among modernizing elites. For examples from India and Iran, see Jean Langford, *Fluent Bodies: Ayurvedic Remedies for Postcolonial Imbalances* (Durham, NC: Duke University Press, 2002) and Cyrus Schayegh, *Who Is Knowledgeable Is Strong: Science, Class, and the Formation of Modern Iranian Society, 1900–1950* (Berkeley: University of California Press. 2009), respectively. For more on Muslim discourses and debates on Islam, see also Ahmed Ragab, "Islam and Science," in *Routledge Companion to Religion and Science*, ed. James W. Haag, Gregory R. Peterson, Michael L. Spezio (London: Routledge, 2011).

31 See for example Yunus Telliel, "Miraculous Evidence: Scientific Wonders and Religious Reasons," *Comparative Studies of South Asia, Africa, and the Middle East*, 39:3 (2019), 528-542.

32 E.g., Mona Abaza, *Debates on Islam and Knowledge in Malaysia and Egypt* (London: Routledge, 2002).

33 For debates around specific biomedical technologies, such as organ transplantation or alternative reproductive technologies, see Hamdy, *Our Bodies* and Marcia Inhorn, *Local Babies, Global Science: Gender, Religion, and In Vitro Fertilization in Egypt* (New York: Routledge, 2003).

34 See, for example, Khaled Fahmy, "Medicine and Power: Towards a Social History of Medicine in Nineteenth-Century Egypt," *Cairo Papers in Social Science* 23:2 (2000), 1-45.

of a separate sphere of "traditional therapies" (*'ilāgāt taqlīdiyya*) or "popular therapies" (*'ilāgāt sha'biyya*) newly reframed as "superstitious," "unscientific," and radically different from biomedicine.[35] In this process, medical professionals and modernizers have been joined by those Muslim scholars who have argued for the compatibility of Islam and science to reject such "superstitious" therapies, including those dealing with jinn.[36] Yet, the state's exclusive legalization of trained physicians to practice medicine[37] has not been accompanied by the outlawing or regulation of "traditional therapies," allowing them to survive and transform, often in a complex dialogue with biomedicine, as anthropologists have shown.[38]

Qur'anic healers' normative scientization of healing is shaped both by the specific context of this therapy's emergence and by the history of debates and transformations I have delineated here. Their double claim of orthodoxy and scientificity can be read as a response to the recurrent framing of therapies around the jinn as both unorthodox and unscientific. To put it differently, Qur'anic healers' modern science of orthodox healing is an attempt, if not to dismantle, at least to destabilize the science/religion/superstition trio that has long dominated modern epistemologies.[39] Taking a longer, medieval and early modern, historical perspective, these practitioners' efforts can be interpreted as a way, even if an un-witting one, of recuperating the scientific status that forms of engagements with the jinn had throughout Islamic history, as recent studies that have revitalized the study of the Islamic occult have authoritatively demonstrated.[40]

---

[35] E.g., Richard Keller, *Colonial Madness: Psychiatry in French North Africa* (Chicago: The University of Chicago Press, 2007) and Ellen Amster, *Medicine and the Saints: Science, Islam, and the Colonial Encounter in Morocco, 1877-1956* (Austin: University of Texas Press, 2013).

[36] See footnote 31, as well as Sherine Hamdy, "Blinding Ignorance: Medical Science, Diseased Eyes, and Religious Practice in Egypt," *Arab Studies Journal*, 12-13 (2004/2005), 26-45.

[37] See Law no. 415 from 1954 concerning the practice of the medical profession, published in *The Egyptian Gazette* (*Al-Waqa'i'a al-Misiryya*), no. 58, July 22, 1954.

[38] E.g., Hania Sholkamy, "Conclusion: The Medical Cultures of Egypt," in *Health and Identity in Egypt*, ed. Hania Sholkamy and Farha Ghannam (Cairo: The American University in Cairo Press, 2004).

[39] See, for example, Peter Harrison, *The Territories of Science and Religion* (Chicago: The University of Chicago Press, 2015).

[40] E.g., Matthew Melvin-Koushki, "Is (Islamic) Occult Science Science?" *Theology and Science* 18:2 (2020), 303-324.

Egyptian Qur'anic healers are not singular figures in these attempts. In fact, Qur'anic healing itself is far from being only an Egyptian formation. Like Salafism itself, the orientation with which Qur'anic healers have most doctrinal affinities, revivalist forms of Islamic exorcism with similar features have emerged transnationally both in the Middle East and its diaspora. [41] Moreover, forms of normative scientization not just of jinn therapies, but of the occult more broadly have flourished in the modern Middle East, as Alireza Doostdar has demonstrated in his fascinating analysis of such rationalizations in modern-day Iran.[42]

IV. Reconfiguring Qur'anic Ingestion in Today's Egypt

Qur'anic healers' attempts to create a normative modern science of healing have also shaped their approach to the practice of ingesting the Qur'an, to which I now turn. As Shaykh Khalil did in Marwa's jinn exorcism session, many Qur'anic healers frequently use the recited-upon-water as a staple component in their therapeutic repertoire. For them, the Qur'an-imbued water, like Qur'anic recitations more broadly, functions as a diagnostic, therapeutic, and prophylactic tool. It is used to sprinkle patients during healing sessions to bring forth the jinn, only to weaken them, forcing or convincing them to exit the body of the possessed, and then it is used to strengthen and nourish the person, preventing further jinn incursions.

For Qur'anic healers, the practice of imbuing water (or other substances) with the Qur'an is normative, as the evidentiary proof of the Qur'an and of various hadiths demonstrates. [43] Moreover, Qur'anic

[41] E.g., Emilio Spadola, *The Calls of Islam* for Morocco, Bille, "Seeking Providence" for Jordan or Moussa Khedimellah, "Une version de la *ruqiya* de rite prophétique en France. Le cas d'Abdellah, imam guérisseur en Lorraine," in *Coran et talismans: Textes et pratique magiques en milieu musulman*, ed. Constant Hamès (Paris: Karthala, 2007) for France.

[42] Alireza Doostdar, *The Iranian Metaphysicals: Explorations in Science, Islam, and the Uncanny* (Princeton: Princeton University Press, 2018).

[43] Besides the cure verses mentioned above, Qur'anic healers also bring as evidence verses that show the tremendous impact of the Word of God on all of creation (*al-ḥashr*: 21), as well as verses that present jinn as sentient, intelligent creatures who have the ability to understand the Qur'an and hence be convinced to remove their hold on the possessed body (*al-aḥqāf*: 29, *al-jinn*: 1, 13). For more on various hadiths related to the practice and the way they have been approached by religious scholars, see Zadeh, "An Ingestible Scripture."

healers ground the normativity of the practice in its support by medieval religious scholars like Ibn Taymiyya and Ibn al-Qayyim al-Jawziyya that are central in the Salafi orientation that Qur'anic healers follow. That important figures in the contemporary Saudi religious establishment also see Qur'anic ingestion as orthodox, and are invoked as authorities by Qur'anic healers themselves, attests not just to these practitioners' religious proclivities, but also to the insertion of this practice in broader contemporary normative configurations and debates.[44] Aware of the long medieval and modern history of this practice, Qur'anic healers are interested in it only insofar that is shows Qur'anic ingestion normativity. For them, Qur'anic ingestion is without a doubt a normative tradition-bound practice.

Within this broad framing, some Qur'anic healers further distinguish between the two main forms it takes in today's Egypt. Thus, several Qur'anic healers, as Shaykh Khalil himself briefly alluded to in our conversation, expressed a clear preference for directly reciting the Qur'an over water, distrusting the method of writing verses on paper and dissolving them in water. Without affirming that the latter practice is forbidden, some of my interlocutors argued nevertheless that the use of an intermediary material, like the piece of paper, is unnecessary, and explained it with reference to the general higher evaluation given to the oral versus the written Qur'an in the Islamic tradition. "The Qur'an originally was recited, not written, so it is better to follow this in healing as well," one of my interlocutors explained.

This expressed preference for one form of Qur'anic ingestion speaks to a broader concern of Qur'anic healers with the materiality of specific therapeutic techniques and their normative status, especially manifested in these practitioners' rejection of amulets mentioned above.[45] Yet, as both scholars investigating Qur'anic ingestion and medieval Muslim scholars concerned with the practices have shown drinking the Word of God itself, even when the Qur'an is directly recited over water, is a form of materializing the Qur'an in a physical substance and incorporating it

---

[44] For more on Saudi's religious establishment approaches to this and other matters of healing, see Zadeh, "An Ingestible Scripture," 99-102.

[45] In their rejection of amulets, Qur'anic healers join Saudi religious scholars who have similarly opposed the use of amulets as posing the danger of polluting the Qur'an through contact with the human body or of leading to polytheism (known as *shirk*) (Zadeh, "An Ingestible Scripture," 99-102).

into the human body. This suggests that at stake in these preferences is not a generalized rejection of materiality as the opposite of immateriality, but an attention to forms and degrees of materiality and their potential normative implications.

If questions of normativity have shaped to a certain degree the use of Qur'anic ingestion by Qur'anic healers, what has most persistently attracted their attention, making Shaykh Khalil's voice to vibrate and his eyes to sparkle with excitement, is the idea that modern science demonstrates the effects of reciting the Qur'an over water, providing an additional form of evidence that confirms, in the language of science, what is already established from within the Islamic tradition. That evidence, as Shaykh Khalil told me that April day comes from the "scientific experiments of a Japanese scientist."

The Japanese scientist Shaykh Khalil was referring to is Masaru Emoto, whose name and work have become the most invoked source of evidence and explanation for the benefits of Qur'anic ingestion in today's Egypt. Born in 1943 and dying at the age of 71 in 2014, Emoto first studied International Relations in Japan and later earned the title of Doctor in Alternative Medicine from the Open International University in India, a fake institution which was shut down in 2019 after twelve years of functioning.[46]

His international reputation is tied to a series of experiments conducted since the mid-1990s, that demonstrate, he claims, that states of consciousness, words, music, or prayers influence water's molecular structure, as proven by the form of the resulting crystals after freezing the water so "treated." On this basis, Emoto argues that there is a direct, energy-based connection between the aesthetic or affective qualities of the influencing agent and physical matter, particularly the shape of frozen water crystals, positing in this way the influence of mind over physical matter.[47] The results of these experiments, including photographs of the crystals obtained in this way, have been published by Emoto in his books, *The Hidden Messages in Water* and *The Healing Power of Water*, translated into

---

[46] On Emoto's life and work, see his website: https://masaru-emoto.net/. Last accessed October 27, 2021.

[47] See Hado – Office Masaru Emoto, here: https://masaru-emoto.net/en/hado/. Last accessed October 28, 2021.

multiple languages.[48] On his website, one can submit water samples to obtain crystal photographs for $550 per sample, as well as purchase a variety of merchandise.[49]

The work of Masaru Emoto, popular in Japan and beyond, is considered by the scientific community as pseudoscience and New Age gibberish.[50] His experiments have been debunked as not meeting scientific standards, not carried out under controlled conditions, not replicable, and rooted in ideas incompatible with basic physics; in other words, not scientific experiments at all.[51] Of course, scientific debunking of what science itself designates as "pseudoscience" does not always work in practice, not only because the act of debunking is rejected by proponents of pseudoscience, but also because it ignores the social bonding around the supposed "bunk."[52]

Emoto is a case in point. Despite attempts to discredit his experiments, his claims of scientificity linger internationally, including in Egypt, where he is widely known as the Japanese researcher who has scientifically demonstrated the power of the Qur'an to change the structure of water.[53] Framed in this way, his name and experiments were repeatedly mentioned to me by numerous Egyptians. This emphasis on the scientific status of Emoto's experiments has contributed to spreading

---

[48] See Masaru Emoto's books at https://hado.com/ihm/books. Last accessed November 22, 2021.

[49] See Order – Office Masaru Emoto at https://masaru-emoto.net/en/application/ and Water Crystal Goods at https://hado.com/ihm/product/water-crystal-goods/. Last accessed November 24, 2021.

[50] In the U.S., he became known after the inclusion of his water crystal experiments in a 2004 indie movie, *What the Bleep Do We Know?*, which explores connections between quantum physics and consciousness by combining a fictional narrative plot with computer graphics and interviews. The film was widely criticized by members of the scientific community as steeped in pseudoscience, but this was no obstacle to its making over $15 million at the box office (see "The Minds Boggle," *The Guardian*, 15 May, 2005, at www.theguardian.com/science/2005/may/16/g2.science, last accessed Nov. 24, 2021).

[51] See Harriet Hall, "Masaru Emoto's Wonderful World of Water," *Skeptical Inquirer*, 31:6 (2007), 49-51, as well as the website of retired professor of physical chemistry, Stephen Lower, with one page dedicated to "water crystals quackery," www.chem1.com/CQ/ Last accessed November 24, 2021.

[52] On debunking and its limits, see Emily Ogden, "Debunking Debunked," *Aeon*, Aug. 12, 2019. at https://aeon.co/essays/is-debunking-more-about-the-truth-teller-than-the-truth.

[53] For an example in English, see "Japanese scientist Calls ZamZam Miraculous Water and Cure for Every Illness" at https://theislamicinformation.com/news/japanese-scientist-masaru-emoto-zamzam/. Last accessed November 30, 2021.

the conviction that Qur'anic ingestion is proven as beneficial by modern science beyond immediate Qur'anic circles, even among those opposed to Qur'anic healing. His books have been translated into Arabic and prefaced by Zaghul al-Naggar, an Egyptian geologist known for his publications on the "scientific miracles" of the Qur'an. Al-Naggar's interest in Emoto's work reflects how these two ideas, Qur'an's scientific miracles and Emoto's experiments, pertain to the same discursive framework and share the same logic, both being based on the idea that modern science confirms revealed Islamic knowledge.

Emoto's popularity in Egypt was boosted by his participation in 2008 in an installment of *Cairo Today* (*Al-Qahira al-Yawm*), a widely watched talk show then hosted by the media figure 'Amr Adib.[54] Invited to the studio was also Dr. Ibrahim Karim, a well-known Egyptian New Age figure. Each of the crystals presented during the show, resulting after reciting the names of God, playing a recording of *athan* (the call to prayer), and putting a printed copy of the Qur'an over water, was received by participants with exclamations of surprise, admiration, and praises to God - *subḥān allah*! Explaining the process behind each crystal, Dr. Ibrahim Karim translated Emoto's notion of energy *hado* with the Arabic term *ṭāqa*, but also argued that the energetic resonance of words, images, or letters is enhanced by one's faith (*īmān*) and good intention (*niyya*). This blend of New Age-inspired concepts like energy and Islamic ones has gained some popularity in the past decades through the influx of new forms of spirituality, parapsychology, popular psychology, and self-help manuals.[55] In line with how Emoto's experiments have circulated in Egyptian society, all participants in the show repeatedly underlined that these experiments provide "scientific evidence" (*ithbāt/dalīl 'ilmī*) of the Qur'an's "material/physical effect" (*ta'thīr māddī*) over water.

Like the participants in this TV show, Qur'anic healers also frame Emoto's experiments as the scientific evidence, or the reason-based evidence (*dalīl 'aqlī*), for the therapeutic efficacy of Qur'anic ingestion for the therapeutic efficacy of Qur'anic ingestion that corroborates the revealed evidence (*dalīl naqlī*) provided by the Qur'an and hadith. In this way, the practice of reading the Qur'an over water and the curative

[54] Although Masaru Emoto was present in the studio, he did not say a word for the entire duration of the show.

[55] On New Age beliefs in the Middle East, see Doostdar, *The Iranian Metaphysicals*.

qualities of the resulting water are doubly authorized, by science and by revelation. Here, science confirms in a different language what is already established within the Islamic tradition.

The fact that this evidence is called "scientific" is particularly significant for Qur'anic healers. This is because in their eyes this is a form of evidence that is credible to Muslims and non-Muslims alike. For Qur'anic healers, as for many other Egyptians, modern science is understood to be universally true, objective, unbiased, and neutral (*muhayid*), a positivist framing of science that goes back to the nineteenth-century reformist reactions to colonial attacks on Islam. Emoto's experiments' scientific character is further enhanced by their author's religion. Adopting what could be seen as a form of reverse identity politics, Qur'anic healers argue that the fact that Emoto is not a Muslim means he has no interest (*maṣlaḥa*) in either proving or disproving the therapeutic capacities of Qur'anic ingestion. His work is twice unbiased – because it is scientific and because it is produced by a non-Muslim.

For Qur'anic healers, the significance of Emoto's experiments does not end with their scientific status. It also lies in what this evidence reveals, namely the specific mechanisms through which the Qur'an transforms water. Moreover, some Qur'anic healers have taken these experiments as a springboard for further developing their therapeutic practice and providing an explanation of how the Qur'an cures in general. For example, Shaykh Mamduh, another Qur'anic healer and main interlocutor, elaborated:

> Because of the Qur'anic recitation, the water is changed in its composition (*fī tarkībihā*) even if we don't see this change with our eyes. So when we drink it, our bodies absorb this transformed water and this is how it affects our bodies. Moreover, our bodies are 70 percent water, so when we recite the Qur'an it affects this water that we are made of. In this manner, the Qur'an directly affects (*yu'athir 'alā*) our bodies.

Here, Shaykh Mamduh merges Emoto's claims with a biomedically-rooted knowledge of the body's chemical composition and the process of liquid absorption. In other words, he invokes science twice. This recourse to human physiology can also take other forms, as another Qur'anic healer I interviewed suggested:

> When we drink water, this water goes directly to the kidneys, the center from where water spreads in the body. If, for example, I have jinn possession (*mass*), the jinni is walking in the blood as the Prophet said (*al-ginn yimshī fī al-damm*).[56] The Qur'anic water (*mayya maqrū'a*) from the kidneys is also spread in the blood. The jinni stays there, in the blood, while the water is coming from the kidneys. The water is advancing until it arrives in front of the jinni, blocks him, and forces him out.

Dramatizing an encounter between the jinn and the Qur'anic water in the blood into what reads almost like a duel, Shaykh Said's account similarly combines Emoto's ideas with specific interpretations of hadith and with a view of the human body that bears the imprint of biomedical knowledge even it is incorrect. In other words, Shaykh Said's explanations are rooted in an anatomo-physiological understanding of the human body as composed of organs and systems with specific functions. The possessing jinn, once inside the body, follows the basic principles of these systems, such as the circulatory one.

Through these examples, we can see how Emoto's experiments have fueled the increased interest of Qur'anic healers in providing explanations for their therapies that emphasize physiological mechanisms and proofs. For some Qur'anic healers, these kinds of explanations are even taking precedence over the longstanding understanding of the Qur'an's force through the notion of *baraka*. A complex term in the Islamic tradition, *baraka* can be translated as blessing, a divine beneficial force for the physical and psychic realm at once that can reside in various people or things, especially in the Qur'an.[57] Indeed, for many lay Egyptians whom I encountered during my research the benefits of Qur'anic ingestion and the curative role of the Qur'an more generally were typically framed through the notion of *baraka*, and they seemed uninterested in further unpacking and dissecting

---

[56] This is in reference to a well-known hadith that mentions that the devil flows, literally runs, in humans like blood, *al-shayṭān yajrī min ibn ādam majrā al-damm*. While some interpretations take the devil as a metaphorical way of describing humans' innate evil tendencies, others understand the hadith literally.

[57] See G. S. Colin, "Baraka," in *Encyclopaedia of Islam*, second edition, ed. P. Bearman et al. Consulted online on 18 October 2022 <http://dx.doi.org/10.1163/1573-3912_islam_SIM_1216> . First published online: 2012.

the specific mechanism of the Qur'an's curative effects. Yet these are precisely the questions that animate many, though not all, Qur'anic healers. Such an interest reflects these practitioners' attempts to scientize healing, here through their embrace of a positivist mode of reasoning, bearing the imprint of a modern scientific epistemology favoring empiricism.

For Qur'anic healers, Emoto is important not only for what his work says about Qur'anic ingestion, but also for what it says about them as healers – by invoking his experiments they simultaneously demonstrate their epistemic knowledge and therapeutic authority. Embracing Emoto is a testament to their openness and commitment to modern science and to the goal of creating a modern orthodox science of healing.

Beyond Emoto and Qur'anic ingestion, some Qur'anic healers have expanded the recourse to modern science to call for collaborative experiments with psychiatrists, physicians, and other scientists aimed at scientifically determining the effects of Qur'anic healing. Such calls are based on the view delineated above that science confirms what is already known from the Islamic tradition, the same view on which the literature on the "scientific miracles" of the Qur'an is based.

While all the psychiatrists I encountered during my research rejected Emoto's experiments as pseudoscience, a few religiously inclined ones shared with Qur'anic healers an interest in scientifically determining the influence of Qur'anic recitation on the human body. This is the case of Dr. Al-Altorni, whose mention of such an experiment carried out in the United States sparked a contentious debate among the participants at an international psychiatric conference I attended in spring 2011.[58] In our conversations, a few other psychiatrists also invoked such studies from other countries, which, unlike those of Emoto, they considered scientific.[59] In this manner, even though psychiatrists and Qur'anic healers might disagree on what counts as scientific and what does not, they do share a belief in the authority of modern science and concur that it can be used as evidence for elucidating practices belonging to the Islamic tradition.

Yet, there are discordant voices. Invoking Emoto and science in support of Qur'anic ingestion, and Qur'anic healing more generally, is

[58] To my knowledge, experiments of this kind have not been carried out in Egypt.

[59] When I say "invoked," I do not mean that they referenced specific studies, only that they pointed out that such studies exist, as a quick Internet search easily proves.

not universally embraced by all Qur'anic healers or by other actors interested in these debates, even if such critical, or at least cautious voices seem to be in minority. A couple of interlocutors among Qur'anic healers expressed a sense of unease in what concerns the employment of modern science and of experiments as tools for proving the healing capacity of the Qur'an. This is what Shaykh Ibrahim had to say:

> Science is based on hypotheses, on experiments to confirm or refute such hypotheses. Science is a form of doubt (*al-'ilm nū' min al-shakk*). But I, as believer, am not supposed to doubt the Qur'an. What if these experiments show that the Qur'an does not cure, am I going to stop believing it is a cure? Science changes, but religion is unchanging (*al-'ilm mutaghayyir bass al-dīn thābit*).

Here, Shaykh Ibrahim argues that science cannot take precedence over the Qur'an and *sunna*, the two main sources of authority in the Islamic tradition. Putting the Qur'an under the investigative lens of science, which favors doubt, troubles this basic assumption and should therefore be avoided.

An opposition to experimenting with the Qur'an was also expressed by some self-described religious psychiatrists who were concerned that such experiments "devalue the Qur'an." Similar ideas were articulated by several participants in a conference on Qur'anic healing organized in 2007 in Abu Dhabi, as Dr. Mohammad al-Mahdi mentions in a report:

> Warnings were raised [by some participants] against considering the Qur'an only as a therapeutic method we subordinate to scientific research using the standards of experimental science and we compare with other therapeutic methods, as it happens in studies focusing on drugs and other treatments. This is because the Qur'an has goals, purposes, levels, and outlooks which the tools of experimental scientific research cannot perhaps capture in an appropriate manner.[60]

[60] Muhammad al-Mahdi, "Mu'tamar al-'Ilaj bi-l-Qur'an bayn al-Din wa-l-Tibb" [Conference: Qur'anic Healing between Religion and Medicine], *Majanin*, April 12, 2007. http://www.maganin.com/content.asp?contentId=12082.

Such reservations towards submitting the Qur'an to scientific experiments are based on a perspective according to which the epistemological bases of modern science are different from those of religion. Hence, the former cannot be brought to bear on the latter. In this manner, these critiques echo the stance of the Muslim thinkers interested in the "Islamization of science and knowledge," a project that, when extended to psychology and psychiatry, is a domain of interest for some religious Egyptian psychiatrists such as Dr. Al-Mahdi.

The concern with such epistemological differences is intertwined for these critics with a concern for the sensibilities, dispositions, and attitudes that accompany or should accompany science and religion. For them, what the scientific approach lacks first and foremost is the proper attitude of humility and awe believers should have when dealing with the Qur'an, including when using it as a therapeutic tool. Instead, science calls for hypotheses, which are by definition falsifiable, and it calls for doubt – all improper dispositions towards the Word of God. For these critics, science and religion elicit and require contrasting, mutually exclusive epistemic affects.

It is not that these critics deny the authority of modern science in and of itself – on this they are in agreement with the majority position I discussed in this essay. What they deny is its authority to speak about Islam, specifically opposing its employment as evidence for elucidating one aspect of the Islamic tradition – the practice of imbuing water with the Qur'an and the use of the Qur'an in healing more broadly. Thus, while those who support the recourse to modern science adopt a view whereby the realms of science and Islam are seen as complementarily different, the opponents disentangle the two realms, and see them as exclusively different, if equally valid.

V. Conclusion

Qur'anic healers, the practitioners of the revivalist form of exorcism I focused on in this essay, have reconfigured the longstanding practice of Qur'anic infusion and ingestion in ways that emphasize the normativity and especially the scientificity of this therapy. Arguing that Qur'anic ingestion is doubly authorized, from within the Islamic tradition and from without, by modern science, these practitioners have furthermore invoked modern science to elucidate and emphasize the specific mechanism of this therapeutic technique. In this way, they have also employed science to expand Islamic therapeutic knowledge into new directions.

Yet, readers might wonder how the perspective I adopted here, taking Qur'anic healers' framing of Emoto's work as science at face value, squares with the fact that its pseudoscientific status is not in doubt in the scientific community. Indeed, some scholars who have focused on kindred employments of science, most notably the idea of the Qur'an's scientific miracles, have seen them as rooted in a misunderstanding of modern science or as apologetics, mere rhetorical and not substantive engagements with science.[61] Outside academic perspectives, the idea that Islam is anti-scientific and hence stuck in a medieval past of magic practices, a framing akin to an Orientalizing medievalism, continues to dominate many cultural productions.[62]

My analytical concern in this paper is not that Qur'anic healers embrace as scientific what scientists see as pseudoscientific, but the ways in which science is invoked and privileged in support of Qur'anic healers' therapeutic knowledge and authority; in other words, in the work that science does in Qur'anic healing. The existence of pseudoscience itself, fake knowledge that wants to be science, speaks about the prestige of science. The two categories are not opposites, but dependent on each other. Thus, the adoption by Qur'anic healers of Emoto's pseudoscientific experiments as science is indicative of the latter's hegemonic status in today's Egypt. In that sense, Qur'anic healers are just men of their time for whom science is a value and a tool at once.

In this case, a more suitable question to understand Qur'anic healers' reconfiguration of Qur'anic ingestion is: what might be lost by not taking practices and statements like those of Qur'anic healers as modes of serious inquiry, regardless of how they might look to scientists themselves? What would be lost, I suggest, is the ability to analyze the social life of science beyond its disciplinary confines including its role in

---

[61] E.g., Stefano Brigliardi, "The 'Scientific Miracles of the Qur'an': Map and Assessment," in *Islamic Studies Today: Essays in Honor of Andrew Rippin*, ed. Majid Daneshgar and Walid A. Saleh (Leiden: Brill, 2017) and Dallal, *Islam, Science*.

[62] April Harper, "Misdiagnosing Medieval Medicine: 'Magical' Muslims, Metanarrative, and the Modern Media," in *The Middle Ages in Modern Culture: History and Authenticity in Contemporary Medievalism*, ed. Karl C. Alvestad and Robert Houghton (London, New York: Bloomsbury Academic, 2021), 58-73.

sustaining and transforming a long-standing religious practice such as Qur'anic ingestion.

SECTION II

Doctors at Work in Medieval Worlds

EARLY MEDIEVAL SURGERY: CHALLENGING POPULAR STEREOTYPES WITH ARCHAEOLOGICAL EVIDENCE

CLAIRE BURRIDGE*

I. Introduction: Popular Perceptions of Early Medieval Medicine[1]

The proliferation of television shows, films, games, books, comics, and other media based, albeit loosely, on the history and literature of the early Middle Ages bears witness to the public's enduring fascination with this period. Two recently concluded television series exemplifying this trend, *The Last Kingdom* and *Vikings*, for example, have proven to be such successes that the former has spawned a film, *Seven Kings Must Die*, and the latter a second series, *Vikings: Valhalla*.[2] Matters of health come up

* Department of History, University of Sheffield.

[1] First and foremost, I would like to thank Lucy Barnhouse and Winston Black for their work in organising this volume and for their generous, constructive feedback on my contribution. My thanks, too, to the anonymous reviewers, my fellow contributors, and the organisers of the 36th Annual International Conference on Medievalism in 2021 for aiding in the development and revision of this piece. Finally, I would also like to extend my gratitude to various non-medievalist friends and family members who shared their perceptions of medieval medicine with me.

[2] For a sense of the programme's popularity, discussions among fans, and the excitement generated by the spin-offs, see dedicated fan sites, such as *The Last Kingdom* Wiki,

with great frequency in these and similar programmes: consider, for example, the inclusion of King Alfred's chronic illness in *The Last Kingdom* or the serious, often fatal, injuries seen throughout both series. Indeed, as some of the "bloodiest epics on TV", *The Last Kingdom* and *Vikings* feature everything from massive, pitched battles to gruesome acts of interpersonal violence.[3] Yet, despite the frequent depiction of injuries in these shows, attempts at healing are rarely given screentime.[4] This is especially true for complex medical interventions such as surgical procedures. In other words, although health is often in the spotlight, healthcare is usually out of sight.

While there is abundant evidence, both textual and archaeological, testifying to the existence of medical knowledge and practices in the early Middle Ages (a selection of which will be detailed below), popular programming would suggest otherwise. This absence of medicine, however, is unsurprising. Crucially, this is not because scenes involving healthcare would not align with these shows' storylines; given the above-mentioned frequency with which injuries (and, to a lesser extent, illness) appear, some mention or visualisation of healing practices, even if it were simply included as background material, could have been easily integrated. Rather, the near total absence of medicine, and especially surgery, in popular media set in the early Middle Ages speaks to and, in turn, reinforces stereotypes regarding the state of medicine in early medieval Europe.[5]

---

https://the-last-kingdom.fandom.com/wiki/The_Last_Kingdom_Wiki (last accessed 2 May 2022) and *Vikings* Wiki, https://vikings.fandom.com/wiki/Vikings_Wiki (last accessed 2 May 2022).

[3] Kari Croop, *The Last Kingdom* – TV Review, *Common Sense Media*, www.commonsensemedia.org/tv-reviews/the-last-kingdom (last accessed 2 May 2022).

[4] There are, of course, some exceptions to this general absence, such as *Game of Thrones*' inclusion of amputations resulting from war wounds or *Vikings*' depiction of Ragnar's addiction to painkilling drugs provided by Yidu, a slave from Asia, in Season 4 – a highly problematic storyline riddled with Orientalist stereotypes. For a deeper analysis, see Helen Young and Kavita Mudan Finn, *Global Medievalism: An Introduction* (Cambridge: 2022), 20-21. And for more on the lack of medical storylines in other types of popular media, see Lucy Barnhouse's chapter in this volume, and for more on medievalism, medicine, and Orientalism, see Robin Reich's chapter in this volume.

[5] On popular culture's general buttressing of stereotypes, especially in terms of race, see, for example, Young and Mudan Finn, *Global Medievalism: An Introduction*; significantly, *Vikings* is highlighted as a case study (pp. 12-25).

Collectively, medieval medicine is often cast as equal parts irrational and ineffective, backwards and bloody, but this imagery is more typically based on misrepresentations of later medieval medical knowledge and practices. Take, for example, the incessant bloodletting and reliance on superstition displayed by a classic *Saturday Night Live* skit in which Steve Martin plays Theodoric of York, a barber-surgeon working in fourteenth-century England.[6] Negative portrayals of medieval medicine are not hard to find.[7] Turning to the early Middle Ages, however, medicine generally disappears from view – even in plotlines that highlight health conditions and injuries or showcase warfare and combat.[8] The absence of medicine in these contexts reveals that this body of knowledge is not seen to fit into the early Middle Ages as the period is popularly imagined. The provision of healthcare, and particularly the successful deployment of sophisticated medical interventions such as surgical procedures, is hard to square with the standard depiction of this period.

This chapter confronts these outdated stereotypes by answering two related questions: is there evidence of surgery in early medieval Europe?[9] If so, is there also evidence to suggest that individuals survived these surgeries?

Part of the reason for the continuation of these negative stereotypes concerns the nature of the evidence: the written sources preserve almost no record of surgery in the early medieval West, presenting a stark contrast with classical, Byzantine, Islamic, and later medieval European medical texts and other documentary evidence that bear witness to the

---

[6] "Theodoric of York, Medieval Barber," *Saturday Night Live* Season 3, Episode 18 (22 April 1978). See Luke Demaitre's chapter in this volume for more on how "supposedly lowbrow and momentary humor can offer food for serious reflection" (p. 31) as well as Robin Reich's comments, also in the present volume, on this particular skit (pp. 95-96).

[7] On stereotypes of medieval history, see Winston Black, *The Middle Ages: Facts and Fictions* (Santa Barbara, California: ABC-CLIO, 2019); for topics relating to medicine and science, see Chapters 3, 6, 9, and 11.

[8] Consider, for example, the lack of surgery in popular television programmes and films theoretically set in the early Middle Ages, such as *The Last Kingdom* (2015-22), *Vikings* (2013-20), *Tristan and Isolde* (2006), *King Arthur* (2004), or even *Monty Python and the Holy Grail* (1975).

[9] In this chapter, "surgery" is defined as "the treatment of injuries or disorders of the body by incision or manipulation, especially with instruments," following Angus Stevenson (ed.), *Oxford Dictionary of English* (Oxford: Oxford University Press, 2010), www.oxfordreference.com/view/10.1093/acref/9780199571123.001.0001/m_en_gb0832630 (accessed 13 Dec. 2019).

knowledge and practice of surgery.[10] This lack of textual evidence has been interpreted as the disappearance of this knowledge in the post-Roman West, an assumption that stems from and reproduces traditional views regarding the stagnation, if not retrogression, of medicine in the "dark ages."[11] While this understanding of early medieval medicine has been overturned, the lacuna in the written record has meant that the question of surgery has been largely ignored.[12] In this chapter, therefore, I shall turn to the osteological record, using evidence from skeletal remains to supplement the texts. Markers of surgical intervention, including significant, invasive procedures such as trepanation (the removal of sections of the skull), reveal that, despite the absence of written evidence, surgical practices certainly continued during this period. Furthermore, evidence of healing and long-term care, such as the incredible discovery in 2013 of a lower leg and foot prosthesis associated with the skeleton of a sixth-century individual, speaks to the sophistication and success of some surgical treatments. A third goal of this chapter is to emphasise the importance of interdisciplinary research

---

[10] For a general overview, see: Lawrence I. Conrad, Michael Neve, Vivian Nutton, Roy Porter, and Andrew Wear, eds., *The Western Medical Tradition: 800 BC to AD 1800* (Cambridge: Cambridge University Press, 1995); see also: Tony Hunt, *The Medieval Surgery* (Woodbridge: Boydell, 1992); Michael McVaugh, *The Rational Surgery of the Middle Ages* (Florence: SISMEL, 2006); Piers D. Mitchell, *Medicine in the Crusades: Warfare, Wounds, and the Medieval Surgeon* (Cambridge: Cambridge University Press, 2004); Vivian Nutton, *Ancient Medicine*, Second Edition (London: Routledge, 2013); Peter E. Pormann and Emilie Savage-Smith, *Medieval Islamic Medicine* (Edinburgh: Edinburgh University Press, 2007).

[11] Simon A. Mays, "A Possible Case of Surgical Treatment of Cranial Blunt Force Injury from Medieval England," *International Journal of Osteoarchaeology* 16 (2006), 95-103, at 99. For the early, highly negative and dismissive scholarship on medieval medicine, see especially Charles Singer, "A Review of the Medical Literature of the Dark Ages, with a New Text of about 1110," *Proceedings of the Royal Society of Medicine* 10 (1917), 107-60, and John Henry Grafton Grattan and Charles Singer, *Anglo-Saxon Magic and Medicine: Illustrated Specially from the Semi-Pagan Text* Lacnunga (Oxford: Oxford University Press, 1952).

[12] There is not sufficient space to address the extensive body of scholarship that has rehabilitated early medieval medicine; in brief, see the work of pioneers Loren C. MacKinney and Henry E. Sigerist; a second wave of scholars headed by John M. Riddle, Jerry Stannard, and Linda E. Voigts; and, more recently, Maria Amalia D'Aronco, Florence Eliza Glaze, Monica H. Green, Meg Leja, Peregrine Horden, Anne Van Arsdall, etc. For a notable exception regarding the general lack of scholarship on early medieval surgery, see: Debby Banham and Christine Voth, "The Diagnosis and Treatment of Wounds in the Old English Medical Collections: Anglo-Saxon Surgery?," in Larissa Tracy and Kelly DeVries, *Wounds and Wound Repair in Medieval Culture* (Leiden: Brill, 2015), 153-74.

and offer a model for incorporating non-textual evidence in the study of medieval medicine and surgery. I conclude with a consideration of how the integration of osteological evidence can help us to reflect on questions relating to the transmission and production of knowledge, both medieval and modern, returning to the opening examples of current forms of popular media. I consider viewers' perceptions of and interest in the historical accuracy of this type of programming, identifying possible ways to incorporate richer, more representative histories of the early Middle Ages in media designed for the general public.

II. The Big Lacuna: The Absence of Surgery in the Written Record

Historians of early medieval medicine have traditionally relied on textual evidence. Both medical literature and documentary sources, such as charters or the famed *Plan of St. Gall* (a ninth-century diagram thought to represent an idealised vision of a monastic centre which, significantly for this context, includes a medical area),[13] have provided a wealth of information concerning health and medicine in this period. Writings that can be considered "medical" cover a variety of styles and genres, and include treatises on hygiene and preventative medicine, dietetics, obstetrics and gynaecology, collections of pharmaceutical prescriptions, and medical glossaries.[14] The manuscript evidence showcases the diversity of medical knowledge in circulation and illustrates the sustained interest in medicine during this period. On the other hand, the study of hagiographical writings, letters, histories, charters, law codes, and other documentary evidence, such as the aforementioned *Plan of St. Gall*, has shed light on perceptions of health and healing, significant health-related events (such as outbreaks of epidemics), the complexity of the "medical

[13] For more scholarship on the *Plan of St Gall*, see Barbara Schedl, *Der Plan von St. Gallen: Ein Modell europäischer Klosterkultur* (Vienna: Böhlau Verlag, 2014) as well as Walter Horn and Ernest Born, *The Plan of St Gall: A Study of the Architecture and Economy of, and Life in, a Paradigmatic Carolingian Monastery*, 3 vols (Berkeley: University of California Press, 1979).

[14] On the variety of medical texts, see Augusto Beccaria, *I codici di medicina del periodo presalernitano (secoli IX, X e XI)* (Rome: Edizioni di Storia e Letteratura, 1956) and Faith Wallis, "The Experience of the Book: Manuscripts, Texts, and the Role of Epistemology in Early Medieval Medicine," in Don G. Bates (ed.), *Knowledge and the Scholarly Medical Traditions* (Cambridge: Cambridge University Press, 1995), 105-43 (see especially 112, n. 30).

marketplace," and so on.[15] Although there are a few key exceptions, such as writings on bloodletting, cautery, and scarification and a handful of treatments in Old English medical texts that involve surgical procedures, the vast majority of sources preserve no evidence of surgery.[16] This absence is particularly striking since surgical treatises continued to circulate in the Greek East and Islamic world via physicians and medical authors such as Paul of Aegina, Hunayn ibn Ishāq, and Abū Bakr al-Rāzī.[17]

Given that the study of medicine in early medieval Europe has been so strongly based on textual evidence, it is not surprising that surgery has been overlooked. Indeed, early twentieth-century scholars' disdain for and derision of early medieval medicine have been effectively countered by highlighting the diversity and dynamism of the medical texts in circulation and the importance of analysing them within their social and cultural context. The lack of surgery in the written record, therefore, has meant that this topic has been largely left out of the general rehabilitation and development of the field. This relative absence of evidence for surgery, however, should not be read as evidence of absence, especially since the evidence in question is based solely on the written record. Instead, the lack of textual evidence suggests that, if surgical procedures were employed during this period, knowledge of these practices was transmitted through non-textual means.[18] Here, the osteological record

[15] On the use of multiple types of textual evidence beyond the strictly medical literature, see, for example, Valerie J. Flint, "The Early Medieval *Medicus*, the Saint – and the Enchanter," *Social History of Medicine* 2 (1989), 127-45, and Clare Pilsworth, *Healthcare in Early Medieval Northern Italy: More to Life than Leeches?* (Turnhout: Brepols, 2014).

[16] Beccaria, *I codici* ; Banham and Voth highlight several examples of surgical procedures in *Bald's Leechbook* and *Leechbook III* as well as an anecdote from Bede, see "The Diagnosis and Treatment of Wounds," 153-74; see also Charlotte A. Roberts, "Surgery," in Michael Lapidge, John Blair, Simon Keynes, and Donald Scragg (eds), *The Wiley Blackwell Encyclopedia of Anglo-Saxon England*, Second Edition (Chichester: Wiley, 2014), 445-7.

[17] Peter E. Pormann, *The Oriental Tradition of Paul of Aegina's* Pragmateia (Leiden: Brill, 2004), Fuat Sezgin, *Ḥunain Ibn Isḥāq (d. 260/873): Texts and studies* (Frankfurt am Main: Institute for the History of Arabic-Islamic Science at the Johann Wolfgang Goethe University, 1996); Fuat Sezgin, Mazin 'Amāwī, Carl Ehrig-Eggert, and Eckhard Neubauer, *Muḥammad ibn Zakarīyā' ar-Rāzī (d. 313/925): Texts and studies* (Frankfurt am Main: Institute for the History of Arabic-Islamic Science at the Johann Wolfgang Goethe University, 1999).

[18] Banham and Voth, "The Diagnosis and Treatment of Wounds," 153-74. For more on gaps in the surviving textual record, see also Robin Reich's chapter in this volume.

can help to answer this chapter's underlying questions concerning the existence of surgery and survival of patients in early medieval Europe.

III. Osteological Evidence for Surgery – and Survival

As Robin Fleming has shown, archaeological evidence, and especially the evidence preserved by skeletal remains, can effectively complement the textual sources traditionally relied upon by historians, helping counteract the biases of the written record and "re-animate the historical dead."[19] Bones and teeth react to various stresses and age-related processes, including infection, injury, repeated use, and surgery, and, in some cases, these changes leave indicators on the skeleton.[20] The analysis of skeletal remains thus has the potential to provide information on many aspects of an individual's life, including their diet, activity patterns, and experience of disease and surgery. It must be remembered, however, that the osteological record only preserves indicators of certain types of surgery (namely, surgeries that involve bones), and surgical procedures that affect soft tissue exclusively, such as bloodletting or scarification, would leave no trace in the skeletal remains.

In addition to exhibiting signs of skeletal surgery, bones can offer insights into the postoperative healing process based on the presence or absence (and, if present, extent) of remodelled bone at the site of the surgery.[21] If there is no sign of remodelling, then the surgical intervention

---

[19] Robin Fleming, "Bones for Historians: Putting the Body Back into Biography," in David Bates, Julia Crick, and Sarah Hamilton (eds), *Writing Medieval Biography, 750-1250: Essays in Honour of Frank Barlow* (Woodbridge, 2006), 29-48, at 29. See also Robin Fleming, "Writing Biography at the Edge of History," *The American Historical Review* 114 (2009), 606-14. This type of approach integrating osteological and textual evidence has proven particularly useful when considering individuals' experiences of health, disease, injury, and surgical interventions in the past; for a later medieval example, see Mitchell, *Medicine in the Crusades.*

[20] Charlotte A. Roberts, *Human Remains in Archaeology: A Handbook* (York, 2012); Donald J. Ortner, "What Skeletons Tell Us: The Story of Human Paleopathology," *Virchows Archiv*, 459 (2011), 247-54.

[21] It must be remembered that bone remodelling can only provide information about the individual's survival and physical recovery; no comment can be made regarding their mental and emotional health, something particularly important to keep in mind in the following discussion of trepanation.

occurred at or very near to the individual's death.[22] In some cases, it can be difficult to distinguish between peri- and post-mortem damage, though the fragmentation of bones due to soil weight or any damage incurred during the excavation process are often recognisable.[23] If the individual survived the surgery, bone repair would have begun almost immediately (evidence of remodelling can be seen within roughly two days) and may continue for several years.[24] The gradation of remodelling can therefore provide a timeframe for understanding the healing process: did the individual make a full recovery or die within a few days or weeks after the surgery? If there are only early signs of bone repair, it suggests that the individual survived the initial procedure but died relatively soon after, perhaps due to infection or other complications.[25]

With this framework in mind, it is possible to investigate the extant osteological evidence for surgery in early medieval Europe, such as examples of trepanation. Trepanation, the removal of a section of skull, is a surgical procedure that has been "performed in many parts of the world from prehistory to the present", and early medieval Europe is no exception.[26] While it generally remains unclear why a piece of skull was surgically removed – and many theories have been proposed, ranging from the release of spirits to the treatment of cranial injuries – this chapter is less concerned with the rationale behind the procedure and more interested in exploring the examples themselves and whether there is evidence that the individuals who underwent this significant surgery

---

22 Adelaide Tosi, Paolo Badino, and Barbara Pezzoni, "Medical Conditions Observed in Osteoarchaeological Remains: Arthropathies, Traumatic Lesions, Tumours, Metabolic Diseases and Dental Pathologies," *Medicina Historica* 1 (2017), 29-34, at 30.

23 Tony Waldron, *Palaeopathology* (Cambridge, 2009), 138; Tosi, Badino, and Pezzoni, "Medical Conditions Observed in Osteoarchaeological Remains," 30.

24 Waldron, *Palaeopathology*, 148; Charlotte A. Roberts and Jacqueline McKinley, "Review of Trepanations in British Antiquity Focusing on Funerary Context to Explain their Occurrence," in Robert Arnott, Stanley Finger, and C. U. M. Smith, *Trepanation: History, Discovery, Theory* (Lisse, 2003), 55-78, at 55 and 64.

25 Waldron, *Palaeopathology*, 148.

26 Roberts and McKinley, "Review of Trepanations in British Antiquity," 55; on trepanation generally, see Robert Arnott, Stanley Finger, and C. U. M. Smith, *Trepanation: History, Discovery, Theory* (Lisse, 2003).

survived (though I shall note a handful of cases in which the trepanation appears to have occurred in response to cranial trauma.)[27]

Trepanations have been identified in early medieval cemeteries both on the continent and in the British Isles. Jochen Weber and Alfred Czarnetzki, for example, conducted a study of head injuries based on a sample of 304 crania from four early medieval cemeteries in southwestern Germany.[28] Located in Alemannic territory, the cemeteries (Neresheim, Kirchheim/Ries, Schretzheim, and Nusplingen) were in use from the sixth to the eighth centuries.[29] Weber and Czarnetzki identified thirty-three skulls (eleven percent of the sample) with cranial fractures, twenty-nine of which were judged to be male and four female.[30] In twenty-two of these cases, the injuries had occurred in the left frontoparietal region, suggesting that the fractures resulted from "face-to-face encounters with the weapon inflicting these wounds held in the right hand".[31] The *Lex Alamannorum*, an Alemannic law code updated in the eighth century, is unique among early medieval law codes in that it not only comments on head injuries, but provides particular detail regarding their treatment.[32] In chapter 57, clauses 6-7 state:

> If, however, a physician loses that bone and cannot present it, then let him call two witnesses who have seen that the bone broke away by that blow, or let that physician prove that the bone broke away by that blow. If, however, the skull is cut through so that the brain appears and a physician can touch it with a *pinna* or a cloth, let him compensate with twelve solidi. If, however, the brain protrudes from the wound, as often happens, so that the physician mends [the skull] with medication or silk and afterwards [the patient]

[27] Grattan and Singer, *Anglo-Saxon Magic and Medicine*; Michael R. Zimmerman, Erik Trinkhaus, and Marjorie Lemay, et al., "Trauma and Trephination in a Peruvian Mummy," *American Journal of Physical Anthropology* 55 (1981), 497-501; Arnott, Finger, and Smith, *Trepanation: History, Discovery, Theory*.

[28] Jochen Weber and Alfred Czarnetzki, "Brief Communication: Neurotraumatological Aspects of Head Injuries Resulting from Sharp and Blunt Force in the Early Medieval Period of Southwestern Germany," *American Journal of Physical Anthropology* 114 (2001), 352-6.

[29] Weber and Czarnetzki, "Brief Communication," 352.

[30] Weber and Czarnetzki, "Brief Communication," 353.

[31] Weber and Czarnetzki, "Brief Communication," 354.

[32] Pilsworth, *Healthcare in Early Medieval Northern Italy*, 108-10.

> recovers, and this is proved to be true, let him [the giver of the blow] compensate with forty solidi.[33]

The *Lex Alamannorum* presents a range of severity within cranial fractures, a picture that accords with Weber and Czarnetzki's analysis of the skeletal remains: their report highlights the relationship between the severity of the trauma (such as the number of injuries and depth of weapon penetration) and chance of survival. The law code also speaks to medical care, describing both surgical intervention (the manipulation of bone and removal of bone fragments as well as the use of instruments) and non-invasive treatments. In the sample studied by Weber and Czarnetzki, three of the injured crania exhibited signs of "circular-shaped trepanations in the proximity of fractures," meaning that roughly ten percent of the fractured skulls exhibited signs of surgical intervention.[34] Moreover, the location of the trepanations in relation to the fracture site suggests that, at least in these cases, the procedure may have been performed as a response to a head injury (perhaps to remove bone fragments, relieve pressure on the brain, etc.), though the authors caution that "a religious or symbolic motive cannot be excluded."[35] That these trepanations may have occurred in relation to cranial trauma seems particularly plausible in light of the medical treatments recorded in the *Lex Alamannorum*.

Finally, the law code also speaks to survival: do the trepanated skulls show signs of recovery? In all three cases, bone remodelling indicative of healing was reported. Significantly, the fracture and trepanation sites display no "signs of postoperative infection," reflecting the effectiveness of the medical care received after the procedure (possibly involving the

[33] "Si autem ipsum ossum perdit medicus et non potest eum presentare, tunc duos testes abhibeat, qui hoc vidissent, quod de illa plaga ossus tullisset, aut ille medicus hoc conprobet, quod verum fuisset, quod de ipsa plaga ossus tullisset. Si autem testa trescapollata fuerit, ita ut cervella appareat, ut medicus cum pinna aut cum fanone cervella tetigit, cum 12 solidis conponat. Si autem ex ipsa plaga cervella exierunt, sicut solet contingere, ut medicus cum medicamentum aut cum sirico stupavit, et postea sanavit, et hoc probatum est, quod verum sit, cum 40 solidis conponat." *Leges Alamannorum,* ed. Johannes Merkel, MGH Leges 3 (Hanover, 1863), Cod. A, LVII, 5-7; Cod. B, LIX, 5-7, 64-5. English translation from Theodore John Rivers, *Laws of the Alamans and Bavarians* (Philadelphia, 1977), 86.

[34] Weber and Czarnetzki, "Brief Communication," 355.

[35] Weber and Czarnetzki, "Brief Communication," 355.

medication and bandaging techniques mentioned in Clause 7).[36] In contrast, four of the non-trepanated crania with evidence of bone remodelling exhibit signs of infection, or nearly twenty percent of the sample.[37]

Overall, the evidence of some degree of bone remodelling in twenty-five of the thirty-three fractured crania speaks to the presence of successful medical care, yet it is the three cases of trepanation that provide the clearest evidence for sophisticated surgical intervention. These three skulls demonstrate not only the existence of a complex surgical procedure, but also the efficacy of this procedure. Still, while these trepanations do provide evidence of early medieval surgery – and survival – they represent a minuscule fraction of the osteological record; the *vast* majority of excavated crania from comparable cemeteries on the continent preserve no signs of surgical intervention. Early medieval England presents a slightly different picture: though the evidence for trepanation remains limited, twenty-four cases have been identified, and we shall now turn to these examples from the Insular context.[38]

In contrast to the three trepanated skulls from southwestern Germany, most of the English examples of trepanation have not been linked to an injury, though there are a number of exceptions. A trepanation from Wharram Percy, a medieval cemetery in Yorkshire, for example, appears to have been performed as part of the treatment for a depressed cranial fracture.[39] According to Simon Mays's analysis of the skull, the individual, dated to the tenth or eleventh century, "suffered a severe blunt injury to the cranial vault as a result of a blow to the left parietal bone," suggestive of face-to-face combat not unlike many of the Alemannic examples of head trauma.[40] Mays notes that depressed fractures must be elevated to relieve pressure on the brain and, in cases where the fractured bone may have impacted, fragments cannot be simply removed; instead, a larger area of the skull must be excised. The presence of remodelled bone at the site of the trepanation and evidence

[36] Weber and Czarnetzki, "Brief Communication," 355.

[37] Weber and Czarnetzki, "Brief Communication," 353. With eight of the thirty-three fractured skulls showing no evidence of healing (suggesting that their injuries were fatal), remodelling can be seen in twenty-five skulls. Twenty-two of these twenty-five skulls did not exhibit signs of trepanation.

[38] Roberts, "Surgery," 445-7.

[39] Mays, "A Possible Case of Surgical Treatment," 95-103.

[40] Mays, "A Possible Case of Surgical Treatment," 99.

of a healed infection indicate that this individual survived not only the initial trauma, but also the resulting surgery and a postoperative infection.[41]

While the above example is unusual in the English material in that the trepanation can be convincingly linked to trauma, it is similar to the other cases with respect to the evidence it provides for the individual's recovery. One of the most notable features of the early medieval English trepanations is that the individuals who underwent these procedures all appear to have survived their surgeries. Of the twenty-four examples known at present, bone remodelling at the site of the surgery is visible in all cases, and this bone growth directly documents the body's postoperative healing processes at work. As Charlotte Roberts explains, "the remarkable success of these trepanations can be seen in the evidence for healing of the edges of the trepanation hole. All the individuals who were trepanned survived their ordeal, some for many years."[42] This record of healing and survival is impressive when the lack of antibiotics and sterile operating facilities are considered, highlighting not only the competence of the surgeons, but the care that the patients received over the following days, weeks, and months as they recovered. Such a success rate speaks to the effective combination of surgery and herbal medicine, suggesting that these different types of medical practice worked in concert and that medical practitioners either had a knowledge of both specialities or that specialists worked together to ensure successful treatments.

The possibility that a single travelling surgeon may have been responsible for several of the trepanations from this period was first raised in 1974 by Calvin Wells, a surgeon-turned-palaeopathologist, who examined five early medieval trepanated skulls found within East Anglia.[43] Wells emphasised the uniformity of these trepanations in terms of their size, shape, orientation, angle of bevelling, and location, all variables that can differ enormously between trepanations.[44] Given the striking regularity of these five examples, Wells argues that they represent the work of one individual; the fact that all five skulls were found within

41 Mays, "A Possible Case of Surgical Treatment," 99.

42 Roberts, "Surgery," 446.

43 Calvin Wells, "Probable trephination of five Early Saxon skulls," *Antiquity* 48 (1974), 298-302; see also Roberts, "Surgery," 446.

44 Wells, "Probable trephination of five Early Saxon skulls," 301.

a relatively close geographical range adds weight to this possibility. Indeed, Wells takes his argument one step further based on his own personal experience in this surgical procedure: he argues not only "that each operation was done by the same surgeon but also that each was done *with the same instrument*."[45] The fact that five of the twenty-four trepanations may represent the work of a single surgeon, termed by Wells the "Master of the Gliding Gouge," does, however, point to the general rarity of this procedure within the wider context of early medieval England. How many surgeons were responsible for these twenty-four trepanations? Might this represent the circulation of specialised surgical knowledge among a small and exceptional circle of medical practitioners? While we shall return to the question of knowledge transmission below, it is important to remember that although these English examples, like the German trepanations, concern a fraction of the excavated skeletal remains, their existence, as well as the evidence for the survival of trepanated individuals, again confirms the successful practice of surgery in early medieval Europe

A comment must also be made regarding the surgical techniques involved in the English finds. While trepanations can be performed using a variety of methods, including drilling, cutting, and scraping, all but one of the extant early medieval English trepanations involved scraping.[46] In this method, the surface of the skull is scraped with a sharp tool, such as a flint, until the bone has been perforated. According to Roberts, "the scraping method was, without doubt, the safest way to perforate the skull," due to the surgeon's control of the scraping tool combined with the lower risk of penetrating the brain (or at least a lower risk relative to other methods, such as drilling).[47] Perhaps the use of this "safe" technique helps to explain the survival rate seen in early medieval examples of trepanation. In contrast, classical medical authorities, such as Galen and Celsus, recommended a combination of drilling and cutting.[48] The writings of surgeons from both the Islamic world and later

[45] Wells, "Probable trephination of five Early Saxon skulls," 302; emphasis original.

[46] Roberts, "Surgery," 446.

[47] Roberts, "Surgery," 446.

[48] Mays, "A Possible Case of Surgical Treatment," 99; Ralph Jackson, *Doctors and Diseases in the Roman Empire* (London: British Museum Publications, 1988); Julius Rocca, "Galen and the Uses of Trepanation," in Robert Arnott, Stanley Finger, and C. U. M. Smith, *Trepanation: History, Discovery, Theory* (Lisse: Swets & Zeitlinger, 2003), 253-71.

medieval West indicate that trepanation techniques similar to those recorded by classical authors were generally favoured over the scraping method.[49] Notably, the early medieval English reliance on the scraping method stands apart from the techniques recommended in the written record. This finding supports Debby Banham and Christine Voth's argument that knowledge of surgery in early medieval England was not transmitted textually, but rather through oral traditions and experience.[50] The evidence recorded in the skeletal remains thus disproves the stereotype that, given the lack of treatises on surgery in early medieval medical literature, knowledge of surgical practices was lost in this period and only re-emerged in the later Middle Ages thanks to the influence of Islamic medical texts and a return to classical traditions.

While early medieval trepanations provide the largest body of evidence testifying to effective surgical procedures in this period, they are not the only type of surgery seen in the osteological record. For the final example, we shall move *a capite ad calcem*, from head to heel, to consider evidence of surgery at the opposite end of the body from a recent excavation in Hemmaberg, Austria. Twenty-nine individuals dated to the sixth century were found in a small cemetery associated with the early medieval church of St. Hemma and Dorothea.[51] One of the skeletons, a male estimated to be between thirty-five and fifty years old at death, was missing the left foot and distal joints of the left tibia and fibula.[52] The skeleton was well-preserved and the point where the tibia and fibula ended was marked by extensive bone remodelling, including the distal fusion of the tibia and fibula. These findings indicate that amputation, rather than poor preservation, had resulted in the loss of the individual's lower left leg and foot. The extent of the bones' remodelling has obscured the "nature of the cuts made during amputation and the implement used to carry it out," so no further comments can be made about the amputation procedure.[53] Although inflammatory changes in

---

[49] Mays, "A Possible Case of Surgical Treatment," 99-100; Hunt, *The Medieval Surgery*; McVaugh, *The Rational Surgery of the Middle Ages*; Mitchell, *Medicine in the Crusades*; Nutton, *Ancient Medicine*; Pormann and Savage-Smith, *Medieval Islamic Medicine*.

[50] Banham and Voth, "The Diagnosis and Treatment of Wounds," 173.

[51] M. Binder, J. Eitler, J. Deutschmann, et al., "Prosthetics in Antiquity – An Early Medieval Wearer of a Foot Prosthesis (6th Century AD) from Hemmaberg/Austria," *International Journal of Paleopathology* 12 (2016), 29-40, at 30-31.

[52] Binder, Eitler, Deutschmann, et al., "Prosthetics in Antiquity," 31-32.

[53] Binder, Eitler, Deutschmann, et al., "Prosthetics in Antiquity," 35-36.

the bone at the site of the amputation suggest that an infection occurred during the recovery process, the full remodelling of the bone reflects that the individual not only survived the amputation, but lived for at least several more years. Once an injury has healed, it is not possible to estimate an individual's long-term survival based on the injury alone; in this case, however, additional evidence provides more information regarding the individual's medical care and recovery after the amputation.

First, an iron band was found in place of the lower leg and foot; this band appears to have been used to connect a wooden prosthesis to the end of the tibia and fibula. Although the wooden attachment has largely disintegrated, the "remains of heavily deteriorated wooden slats on the inside of the ring were preserved," indicating that the individual was buried with the prosthesis.[54] A closer analysis of the physical evidence suggests that the individual relied on the prosthetic attachment after recovering from the amputation. A comparison of the bone density between the right and left legs, for example, suggests that the left leg was initially immobilised for an extended period, resulting in significant atrophy. Other changes in the left leg, including arthritic formations in the knee that reflect an "altered strain on the joint" due to changes in stability, indicate that, after this period of immobilisation, the individual utilised the prosthesis.[55] Asymmetry in the joint degeneration of the arms and shoulders suggests that the individual may have relied on a crutch, as well. These findings reveal that this individual survived for at least several years after the amputation occurred, showcasing not only successful medical treatment with respect to the amputation, subsequent infection, and recovery process, but also continued medical care and support.

It is important to note that the cause of the amputation remains open to speculation given the nature of osteological evidence, and particularly the fact that individual's full recovery (i.e., complete bone remodelling) has erased any clues as to the amputation process. Did the amputation occur for medical reasons, such as the development of a gangrenous infection in the foot? Was it the result of trauma on the battlefield? Could it reflect a judicial mutilation received as punishment? Given the uncertainty surrounding such questions, it remains impossible to confirm

54 Binder, Eitler, Deutschmann, et al., "Prosthetics in Antiquity," 32.
55 Binder, Eitler, Deutschmann, et al., "Prosthetics in Antiquity," 38.

whether surgical procedures were directly involved in the amputation itself but, based on this chapter's definition of surgery, it seems almost certain that, even if the amputation was not the result of a medical intervention, the medical treatment following the amputation would have involved some degree of manipulation as well as surgical procedures.[56] Therefore, this example challenges stereotypes of early medieval medicine despite the lack of adequate evidence to deduce the cause of the amputation. The amputation would have required extensive, immediate, and sophisticated medical care to stop the bleeding and keep the patient alive. The evidence of a healed infection at the site of the amputation as well as the atrophy of the left leg speaks to this individual's lengthy recovery process and long-term treatment, further countering the popular perception of the absence of medical knowledge and practices during this period.

IV. Conclusion: Knowledge Transmission and Production, Past and Present

This chapter has reviewed osteological evidence for successful surgical procedures in early medieval Europe, challenging the pervasive stereotypes regarding surgery – or rather its absence – in this period. Despite a general lack of references to surgery in the textual record, skeletal remains document not only the existence of surgery, but also its success. Signs of healed trepanations, as well as the Frankish leg prosthesis, reflect the competence of early medieval surgeons and the provision of long-term medical care. These successful surgeries reveal that knowledge of complex surgical procedures, though not preserved in the surviving written sources, continued to circulate in early medieval Europe. The clustered nature of the surgical evidence, and its relative rarity, indicates that this highly specialised and technical knowledge may not have been widely disseminated. In line with Banham and Voth's study of wounds in an Insular context, I suggest that knowledge of surgical techniques was likely passed on between individuals and based on extensive training and hands-on experience rather than book learning.[57] Indeed, the use of the scraping method observed in the

[56] See note 9 above for the definition.

[57] Banham and Voth, "The Diagnosis and Treatment of Wounds in the Old English Medical Collections: Anglo-Saxon Surgery?," 173.

English trepanation examples suggests that this surgical tradition may have been distinct from the practices recorded in texts that both pre- and post-date this period, further supporting the individualised nature of this craft.

Evidence for the significant transmission of knowledge outside the written record, moreover, highlights the diversity of medical traditions that circulated within the early medieval healthscape – a diversity that can go relatively unseen when scholars rely exclusively on textual sources. The osteological record thus serves as a valuable reminder of the biases of the written record and the dangers of interpreting the absence of evidence as the evidence of absence. By bringing together different bodies of evidence, such as skeletal remains and documentary sources, it becomes possible to explore questions that neither type of material could effectively investigate in isolation and build a more comprehensive picture overall. Can such work be integrated into popular narratives regarding the early Middle Ages? To what extent are the viewers of films and television series set in early medieval Europe – the drivers of the blossoming of modern medievalism noted at the opening of this chapter – interested in historical accuracy?

An appraisal of discussion boards on fan sites and parental reviews shared on *Common Sense Media* (a non-profit organisation dedicated to reviewing and rating media with a focus on its appropriateness for children) for *The Last Kingdom* and *Vikings* indicates that many individuals are highly interested in these programmes' historicity. In some cases, members of the public posting on these websites have named the shows' perceived historical accuracy as a major draw. A parental reviewer on *Common Sense Media*, for example, described *The Last Kingdom* as a series that "delivered a healthy dose of history," while others have praised *Vikings* for its portrayal of "accurate behaviour" that correctly reflects the historical period.[58] On the other hand, some viewers have pointed out historical inaccuracies in both shows and have sought to correct the

[58] Parental reviews of *The Last Kingdom*, *Common Sense Media*, www.commonsensemedia.org/tv-reviews/the-last-kingdom/user-reviews/adult (last accessed 2 May 2022); parental reviews of *Vikings*, *Common Sense Media*, www.commonsensemedia.org/tv-reviews/vikings/user-reviews/adult (last accessed 2 May 2022).

perception that they accurately depict the historical events and characters upon which they are (loosely) based.[59]

This popular enthusiasm for history – and, crucially, historical accuracy – suggests that the public would readily support a more authentic and nuanced representation of the past in the various types of media that have capitalised on the fashion for all-things-medieval. Yet, disappointingly, when discussing the historical basis of *Vikings* during an interview in *The New York Times*, the series' writer, Michael Hirst, suggested that his intended audiences were unlikely to be seeking a historically accurate rendering of early medieval Europe: "We want people to watch it. A historical account of the Vikings would reach hundreds, occasionally thousands, of people. Here we've got to reach millions."[60]

Moreover, Hirst lamented the lack of evidence that exists for, as he termed it, "the Dark Ages," using an alleged dearth of documentation ("the Vikings … didn't read, they didn't write") to explain the liberties that were taken in the making of the programme.[61] As this chapter has demonstrated, however, there is a rich body of relevant evidence that could have been productively incorporated into programmes such as *Vikings*. This interview was conducted in 2013, the year that the first of the six seasons of *Vikings* was released. While it does not appear that the fans' interest in and engagement with the series' historical background was taken into consideration over the following seasons, perhaps Hirst and others responsible for the new spin-off, *Vikings: Valhalla*, will begin to recognise that, in many cases, better historical portrayals would not hurt their ratings. Rather, the fan discussion boards suggest that attempts to craft a narrative and create visuals that represent the period *more* accurately would likely be very well received.

---

[59] Parental reviews of *Vikings*, *Common Sense Media*, www.commonsensemedia.org/tv-reviews/vikings/user-reviews/adult (last accessed 2 May 2022). One reviewer of *Vikings* even declared: "NOTIFICATION: Even though history channel has shown this, this is a fictitious series, in some reviews i have seen that this is falsely taken as education/documentary ... NO NO NO, it is loosely based on some historical figures, that is it."

[60] Tom Gilbert, "Vikings Come Ashore in a New Light," *The New York Times*, 22 April 2013, www.nytimes.com/2013/02/24/arts/television/vikings-struggles-come-to-life-in-history-channels-series.html?searchResultPosition=1 (last accessed 3 May 2022).

[61] Gilbert, "Vikings Come Ashore in a New Light."

As addressed at the start of this chapter, shows such as *Vikings* and *The Last Kingdom*, given their frequent depiction of violent injuries, provide obvious moments at which the incorporation of elements of healthcare, and perhaps even the types of surgical interventions outlined above, would be fitting. Surely it would be possible to include a glimpse into the potential medical treatments that would have necessarily followed scenes of warfare, hand-to-hand combat, or other forms of violence. Indeed, the horrific cranial injury that plays a key role in the story of Season 4 of *The Last Kingdom* presents one such example where more medical content could have been easily integrated. This is not to suggest overemphasising a medical dimension – it would be inappropriate to, say, introduce the "Master of the Gliding Gouge" as a character or turn one of these shows into a medical drama – but the near total lack of medicine in these types of contexts does seem like a missed opportunity. By introducing more depictions of medical practices, and especially surgery, in the early Middle Ages, the content in question could acknowledge the existence of specialised medical knowledge in this period, thereby combatting the assumption that it was simply forgotten for many centuries. Integrating such information – without overstating it – within popular series, films, and other media would enable the public to access and absorb a better, more accurate representation of early medieval medicine. Popular culture and academic research need not be in opposition: the work of historians and archaeologists can be seamlessly included in content produced for general audiences.

Context, however, remains crucial, and the extent of the evidence involved in this study must be remembered: when considered against the backdrop of all excavated early medieval skeletal remains, the examples of surgery are few and far between. In a period before antibiotics, sterile operating conditions, and other features of modern medicine, it is not surprising that surgery would have been the last resort, turned to only when non-invasive treatments had failed or if surgical intervention was the only possible course of action, as might have been the case with traumatic injuries that occurred in battle.[62] Dietary and pharmaceutical treatments, therefore, would have been the first port of call. Yet the osteological evidence indicates that surgery *did* occur, if only very infrequently. And, despite the small number of examples that document

[62] Mitchell, *Medicine in the Crusades*, 184.

surgical intervention, it is also evident that individuals could survive these surgical procedures. Going under the knife was not necessarily a death sentence.

Ultimately, the violent nature of many popular films and shows set in the early Middle Ages produces settings in which medicine, and especially surgery, could be showcased (or at least alluded to). Based on fan reviews, there appears to be a genuine interest in the history of this period and, in some cases, an assumption that these various forms of popular media accurately portray this history. The current enthusiasm for early medieval content, a "medievalism moment" within pop culture, thus marks an ideal time for historians and archaeologists to work with those involved in producing popular programming set in the early Middle Ages. Through collaboration, we can ensure that not only is the period more accurately depicted overall, but we can also challenge outdated stereotypes about early medieval medicine, and especially surgery, head-on.

AVICENNA, PRINCE OF PHYSICIANS, AND MODERN POLITICAL MEDIEVALISM

WINSTON BLACK*

Abū 'Ali al-Husayn ibn 'Abdullāh Ibn Sīnā (ca.980-1037 CE), known in Western nations by the Latinized version of his name, Avicenna, is rightly regarded as one of the most important intellectual figures in the history of Islam. Experts in his life and thought argue that he should be known primarily as a systematic thinker, the greatest philosopher of the Islamic world.[1] His most voluminous and original writings were philosophical in nature, culminating in his encyclopedia of logic and metaphysics known as *Kitāb al-Shifā'*, that is, *The Book of Healing*. Despite its name, this work was not medical in nature, but directed rather at healing the ignorance of the soul. While scholars of philosophy and of Islamic intellectual culture rightly focus on the importance of this and similar books for understanding Avicenna, he has been known far better among popular audiences, both in the West and increasingly throughout the world, as a physician and author of medical texts, most notably the medical encyclopedia *al-Qānūn fī l-tibb*, or the *Canon of Medicine*.

---

* Gatto Chair of Christian Studies, St. Francis Xavier University.

[1] For example, two of the most recent English-language works on Avicenna are dedicated almost entirely (roughly 90% of each) to his philosophical system, recognizing his medical writings and activity as only a subset of his natural philosophy: Jon McGinnis, *Avicenna* (Oxford, 2010), and *Interpreting Avicenna: Critical Essays*, ed. Peter Adamson (Cambridge, 2013).

Avicenna's reputation as a celebrated physician is hardly new, as it began in his own autobiography, in which he recorded his childhood, education, and first career as a teenage physician correcting his elders. The remainder of his story was completed by his secretary and student al-Jūzjānī, who adored both his master and his master's many books.[2] In Latin Europe, Avicenna was known foremost as *Princeps Medicorum*, "Prince of Physicians," after Gerard of Cremona translated the *Canon of Medicine* into Latin in the later twelfth century. Within a few decades of this translation, the *Canon* became one of the central texts of learned European medicine and remained so for centuries more. Even though other works by Avicenna were translated into Latin in the later Middle Ages, including philosophical texts like *The Book of Healing*, it was the *Canon of Medicine* that remained his defining work in Europe.

This image of Avicenna as a "prince" among physicians and one of the central authorities in medical education dominated the Western reception of Avicenna for the rest of the Middle Ages. Several printed medical texts from the fifteenth and sixteenth centuries are prefaced with engravings of Galen, Avicenna, and Hippocrates as the fathers of learned medicine; only Avicenna is shown wearing a royal crown. In fact, most popular representations of Avicenna to this day come primarily from this Western and Euromedievalist perspective, even when they take place within the Central Asian nations where Avicenna lived and worked.[3]

Unlike most medieval physicians, Avicenna's fame extends far beyond academia. Modern statues of Avicenna have been erected in public squares in both Hamadan, Iran, and Dushanbe, Tajikistan, both of which nations claim Avicenna as a native son. The latter statue is located outside the Avicenna Tajik State Medical University, which was founded and named in his honor in 1939. Avicenna's face, name, and ideas are celebrated not only in the Persian lands that Avicenna called home, but also in other Asian, African, and Western nations, as well as by international organizations such as UNESCO and the World Health

---

[2] The Arabic biography is edited and translated into English by William E. Gohlman, *The Life of Ibn Sina. A Critical Edition and Annotated Translation* (Albany, 1974).

[3] I owe the term "euromedievalist" to Geraldine Heng, who has popularized it in her works, including *The Invention of Race in the European Middle Ages* (Cambridge, 2018) and, more accessibly, "Afterword: Medievalists and the Education of Desire," in *Whose Middle Ages? Teachable Moments for an Ill-Used Past*, ed. Andrew Albin, Mary C. Erler, Thomas O'Donnell, Nicholas L. Paul, and Nina Rowe (New York: Fordham University Press, 2019), 275-290.

Organization, all of which promote Avicenna as part of a common intellectual heritage. Avicenna is embraced not only as a general physician and teacher of medicine, but also as a humanist, scientist and theologian, mystic, poet, psychiatrist, nephrologist, cardiologist, pharmacologist, and so on. Whatever area of the medical sciences or humanities that interests a modern author (particularly those in the Near East and Central Asia), Avicenna is bound to be named as a medieval founder or key figure. In simplest terms, Avicenna is regarded as a medical genius who supposedly developed physiological theories, disease etiologies, and treatment far ahead of his time. It is this composite and mostly ahistorical image of Avicenna that is promoted in modern medievalisms and which serves as the focus of this essay.[4]

As with so many medieval figures, when Avicenna appears in modern media, he is stripped of historical context and serves rather as a symbol for political, scientific, or religious agendas. Modern nations and organizations use Avicenna's face or name as a powerful symbol for a complex set of popular ideas about medieval medicine, medieval Islam, the history of Iran, and historical relations between West and East.[5] Unlike many of the "medical medievalisms" discussed in this volume, which frequently hinge on the supposed barbarity and ineffectiveness of medieval medicine, Avicenna is an almost universally positive symbol, as he is used to represent a rare light of medical and scientific progress in

[4] Most scholars of medievalism focus on the modern appropriation of ideas and imagery from medieval European society. According to Larry Scanlon, in his "Introduction" to a special issue on "Medieval America" of *American Literary History* 22:4 (2010), 715: "Medievalism is an umbrella term for any engagement with the medieval past, including ideas about the Middle Ages, conscious revivals of medieval motifs, narratives, forms and genres, repressed continuities, perhaps even the scholarly study of the Middle Ages itself." A narrower, yet still very broad, definition is given by Tison Pugh and Angela Jane Weisl, *Medievalisms: Making the Past in the Present* (Routledge, 2013), 1: "In its simplest sense, *medievalism* refers to the art, literature, scholarship, avocational pastimes, and sundry forms of entertainment and culture that turn to the Middle Ages for their subject matter or inspiration…"

[5] A significant and still under-studied area of medievalism is Islamic medievalism, the modern incorporation of people and ideas from medieval Islamicate cultures. Recent exceptions to this trend include Nadia Altschul's discussion of alternate medievalisms, including Islamic medievalism, in *Politics of Temporalization: Medievalism and Orientalism in Nineteenth-Century South America* (University of Pennsylvania Press, 2020), 12; and Shamma Boyarin, "The New Metal Medievalism: Alexander the Great, Islamic Historiography and Nile's 'Iskander Dhul Kharnon'," in *Medievalism and Metal Music Studies: Throwing Down the Gauntlet*, ed. Ruth Barratt-Peacock and Ross Hagen (Emerald Publishing, 2019), 81-91.

an otherwise hopelessly backward Middle Ages. For example, in a brief article about Avicenna in a 2002 issue of the *Singapore Medical Journal*, the author S.Y. Tan (a physician and lawyer, not a historian) reproduces popular misconceptions about the differences between European and Islamicate medicine in the Middle Ages: "Even as monks, quacks, barbers, and bloodletters littered the medical landscape of Europe's Dark Ages, Islam strove to restore the intellect of the past and inject fresh inspiration."[6] Here, medieval Muslim physicians and Islam are conflated into a single, progressive ideal, in which "Islam" means not the global religion but the best and brightest individuals who lived in the medieval Middle East. The author uses a single image to represent Avicenna, a 1954 Iranian postage stamp (seen in the middle of the three stamps in Figure 1), as if this were a valid historical source or in any way an accurate representation of the historical physician, for whom no contemporary portrait survives.

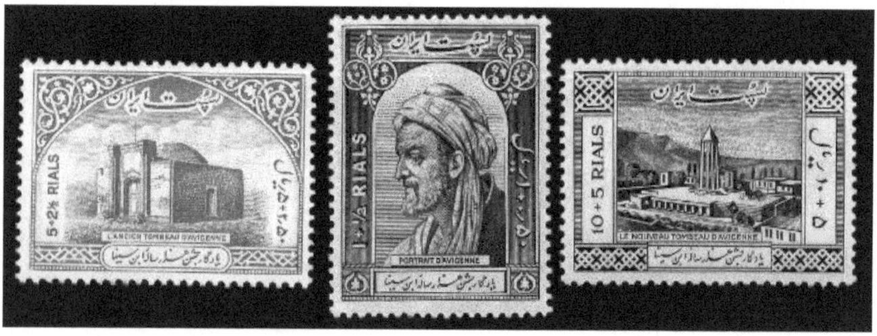

Fig. 1. A series of three postage stamps issued by the nation of Iran in 1954 showing (from left to right) Avicenna's medieval mausoleum, demolished in the 1940s; a modern portrait of Avicenna; and the new mausoleum of Avicenna, completed in 1954. Image courtesy of the Wellcome Collection, Creative Commons Attribution (CC BY 4.0).

This postage stamp, to which I will return, is only one of many examples of how Avicenna has been appropriated in modern contexts. These appropriations are as diverse as the minting of a commemorative medal by UNESCO in 1980 to honor the millennium of Avicenna's

[6] S.Y. Tan, "Medicine in Stamps. Avicenna (980-1037): Prince of Physicians," *Singapore Medical Journal* 43:9 (2002), 445-446, at 445.

birth; the 2009 donation and construction by the Islamic Republic of Iran of the "Scholars Pavilion" (or "Chartagi") at the United Nations offices in Vienna, which features statues of the Persian scholars Al-Biruni, Omar Khayyam, Al-Razi, and Avicenna; a chain of pharmacies in the United Kingdom called "Avicenna" and their website at www.avicenna.org; the portrayal of Avicenna as a main character in Noah Gordon's 1986 novel *The Physician*, as well as in the 2013 feature film based on that novel, starring Sir Ben Kingsley as Avicenna; or the character "Avicenna, Mercenary Doctor," in the miniature wargame *Corvus Belli: Infinity*, in which Avicenna is no longer a male, medieval physician, but a female-presenting rogue AI cyborg medic.

What these examples have in common is that they all depend on a deep cultural memory of Avicenna's expertise in medicine, a memory with roots in both the European and Islamicate Middle Ages. As the United Nations Scholars Pavilion makes clear, Avicenna can also serve as a symbol of peace and cooperation between contemporary Europe and Islamic nations, like Iran, because of their shared devotion to the Persian physician. There are likely thousands of different representations of Avicenna in modern culture that could be explored for understanding medical medievalism and Islamic medievalism, but for the purpose of this essay, I discuss the role of Avicenna, Prince of Physicians, in political medievalism, that is, the appropriation of medieval imagery and ideas in the expression of national identities and international relations.[7] I focus on the manipulation of Avicenna's image as a brilliant and trendsetting medieval physician through public media and propaganda in the twentieth century such as postage stamps, currency, and national monuments.[8]

---

[7] Political medievalism is an important subset of the field of medievalism. See *e.g.*, Bruce Holsinger, *Neomedievalism, Neoconservatism, and the War on Terror* (Chicago, 2007); Bruce Holsinger, "Medievalization Theory: From Tocqueville to the Cold War," *American Literary History* 22:4 (2010), 893-912; Daniel Wollenberg, *Medieval Imagery in Today's Politics* (Arc Humanities Press, 2018); Andrew B.R. Elliott, *Medievalism, Politics and Mass Media: Appropriating the Middle Ages in the Twenty-first Century* (Cambridge: D.S. Brewer, 2017).

[8] One of the most complete repositories of images of Avicenna postage stamps, without which this essay could not have been written, is maintained by Jeff Miller, a retired mathematics teachers in Florida, at "Jeff Miller's postage stamps," https://mathshistory.st-andrews.ac.uk/Miller/stamps/, with a page on just Avicenna at https://mathshistory.st-andrews.ac.uk/Miller/Store/avicenna.html, accessed May 30, 2022.

I. Avicenna and Orientalism

Avicenna's *Canon of Medicine* was a central fixture of medical education in Europe and European colonies for half a millennium, between the thirteenth and the eighteenth centuries. During that period, the name "Avicenna" was nearly synonymous with "medical education," and he was invoked along with Hippocrates and Galen in a trinity of learned medicine. The popularity of the *Canon* persisted or even increased in the age of print, as witnessed by the sixteen different editions of the work printed in Europe during the last decades of the fifteenth century and more than twenty editions throughout the sixteenth.[9] Not only was the work printed, but it was also taught and read closely at this time. As Nancy Siraisi has demonstrated, the *Canon* retained its authority in medical debates throughout the Early Modern period.[10] Writing a commentary on passages of the *Canon* became as much a rite of passage for educated physicians as writing a biblical commentary was for a theologian. It is through this learned medical tradition that Avicenna became an intellectual hero as much for the West as for the Middle East.

Yet over the course of the eighteenth and nineteenth centuries, Western medicine was revolutionized in terms of practice and its theoretical foundations. With the widespread acceptance of germ theory and biomedical approaches to diagnosis and treatment, modern physicians jettisoned almost all the ancient and medieval texts that had once defined their field, including the *Canon of Medicine*. Within just a few generations in the nineteenth century, Avicenna's importance to medicine was forgotten in the West and he became little more than one of many historical figures in an exoticized Middle East. The touchstones for his memory became not his most famous medical text, but his poetry and his tomb in Hamadan, Persia. Avicenna is remarkable among medieval physicians for having a well-marked tomb, which has served as a site of devotion and tourism for centuries. By the nineteenth century, however, the medieval building was in serious disrepair. The tomb was restored in 1877 by Negar Khanum, the granddaughter of the ruling

[9] Soheil M. Afnan, *Avicenna: His Life and Works* (George Allen & Unwin, 1958), 205.

[10] Nancy Siraisi, *Avicenna in Renaissance Italy: The Canon and Medical Teaching in Italian Universities after 1500* (Princeton University Press, 1987); Nancy Siraisi, "Avicenna and the Teaching of Practical Medicine," in *Medicine and the Italian Universities 1250-1600* (Leiden: Brill, 2001), 63-78.

Qajar shah, but the Qajars do not seem to have planned for long-term maintenance of the structure.[11]

A popular history and travel guide from 1906, *Persia Past and Present*, includes Avicenna's tomb as one of the must-sees of Persia, along with a brief and florid biography of Avicenna himself. The author, A.V. Williams Jackson, a professor of Indo-Iranian languages at Columbia University, validates the importance of Avicenna for his American readers by reference to Chaucer's *Pardoner's Tale*, which mentions the *Canon*. But even though Jackson acknowledges Avicenna's influence on medicine in both East and West, the real importance for him (and apparently for his American readers at that time) is Avicenna's mystic poetry, which is said to rival that of the *Rubaiyat* of Omar Khayyam (1048-1131).[12] The *Rubaiyat*, as translated into English in 1859, became one of the most popular works of later nineteenth- and early-twentieth-century Orientalism. Professor Jackson was a key figure in this movement, as his Persian history is divided not, for example, into the ancient, Islamic, and modern empires of Persia/Iran, but rather into two periods of Persian literature: pre- and post-Omar Khayyam. Jackson takes his readers on a timeless journey through the "poetical shrines" around Hamadan, which include the ancient stone lions of Ecbatana, one of the many supposed tombs of Alexander the Great, and the crumbling tomb of Avicenna.

The fact that Avicenna's tomb was falling apart did not seem to bother Jackson, for whom its dilapidated state only confirmed his view of Persia as an ancient land of poetry. But another North American contemporary of Jackson took a different view on the tomb. This was Sir William Osler, one of the most important figures in modern medicine, renowned as a diagnostician and medical author, professor of medicine at McGill University, co-founder of the Johns Hopkins Hospital in Baltimore and of the Medical Library Association of North America. He was also an active historian of medicine and helped found the History of Medicine Society as part of the Royal Society of Medicine in London. His education and interests led him to a greater appreciation of medieval

[11] Talinn Grigor, *Building Iran: Modernism, Architecture, and National Heritage under the Pahlavi Monarchs* (New York: Periscope Publishing, 2009), 114.

[12] A. V. Williams Jackson, *Persia Past and Present: A Book of Travel and Research* (Macmillan, 1906), 165-167. Available online at https://archive.org/details/persiapastpresen00jackuoft.

medicine, Avicenna especially, than was common in the later nineteenth century. Osler's positive attitude toward Avicenna is also mirrored in the inclusion of Avicenna among the gallery of medical authorities in the original reading room of the Wellcome Library for the history of medicine in London (finished in 1949 but reflecting the ideas of its founder Henry Wellcome, 1853-1936, another American immigrant to England). Avicenna is one of the few non-Western and premodern figures included there among the greats of medical history. Osler saw himself as the heir of Avicenna, as he also wrote a highly influential medical textbook, *The Principles and Practice of Medicine*, which, like the *Canon of Medicine*, was widely translated, reprinted, and read long after its author's death. Osler praised the *Canon* as "the most famous medical text-book ever written," and this attitude likely inspired his campaign to restore both Avicenna's reputation in the West and his tomb in Persia.[13]

Osler viewed the sad state of Avicenna's tomb as an insult to the long history of medicine, an insult that could be remedied only by Western outsiders, with the approval of the Persian government under the Qajar shahs, now reduced to pawns between the British and Russian Empires and encroaching French and American spheres of influence. At a 1914 meeting of the Historical Section of the Royal Society of Medicine, Osler proposed a "Suggested Scheme for the Restoration of the Tomb of Avicenna."[14] This announcement came after many months of letters between Osler and his Persian correspondent Dr Mohammed Sa'eed, a Christian Kurd living in Tehran, who supplied him with manuscripts of

---

[13] William Osler, *The Evolution of Modern Medicine: A Series of Lecture Delivered at Yale University on the Silliman Foundation in April, 1913* (Yale University Press, 1921), 99-100.

[14] William Osler, "Suggested Scheme for the Restoration of the Tomb of Avicenna," *Proceedings of the Royal Society of Medicine* 7 (Sect Hist Med) 1914, 280: "SIR WILLIAM OSLER called attention to the need for restoring the tomb of Avicenna. He stated that the sarcophagus still exists and that from time to time the tomb itself had been repaired. The present cost of repair and the expense of keeping a watchman would be from £500 to £600, a sum which might perhaps be raised without much difficulty by the combined action of the Société Française d'Histoire de Médécine with the Royal Society of Medicine, these two societies being especially named because they represented the two European nations most interested in the state of medicine in Mohammedan countries. He suggested that the Persian Government should be first approached and, if a favourable reply were received, that a subscription list should afterwards be opened." https://journals.sagepub.com/doi/pdf/10.1177/00359157140 0701618.

Avicenna's works as well as photographs and descriptions of the tomb.[15] Sa'eed was sympathetic to Osler's plan, at one point complaining that the tomb was now inhabited by wandering Dervishes whose opium and hashish smoke had blackened the building's interior and dome.[16] Osler estimated that the cost of repairing the sarcophagus and the building, as well as hiring a watchman on a permanent basis, would come to between 500 and 600 British pounds.

Later in the summer of 1914, the *British Medical Journal* reported on Osler's plan with approval but echoed the orientalist attitude of Prof. Jackson. The anonymous author imposes a timelessness on Avicenna's homeland, tying together Avicenna's dramatic life and the sad state of his tomb in the early twentieth century, which is blamed on the instability of the Persian Empire itself: "The sea of Persian politics has always been particularly stormy," claims the author.[17] It is hardly a coincidence that both Jackson's travel guide and Osler's campaign take place against the background of the establishment of the first Middle East oil refineries in Persia by the British, Russian, French, and Americans. Persia had quickly become important to the Western powers, who were dedicated to keeping the Persian Empire simultaneously weak and interesting, which could feed the West's growing demand for both oil and tourist destinations.[18]

There is no indication that any monies were collected for the tomb restoration project, as the Great War broke out in Autumn 1914 and Persia was drawn violently into the war, despite declaring neutrality. In fact, in a 1916 letter to Osler, Dr. Sa'eed describes the devastation of the so-called Persian campaign between the Ottomans and the British, which forced his family to flee Hamadan.[19] Osler himself was also struck

[15] Anand Date, "Sir William Osler's Arab and other Middle Eastern contacts," *The Ulster Medical journal* 60:1 (1991), 120-128. For more on Sa'eed, see Jay M. Rasooli and Cady H. Allen, *The Life Story of Dr. Sa'eed of Iran: Kurdish Physician to Princes and Peasants, Nobles and Nomads* (William Carey Library, 1983, reprint of 1958 Second Edition).

[16] Date, "Sir William Osler's Arab…", 127.

[17] "The Tomb of Avicenna", *British Medical Journal* July 25, 1914. https://profiles.nlm.nih.gov/spotlight/gf/catalog/nlm:nlmuid-101743406X258-doc.

[18] See Ervand Abrahamian, *A History of Modern Iran* (Cambridge University Press, 2008), 34-41, on oil treaties and Western intrusions into Qajar Persia in the 1890s-1920s.

[19] Letter from M. Sa'eed to William Osler, October 19, 1916. William Osler Letter Index, McGill Library, CUS417/39.80, https://osler-letters.library.mcgill.ca/record/ cus417-3980.

terribly by the war, losing his only son, Edward Revere Osler, to battlefield injuries in Belgium in 1917. Two years later we find Sa'eed back in relative safety, continuing his correspondence with Osler. In 1919, Osler attempted, with Sa'eed's assistance on the ground in Persia, to restart the campaign to rebuild Avicenna's tomb, but this attempt foundered with Osler's death in December of that year.

II. Avicenna and Nationalism in Pahlavi Iran

The care of Avicenna's tomb and the promotion of his memory gained dramatic and successful support under the new Pahlavi dynasty of Iran, which was eager to remove the maintenance of their own history from Western imperialists and keep it in Persian hands. The modern Imperial State of Iran was formed out of the chaos left in Central Asia after World War I and influenced by the contemporary Bolshevik Revolution in Russia and dissolution of the Ottoman Empire.[20] The Pahlavi shahs, taking their name from the ancient Pahlavi language of Persia, established in 1925 the last monarchy in Iranian history, which lasted until their overthrow in the Revolution of 1979. The first Pahlavi ruler, Reza Shah (formerly General Reza Khan under the Qajars), ushered in an era of modernization, centralization, and secularization of Iranian society, closely following the model of his contemporary Kemal Atatürk in the new Republic of Turkey. It was Reza Shah who asked the world, in 1934, to start referring to his nation as "Iran" rather than "Persia,"[21] at the same time as his government was promoting Iran's glorious Persian past.[22]

Like many twentieth-century states, Pahlavi Iran was highly nationalistic and spent vast sums of money to promote figures from their

---

[20] Mohsen M. Milani, *The Making of Iran's Islamic Revolution: From Monarchy to Islamic Republic.* Second Edition (Westview Press, 1994), 31.

[21] Ervand Abrahamian, *Iran Between Two Revolutions* (Princeton University Press, 1982), 86-87.

[22] "Two features of Reza Shah's...efforts for the modernization of Iran were related to the architectural construction of the period. One was his reference to the country's ancient history, which inspire the present generation to achieve new glories. The other was his desire to adopt aspects of Western civilization in such a fashion that Iran would become equal to the West." D.N. Wilber, "Architecture VII. Pahlavi, before World War II," *Encyclopædia Iranica* II/4, pp 349-351; available online at https://iranicaonline.org/articles/architecture-vii, accessed 16 October 2021.

past to inspire Iranian pride, while also demonstrating the nation's industrial capabilities and modern infrastructure. This was done in a markedly Western fashion, through the printing of new currency and postage stamps along with the construction of modern buildings in French and American style to replace older Persian structures. Both the modern construction and the Persian past are celebrated on stamps issued by Iran under Reza Shah in the 1930s. These include images of newly constructed roads, cement factories, hospitals, airports, and gunboats of modern Iran, alongside other stamps showing the ruins, art, and rulers of ancient Persepolis.[23]

Much of Iran's historical propaganda focused on their pagan past rather than on figures or events of the medieval Islamic era. A key exception is Avicenna, whom the Pahlavis considered to be a particularly useful figure to promote from Iran's past, as his achievements appealed to modern and Western sensibilities, especially among physicians like William Osler and Henry Wellcome. According to the architectural historian Talinn Grigor, Avicenna's importance "for the Pahlavi state…rested on his scientific contributions in medicine and philosophy, not necessarily as a Muslim scholar but as an Iranian."[24] The idea that Avicenna could be used to promote both education and Iranian identity is also made clear in the renaming of an American boys' school in the city of Rasht as the "Avicenna School."[25]

The promotion of Persian cultural heritage through the construction of new buildings and monuments was made possible with significant Western involvement, especially from English and French architects and archaeologists.[26] This involvement came primarily through the Society for the National Heritage of Iran (SNH), a panel of 15 scholars, Western and Iranian, that was formed in 1922 to oversee archaeological sites, promote the achievements of pre-Islamic Persian empires, and to

[23] Reproductions of these stamps can be seen in Abrahamian, *Iran Between Two Revolutions*, 78-81.

[24] Grigor, *Building Iran*, 114.

[25] Rudi Matthee, "Transforming dangerous nomads into useful artisans, technicians, agriculturalists: education in the Reza Shah period," in *The Making of Modern Iran: State and Society under Riza Shah, 1921-1941*, ed. Stephanie Cronin (Routledge, 2003), 123-145, at 141.

[26] Saha Mahdizadeh and Reyhaneh Sadat Shojaei, "The involvement of Western Orientalists in cultural heritage affairs during the Pahlavi Era, Iran (1925-1979)," *Journal of Architectural Conservation* 24:3 (2018), 169-184.

maintain or build various monuments dedicated to Persian and Islamic heroes.[27] The first of these was a monumental new mausoleum for the Persian epic poet, Ferdowsi (940-1025 CE), built in the early 1930s in Tus, Iran. The SNH oversaw the construction of some forty different mausoleums in their half century of activity, apart from numerous other museums, libraries, and preservation projects.[28] Next to Ferdowsi, one of the most important Persian national heroes was Avicenna, whose image and mortal remains played a major role in Iranian nationalism. He became for the Pahlavi dynasty and the SNH the central mascot for promoting Persian contributions to world culture. Paradoxically, the Pahlavis planned to use Avicenna "to divorce Iran from its Islamic past,"[29] because he died and was buried in Hamadan, one of the most ancient of Iran's pre-Islamic cities. This agenda began with Reza Shah, whose government proposed in 1937 to rebuild Avicenna's tomb, ostensibly to celebrate the 900th anniversary of his death. These plans were delayed first by the temporary closure of the SNH in 1938,[30] then by the outbreak of World War II, and finally by internal political turmoil in Iran, leading to Reza's forced abdication in 1941 at the hands of occupying Allied forces.

Reza's son, Mohammed Reza Shah, replaced him and eventually succeeded, where his father's government had not, in promoting Avicenna through architecture and propaganda. After the end of World War II Iran, with American and British aid, began to rebuild in earnest, which included completing a new tomb for Avicenna. The SNH was reformed in 1944 and hired a radical, young, Beaux-Arts trained Iranian architect, Hooshang Seyhoun (1920-2014), to design a monumental mausoleum. The tower of the new mausoleum, which looms over Avicenna's actual tomb in the gardens below, is Seyhoun's modernist take on a famous Persian medieval structure erected during Avicenna's lifetime: a cylindrical tomb tower for the Ziyarid shah Qābūs (d. 1012), built around the year 1006 CE. Once again, political turmoil in the period 1951-1953 slowed construction, but the demolition of the old tomb and construction of the new were completed by 1954.

---

[27] Mahdizadeh and Shojaei, "The involvement," 171.

[28] Talinn Grigor, "Recultivating 'Good Taste': The Early Pahlavi Modernists and Their Society for National Heritage," *Iranian Studies* 37:1 (2004), 17-29.

[29] Grigor, *Building Iran*, 117.

[30] Mahdizadeh and Shojaei, 175.

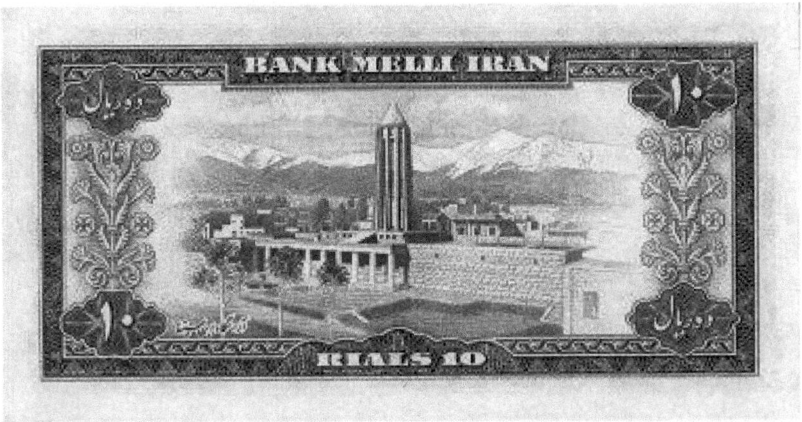

Fig. 2. The reverse of a 1954 10-rial banknote from Iran, showing the newly constructed mausoleum complex for Avicenna in Hamadan, Iran. Image courtesy of Wikimedia Commons, Creative Commons license.

Avicenna, in a portrait that has come to define popular representations of him to this day, his old tomb, and the new tomb were depicted in a series of Iranian stamps issued in 1954 (see Fig. 1). The message was clear: the old empire of Persia, a crumbling edifice like Avicenna's old tomb, was to be replaced by the twentieth-century nation of Iran, sleek and modern, well-maintained, and open to all, just like Avicenna's new mausoleum. This achievement was also celebrated on a 10-rial banknote of 1954 in which Mohammed Reza Shah's historical-political aspirations were made clear. The binary symbolism of the postage stamps, with old giving way to new, is replaced by a more complex historical hermeneutic. The obverse of the banknote shows Mohammed Reza Shah in profile, looking towards the ruined pillars of Persepolis. The reverse (see Figure 2) shows Avicenna's new mausoleum complex, surrounded by gardens and set against the background of the snow-capped Zagros Mountains. Through the imagery of this banknote, Mohammed Reza Shah's reign is represented as the third great era of Iran, following those of the ancient Persian Empire (represented by Persepolis) and medieval Islamic Persia (represented by Avicenna). But Avicenna's new tomb also serves as a bridge between the second and third eras of Persian history, as one of Persia's greatest medieval figures is reburied in one of Iran's most prominent modern buildings.

Half a century later, in 2004, Avicenna and his modern mausoleum were celebrated once again in Iranian postage. This might not seem a surprising commemoration on the fiftieth anniversary of this important monument, but the current Islamic Republic of Iran was founded through an explicit and violent rejection of the Pahlavi dynasty and its Western-inspired secularism. In 1979, the new spiritual leader of Iran, the Ayatollah Khomeini, called for the abolition or destruction of cultural elements that had been embraced by the Pahlavis, most obviously the mausoleum of the first Pahlavi ruler, Reza Shah, which had been built by his son and modelled after the new mausoleum of Ferdowsi. The revolutionaries destroyed this and other buildings in the Iranian Revolution of 1979-1980. At the time, it was feared that Avicenna's mausoleum would also be targeted by the revolutionaries, as it was a favorite site of the Pahlavis and a key image in their propaganda, as we have seen. But the new supreme ruler, the Ayatollah Khomeini, admired Avicenna and ordered that his mausoleum and public square be spared.

III. Avicenna: Medical Hero for Secular and Islamic Iran

In fact, one of the only continuities between Pahlavi Iran and the Islamic Republic of the Ayatollahs is their shared devotion to Avicenna. If we look at the other Iranian stamps featuring Avicenna in the last half century, it can be hard to distinguish any change in attitude to the medieval physician between the two dramatically different governments. Whereas the focus of the 1954 postal series was the replacement of Avicenna's mausoleum, most of the later Iranian stamps featuring Avicenna place him in a more explicitly medical context. On stamps from 1962 to 2013, Avicenna is named or depicted as a physician, portrayed with other important figures in the history of medicine, and used to celebrate the convening of international medical conferences and seminars in Iran.

Yet there are some differences between the Avicenna stamps of the Pahlavis and those of the Islamic Republic that point to changing conceptions of Avicenna's place in Iranian ideology. A Pahlavi stamp of 1962 situates Avicenna in a teleological history from the ancient Greeks to modern biomedicine. He is shown facing Hippocrates, the father of Western medicine, with the Rod of Asclepius between them. Their equal size and locked gaze reinforce an idea that was already centuries old in both Western and Islamicate medical traditions: Avicenna should be regarded on an equal footing with Hippocrates as a premodern medical authority, as their writings equally shaped the humoralism that continued to dominate European and Islamic medical practice into the modern era. These two figures appear again on a 1974 stamp, lending that joint authority to a medical conference held in Isfahan and sponsored by the *Journées médicales du Proche et du Moyen-Orient*, a French-language medical journal published in Lebanon.

In the wake of the Iranian Revolution, however, Avicenna was appropriated in a new way to represent the overt religious ideology of the new Islamic Republic. One of the first stamps of the new Iran, issued in 1980, celebrates the start of the fifteenth century of the Islamic calendar, 1400 lunar years since the *Hijra* of Muhammad in 622 CE.[31] The influence of the Prophet is represented through some of the most important medieval Muslim philosophers: Al-Farabi, Al-Biruni, and Ibn Sina (see Figure 3).

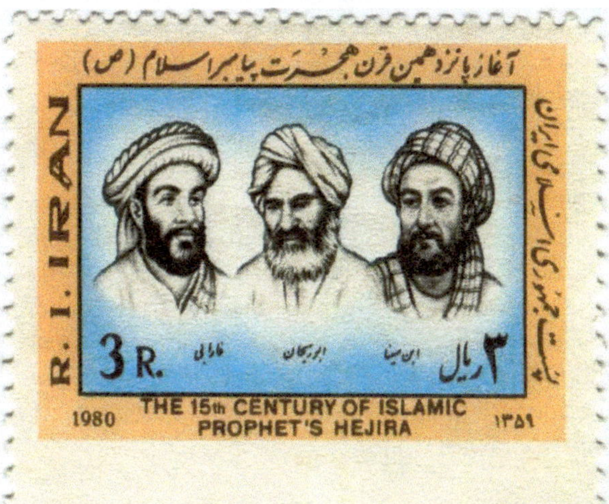

Fig. 3. 1980 postage stamp issued by the Islamic Republic of Iran, showing Al-Farabi, Al-Biruni, and Ibn Sina to celebrate the fifteenth century of the Islamic calendar. Image courtesy of Wikimedia Commons, Public Domain.

[31] My thanks to Professor Nahyan Fancy of DePauw University for discussing this stamp with me.

To those familiar with the Avicenna stamps issued by the government of Pahlavi Iran, the message couldn't be clearer: Avicenna is no longer part of the Western, secular tradition of Hippocrates and French-language medical conferences but should be revered within a specifically Islamic tradition as a spiritual and intellectual descendant of Muhammad. The focus of the postage stamp is not medicine, like most stamps with Avicenna, but rather the Islamic calendar and the *hijra* of Muhammad.

Despite the firm religious message of this stamp and its redefinition of Avicenna as firstly a Muslim philosopher, the postal service of the Islamic Republic of Iran has since returned to the Pahlavi model of representing Avicenna as a physician and linking him visually with important figures from the Western medical tradition. This can be seen in a 1989 stamp celebrating the World Philatelic Exposition in Paris, showing Louis Pasteur and Avicenna together, thereby re-establishing Avicenna's place in Western medicine and suggesting that Pasteur's achievements in microbiology, medical chemistry, and germ theory are dependent in some way on the genius of Avicenna. This anachronistic claim has been made more explicitly in the age of COVID-19, as multiple popular websites from the Near and Middle East state that it was Avicenna who discovered that germs caused disease, eight centuries before the modern Europeans Robert Koch and Pasteur.[32] These claims are based on a misunderstanding or exaggeration of Avicenna's discussion of contagion and quarantine found in his *Canon of Medicine*. Recently, in 2013, Iran celebrated the millennium of this book's completion with another stamp. Unlike the stamps and other propaganda of the Pahlavi era, which sought to disassociate Avicenna from the Islamic Middle Ages, the Islamic theocracy of Iran is seeking to do the opposite: the stamp defines Avicenna and his *Canon* as part of "Islam & Iran's Culture & Civilization."

[32] Ufuk Necat Tasci, "How Ibn Sina's work became a guiding light for scientists facing contagion," *TRT World* 15 April 2020, https://www.trtworld.com/magazine/how-ibn-sina-s-work-became-a-guiding-light-for-scientists-facing-contagions-35440, accessed 3 Nov 2021; K.N. Deya, "The enduring legacy of Ibn Sina's work on contagions," *The Business Standard* 26 April 2020, https://www.tbsnews.net/panorama/enduring-legacy-ibn-sinas-work-contagions-73987, accessed 3 Nov 2021.

IV. Postal Celebrations of Avicenna outside of Iran

After the Pahlavi government completed its dramatic push to promote Avicenna in architecture, sculpture, postage, and currency, the rest of the world was quick to follow suit. It became fashionable for other nations, both Islamic and non-Islamic, to put Avicenna on their own postage stamps, particularly in the 1950s through 1980s.[33] It is not surprising to see Avicenna celebrated on stamps from Dubai, Egypt, Tajikistan, and from Iran, of course, as they are predominantly Islamic nations, and all consider Avicenna part of their cultural and religious heritage. For example, a 1980 stamp from Kuwait makes explicit the idea that Avicenna belongs to all Arab Muslims, stating in English and Arabic, "One Thousandth Birthday of Ibn Sina, Philosopher and Physician of the Islamic Arab State".

But while Iran and other Islamic nations were issuing Avicenna stamps, European nations, especially those of the Communist Eastern Bloc (such as the USSR, East Germany, Poland, and Hungary), also celebrated Avicenna in postage. This is a curious development, as few nations promote the medieval heroes of other nations on their postage. Since the printing of the so-called "Penny Black" in 1840 featuring the new Queen Victoria – considered the world's first modern postage stamp – stamps have always delivered political messages, whether through the overt portrayal of a nation's monarch or head of state, or through subtler promotions of national identity and public interest.[34] This tendency was even stronger during the Cold War in the second half of the twentieth century, when the United States and other global powers used stamps as propaganda to promote national pride and express simplified, pictorial versions of foreign policy.[35] It is against this background that we should

[33] Ahmadreza Afshar, "Honoring Avicenna, the Great Persian Physician on the World's Postage Stamps," *Archives of Iranian Medicine* 13:5 (2010), 447-453. There is also a more recent catalogue of Avicenna stamps online by Jeff Miller, "Images of Mathematicians on Postage Stamps," s.v. "Avicenna," https://mathshistory.st-andrews.ac.uk/Miller/stamps/, accessed October 25, 2021.

[34] Stanley D. Brunn, "Stamps as messengers of political transition," *Geographical Review* 101:1 (2011), 19-36.

[35] Matin Modarressi, "Philatelic Propaganda: U.S. Postage Stamps during the Cold War," *Journal of Cold War Studies* 19:3 (2017), 196-201. Online at https://direct.mit.edu/jcws/article/19/3/196/13676/Philatelic-Propaganda-U-S-Postage-Stamps-during#FN12.

understand the celebrations of Avicenna on stamps in nations well outside of Iran.

Iran, as a wealthy, militarized, and oil-rich nation in central Asia, was a key player in the Cold War and a target for American and Soviet influence. In the wake of World War II, Iran nearly entered the sphere of the Communist Bloc through the rise of the National Front socialist party and the socialist policies of Prime Minister Mosaddegh (1882-1967, also transliterated "Mosaddeq"), serving 1951-53, who sought to nationalize the oil industry, which was controlled primarily by the Anglo-Persian Oil Company, now British Petroleum. This move clearly allied Iran with the interests of the Soviet Union and other communist states. To prevent this potential alliance from ever coming to fruition, the US CIA and British MI6 engineered a military *coup d'état* to overthrow and arrest Mosaddegh, abolish socialism in Iran, and renew the flow of oil to Western nations. For the following 26 years, the United States supported the near absolute monarchy of Shah Mohammed Reza Pahlavi, whose government also controlled most forms of public art and national representation.[36] This was a huge loss to the Soviet Union. The numerous Avicenna stamps printed there and in the Eastern Bloc must be understood in this context. It was a "soft power" move in the Cold War, a means of demonstrating past and potential future Soviet support for Iran, as represented through their celebration of Iran's greatest medieval hero, Avicenna.

Even though the Soviets lost most of their direct influence over Iran after the fall of Mosaddegh, they could continue to claim and promote Avicenna in those other Persianate nations that remained in the USSR or under the influence of the Communist Bloc. These included the Tajik, Uzbek, and Turkmen Soviet Socialist Republics, now the independent nations (since 1991) of Tajikistan, Uzbekistan, and Turkmenistan. As mentioned above, the state medical university of Tajikistan is named after Avicenna, as is the associated International Ibn Sina Hospital. Uzbekistan also proudly claims Avicenna as a native son, as he was born in the Uzbek city of Bukhara.

In some philatelic traditions, Avicenna is represented not just as a physician but as one of a pantheon of historical thinkers, primarily from Western history, suggesting that he should be remembered more as an

[36] Grigor, *Building Iran*, 115.

honorary member of the Western tradition than as a Muslim philosopher-physician belonging specifically to Persian culture. In fact, some of these postal series make little sense in terms of their political or religious message. For example, in 1952, East Germany (the German Democratic Republic) issued one of the earliest stamps showing Avicenna, even before the Iranian stamp in Figure 1. He is included in a set of stamps showing artists and novelists, simply known as the "Famous Men" series, alongside Leonardo Da Vinci, Victor Hugo, and Nikolai Gogol. Equally curious is the selection of famous men for a series of stamps printed in Dubai in 1971: Albrecht Dürer, Isaac Newton, Avicenna, and Voltaire. This grouping problematizes the idea I mentioned before that it is unsurprising for an Islamic state to represent Avicenna on a stamp. What are we to make of his presence among this group of distinctly radical European artists and philosophers? What do the satire and deism of Voltaire have to do with the theology and natural philosophy of Avicenna?

These questions resist easy answers. But what these groups of stamps show us is that in the second half of the twentieth century Avicenna had become a stock figure for the "great thinker of the past", whose name and stereotyped image (in profile with turban, beard, and piercing gaze) various national post offices assumed the public would recognize. Such is also the case with the most recent example of an Avicenna stamp, found on a block of four stamps from the African Republic of Chad, issued in 2015. Avicenna is remembered in this postage set not so much as a physician but as a philosopher as he is grouped in the company of Confucius, Descartes, and Plato. At least in this African context, Avicenna is understood as part of a comprehensive Eurasian tradition of premodern philosophy, and not necessarily just within European history.

An alternate history (or perhaps a local history) of Western medicine is represented on a series of stamps from Hungary, issued in 1987. As noted before, this Hungarian stamp of Avicenna can be understood as part of recurring attempts by the Communist Bloc to claim Avicenna as their own. But this Avicenna stamp can also be seen as part of a specifically Hungarian nationalism celebrating the greatest Hungarian physician, Ignaz Semmelweis. Semmelweis is the most recent of five physicians depicted, after Hippocrates, Avicenna, Ambroise Paré, and William Harvey. Semmelweis's position on the highest-valued stamp in this series emphasizes him as the culmination of over two millennia of medical innovation and discovery in a scientific medical tradition beginning with Hippocrates and shared equally by Western and Middle Eastern cultures. In this case, Avicenna is represented as a physician whose time has passed, but who nonetheless should be celebrated for his contributions to the long history of medicine.

V. Avicenna in Action as Teacher and Healer

What is striking about all the stamps mentioned so far is that Avicenna is not depicted as a physician, although the title is sometimes used, or his position as a healer is made clear through his appearance alongside other physicians like Hippocrates or Pasteur. The Kuwaiti stamp described Avicenna as a physician and the Egyptian stamp used Avicenna to mark the twentieth anniversary of the World Health Organization, but Avicenna is otherwise presented without any clearly medical attributes. Granted, the various national postal authorities that issued these stamps probably assumed that the people who were going to use them had at least a superficial understanding of Avicenna as a great medieval physician.

Yet there were printed other stamps that more clearly depict Avicenna as a physician. These stamps demonstrate a blending of "medical medievalism" and "political medievalism," that is, modern representations of a medieval physician that were designed, printed, and certified by official government services. These stamps show Avicenna in action, working as a practical healer, experimental scientist, revered teacher, and revolutionary author. More than the simple portrait stamps described before, these stamps are designed to teach a quick lesson about who Avicenna was, what he did, and how he should be remembered today. The positive lessons learned about Avicenna are intended to reflect positively on the nations that issued these stamps and the people that used them as postage.

The oldest Avicenna stamp, appearing even before those of Iran and East Germany, was issued by Lebanon in 1948 to celebrate the meeting of UNESCO in Beirut. Avicenna is shown as an alchemist, or even as a medical chemist, with the suggestion that he was preparing his own pharmaceuticals. Avicenna is an excellent mascot for UNESCO, as he could reasonably be used to represent the educational, scientific, and cultural goals of the organization. This stamp is one of the first of many examples of Avicenna transformed from a medieval Persian physician, in the service of warring emirs, into an eirenic symbol of international cooperation. Avicenna is praised in this and other stamps not for his writing of the *Canon* and other books but for his mastery of medicines and medical technology. A stamp from the African nation of Mali in 1980 shows Avicenna with a selection of medicinal herbs and surgical tools, copied from medieval manuscripts. Soon after, in 1982, the nation of Austria issued a stamp showing Avicenna inspecting a jar of urine, just as he recommended in many of his actual medical treatises. This stamp was issued specifically for the European Urology Congress, held in Vienna, and Avicenna is thereby celebrated as a medieval founder of a specific branch of medical science.

I have not had space in this essay to examine closely one of the most important modern representations of Avicenna, and one which has shaped popular understandings of him since the 1980s. This is the novel *The Physician* (1986) by the American author Noah Gordon (1926-2021). The book follows the adventures of an English healer named Rob Cole in the early eleventh century. Rob's many adventures take him to Persia, where he becomes a student of Avicenna ("Ibn Sina" in the book) by pretending to be a European Jew – an idea based on the anachronistic claim that medical establishments in Persia did not allow Christians. In Gordon's version of the Middle Ages, Avicenna is already known during his life as "the greatest physician in the world," even in backward and barbarous Christian England.[37] Gordon portrays Avicenna as a kindly and brilliant, yet sometimes impatient and heavy-handed teacher. He is also shown as a caring and curious practitioner who elevates Rob to his personal apprentice and the heir to all he knows in medicine. In this fashion, Rob supplants the role held by the real figure of al-Jūzjānī, Avicenna's amanuensis, with the implicit conclusion that Avicenna's medical genius will thus pass to the West through this fictional Englishman. Had he lived long enough to read *The Physician*, Sir William Osler might have approved.

In Gordon's version of the history of medicine, Avicenna represents the genius of Islamic medicine, but a genius that Europe (represented by Rob) absorbs and rapidly surpasses. It is a tale of supersession and historical irony, in which Western readers are always aware that their medicine will eventually reign supreme, but not without significant help

[37] Noah Gordon, *The Physician* (Simon & Schuster, 1986), 164.

from the medical cultures of medieval Islam. It is no exaggeration to say that nearly every representation of Avicenna since the 1990s owes something to Noah Gordon's version of him. Even though the book sold poorly at first in the United States, it became an instant hit in Europe, selling millions of copies in multiple translations, especially in Spain and Germany. It was made into a big-budget movie in Germany in 2013 (*Der Medicus*, directed by Philipp Stölzl), starring Ben Kingsley as Avicenna, it was rewritten as a musical in 2016 (again produced by Stölzl), and it was remade as a miniseries on German television in 2022.

I have ended with this brief excursion into *The Physician* franchise because it clearly influenced the portrayal of Avicenna on my last examples of postage stamps. Portugal issued a pair of Avicenna stamps in 2013 to celebrate the millennium of the completion of Avicenna's *Canon*, just like the most recent Iranian stamp. But the knowledge and importance of the *Canon* are represented not with a simple portrait in profile, but with two scenes that look like stills from *The Physician*: Avicenna tenderly touches a young man's jaw, while his mother looks on, and an attendant hovers nearby in the darkness, holding a tray full of medicines and tools. In the other stamp, Avicenna is hard at work writing a book (the *Canon*, presumably) while holding a potentially medicinal plant in one hand. This image teaches us that Avicenna's medical knowledge came not (as historians of medicine tell us) from the rational synthesis of the writings of Hippocrates and Galen, but rather from his patient analysis of nature itself. He is meant to be seen as a forerunner of the best, modern physicians, at once both careful practitioner and learned natural scientist. These "medical medievalisms" do not tell us much about the real Avicenna, nor are they intended to. They instead serve as a window onto the ideals held by the government of present-day Portugal, just as all the other stamps, banknotes, and structures honoring Avicenna in the last century must be understood first as contemporary political statements.

MYSTERIES AND MEDICINES: MEDIEVAL MEDICAL PRACTITIONERS IN CRIME FICTION

Lucy C. Barnhouse*

Medieval medicine is frequently central to whodunits set in the Middle Ages, and has been so since the first examples of medieval crime fiction, appearing at the same time medieval medicine began to emerge from a long tradition of meliorism, in the 1970s. This essay examines why and how this is so, and the ways in which representations of medieval medicine and its practitioners have responded to the rapid growth and diversification of scholarly work on the subject. Previous studies of historical crime fiction have often focused on assessing the accuracy of the series under discussion, a model from which this essay attempts to break. This study draws on over fifty crime novels by over half a dozen authors. Alongside novels featuring medical practitioners as protagonists, I have included other examples of medieval crime fiction for purposes of comparison. Historical crime fiction is a recognized sub-genre, but I argue that medieval sleuths function differently from those solving mysteries in imperial Rome, Tudor England, or eighteenth-century Italy, not only because that rare Benedictine, Brother Cadfael, was a relatively early example of the historical sleuth, predating even William of Baskerville, the perceptive Franciscan of Umberto Eco's *The*

* Department of History, Arkansas State University.

Name of the Rose.[1] Medicine functions in medieval mysteries as a signifier of both knowledge and exoticism. These significations are more important to the genre than detailed evocations of medieval medical practice or ideas. The medical practice of detectives in medieval crime fiction reassures the reader that the protagonist's knowledge and methods are recognizably similar to those of modern sleuths, even as the representation of this practice is used to signal the otherness of the Middle Ages.

Historical crime fiction is used, to an unusual degree, to comment on medieval society, or that society as imagined.[2] This imagined society is almost invariably European.[3] Nearly all the series under discussion here are set in Europe; most, indeed, are set primarily in England. This Anglocentric bias also holds true across a larger sampling of medieval crime fiction made by Anne McKendry.[4] The almost sixty titles I am working with were published from 1977 to 2020, with the 1990s emerging as a particularly fruitful time for new series.[5] European exceptions to the English setting are Caroline Roe's series on Isaac of Girona, set in the Iberian Peninsula, and Indrek Hargla's Apothecary Melchior series, set in fifteenth-century Tallinn (modern Estonia.) Laury Silvers' ongoing Sufi Mysteries quartet features an amateur detective collaborating with the police in tenth-century Baghdad. The first novel in this quartet contains little discussion of medicine or medical practitioners despite the historical identity of Baghdad as an epicenter of medical learning. The second, in which a scholar is murdered at

[1] Ellis Peters, *A Morbid Taste For Bones* (New York, NY: Mysterious Press, 1994), originally published Macmillan London Limited 1977; Umberto Eco, *The Name of the Rose* (New York, NY: Harcourt Brace & Co., 1983), originally in Italian 1980. On historical crime fiction as a sub-genre, see Ray B. Browne and Lawrence A. Kreiser, eds., *The Detective as Historian: History and Art in Historical Crime Fiction* (Madison, WI: University of Wisconsin Press, 2013.)

[2] See Patricia W. Julius, "Margaret Frazer: Sister Frevisse and Medieval Mysteries," in *The Detective as Historian*, 122-132.

[3] See the introduction to this volume by Lucy Barnhouse and Winston Black for a fuller discussion of Eurocentrism in medievalism and medieval studies.

[4] Anne McKendry, *Medieval Crime Fiction: A Critical Overview* (Jefferson, NC: McFarland & Co., 2019), 241-44.

[5] Susanna Gregory, Candace Robb, and C.L. Grace all began medieval series with medical sleuths in the 1990s. The last of the Cadfael novels appeared in 1994.

Baghdad's Barmakid hospital, will be discussed below.[6] Neither Robert Van Gulik's Judge Dee mysteries, set in Tang China, nor I.J. Parker's Akitada series, set in Heian Japan, involve medicine, with their sleuths instead serving as government functionaries.[7]

One of the challenges for detectives in any historical mystery is the unravelling of mysteries without access to the technological apparatus of modern crime-solving. That this is arguably one of the charms for readers of the genre is true across time periods. But unlike their counterparts in other historical periods, medieval detectives are frequently also medical practitioners, and it is on this subset of sleuths that this essay focuses. Even if not skilled in medicine, medieval detectives generally rely on previously acquired professional expertise, *e.g.*, the legal training of Sister Fidelma (Peter Tremayne) or the background of Hugh Corbett (P.C. Doherty), Crowner John (Bernard Knight), and Simon Puttock (Michael Jecks) as legal functionaries. This emphasis on external expertise may be intended to make medieval detectives more plausible to readers. Alan T. Gaylord has referred to the existence of detectives in medieval settings as a "great big anomaly of medievalism," reliant on post-medieval literary tropes.[8] For Anne McKendry, the medieval detective is essentially "a modern interloper," inserted into a medieval landscape to interpret the past for contemporary readers. Thus, "the medieval detective can be disgusted by the offensive smells, rotten food, and appalling sewerage systems that probably would not have affected a 'local.'"[9] Notably, these signifiers of medieval strangeness are all linked to public health. While McKendry has analyzed these reliable background elements as attempts at authentic scene-

[6] Laury Silvers, *The Lover: A Sufi Mystery* (Kindle Direct Publishing, 2019); Silvers, *The Jealous: A Sufi Mystery* (Kindle Direct Publishing, 2020.)

[7] I.J. Parker, *The Rashomon Gate* (New York, NY: St. Martin's Press, 2002) and series. The Akitada mysteries are marketed as taking place in "ancient" Japan despite being set in the eleventh century, late in the Heian period. Robert Van Gulik, *The Lacquer Screen* (New York, NY: Charles Scribner & Sons, 1972); idem, *The Haunted Monastery and the Chinese Maze Murders* (New York, NY: Dover Press, 1977.)

[8] Alan T. Gaylord, "O Rare Ellis Peters: Two Rules for Medieval Murder," in *Studies in Medievalism XX: Defining Neomedievalism(s) II,* ed. Karl Fugelso (Woodbridge: Boydell and Brewer, 2011), 132.

[9] McKendry, *Medieval Crime Fiction*, 239-40.

setting, I read them, rather, as a durable trope of medical medievalism, representing the distance of the Middle Ages.[10]

The otherness of the Middle Ages is rendered explicit in a rhetorical question posed by Edwin Lindsay some thirty years ago in an essay for *Studies in Medievalism*: "What is the validity of a medieval detective?"[11] The question remains one without a single conclusive answer, though the number of novels containing medieval detectives has grown exponentially in the interim. More recent analysis has also suggested that the rational secularism of the detective story genre results in an insoluble paradox at the heart of medieval crime fiction.[12] Even in long-running series of novels, medieval society itself is often represented as a problem to be solved, or as the ultimate insoluble mystery. Medieval detectives are often presented as solving crime against the odds, eccentric – if not always rugged – individualists who are somehow set apart from the world around them. If an "endless circle of violence and misery and fear" is, according to Sherlock Holmes, that which crime-solving attempts to make sense of, and in some sense to resolve, it is also what characterizes many fictional versions of medieval Europe.[13] This image of the Middle Ages – as a place unusually prone to misery, violence, and fear – is arguably one element of what makes medical practitioners, whether infirmarers, physicians, or apothecaries, popular as medieval detectives.

Modern ideas about medicine and about the Middle Ages have often been at odds. Anne McKendry, in her analysis of medieval crime fiction, has argued that representations of medical practice "can challenge a modern reader's sensibilities and, at times, credulity," using a Caesarean section and an "unlikely" appendectomy as examples.[14] Similarly, Sarah

---

[10] These tropes have endured despite the increased attention to medieval public health in the past decade. See, for example, Carole Rawcliffe, *Urban Bodies: Communal Health in Late Medieval English Towns and Cities* (Woodbridge: The Boydell Press, 2013); Guy Geltner, "Public Health and the Pre-Modern City: A Research Agenda," *History Compass* 10:3 (2012), 231-45.

[11] Edwin Ernest Christian Blake Lindsay, "The Habit of Detection: The Medieval Monk as Detective in the Novels of Ellis Peters," in *Studies in Medievalism IV: Medievalism in England*, ed. Leslie J. Workman (Cambridge: D.S. Brewer, 1992), 276.

[12] McKendry, *Medieval Crime Fiction*, 90-91.

[13] Arthur Conan Doyle, "The Cardboard Box," in *The New Annotated Sherlock Holmes*, vol. 1, ed. Leslie S. Klinger (New York, NY: W.W. Norton, 2005), 448. The words are those of Holmes himself.

[14] McKendry, *Medieval Crime Fiction*, 75.

Ifft Decker and Abigail Agresta have commented on Brother Cadfael's remarkable success rate even with severely injured patients.[15] A medieval sleuth's medical practice gives them a claim to what modern readers perceive as enlightenment. C.L. Grace's Kathryn Swinbrooke, for instance, appears in a blurb as being "a Renaissance woman in a Middle Age world," and Cadfael himself has been described as belonging to both the twelfth and twentieth centuries.[16] In Ariana Franklin's *Mistress of the Art of Death*, the physician-practitioner's logic, reason, and trained inference appear as "rare skills in [a] credulous age."[17] But at their best, these medical sleuths can send another message about medieval Europe, asserting that compassion, wisdom, a sense of justice – and, yes, medical knowledge – were not more anomalous than those qualities are in our own societies, however differently they may be manifested. These abstract qualities are more reliably represented in medieval crime fiction than the concrete medical knowledge on which its protagonists ostensibly rely. This enables medieval medicine, as imagined, to accumulate its own tropes. The ways in which medical practice is depicted in historical crime novels have changed very little from Cadfael's first adventures outside the abbey walls, in 1978, to the latest efforts of his successors, such as Adelia Aguilar (Ariana Franklin) and Owen Archer (Candace Robb), in the first two decades of the twenty-first century. This is true even though the amount of scholarship on medieval medicine, and the subfields embraced by this scholarship, have expanded considerably. This stasis is linked, I argue, to the meanings of medieval medicine and medical practice in medieval crime fiction. In examining these meanings, I first discuss the ways in which sickness and disability are represented as an integral part of medieval societies in detective fiction. Secondly, I look at types of practitioners and their expertise; and finally, I turn to representations of *materia medica*, and of how medical knowledge was developed and communicated in medieval Europe. Throughout, I argue that representations of medical knowledge

[15] Sarah Ifft Decker and Abigail Agresta, "Cadfael," Media-eval Podcast August 24, 2019, https://soundcloud.com/user-834389367/cadfael, last accessed February 12, 2022.

[16] C.L. Grace, *A Maze of Murders* (New York, NY: St. Martin's Minotaur, 2003), jacket copy. Edward J. Rielly, "Ellis Peters: Brother Cadfael," in *The Detective as Historian,* 70. See Winston Black, "Avicenna, Prince of Physicians," in this volume, for further discussion of how medieval medical practitioners have been conceptualized.

[17] Ariana Franklin, *Mistress of the Art of Death* (New York, NY: G.P. Putnam and Sons, 2007), 365.

and practice are frequently either vague or absent, despite the centrality of medieval medicine and medical practitioners to historical crime fiction.

I. Sickness and Disability

The centrality of medical practitioners means that the novels in which they feature often examine their interventions in less-dramatic ways than in solving the mysteries behind sudden and violent death. The presence of sickness and disability in these novels is, in a sense, contingent on and conditioned by the professions of these sleuth-practitioners. Parsing the meanings of illness and disability in these imagined Middle Ages, though, is often challenging. Medieval Europe is always-already a time of dirt, disease, and deformity, whose residents are doomed to short lives shadowed by misery and fear. Fourteenth-century Cambridge, where Matthew Bartholomew practices, is described as stinking in summer, from "rotting sewage, festering entrails abandoned by the slaughterhouses, and the rank aroma of unsold fish"; the streets are also described as carpeted in manure.[18] In the opening scene of the second novel of the series, we're told that "mounds of rubbish … lined both sides of the High Street." [19] As the research of Carole Rawcliffe demonstrates, however, civic policies in medieval Europe were designed to prevent such horrific public health scenarios.[20] In C.L. Grace's *The Book of Shadows*, Canterbury, despite being represented as a city of hospitals, is stalked by a sorcerer. This sorcerer is himself described as an "illness" in Canterbury, and he is marked physically, as if with symptoms of evil: a "cloven lip" and rheumy blue eyes.[21] In a different series by the same author, though public health is fairly well represented, medieval England is still a place of endemic violence and disease. [22] The protagonist of Indrek Hargla's Apothecary Melchior series is subject to

[18] The Medieval Murderers [here, Susanna Gregory,] *The Tainted Relic* (London, Simon and Schuster, 2005), 329.

[19] Susanna Gregory, *An Unholy Alliance* (New York, NY: St. Martin's Press, 1997), 1

[20] Rawcliffe, *Urban Bodies*, 12-53; see also Guy Geltner, "Healthscaping a Medieval City: Lucca's *curia viarum* and the Future of Public Health History," *Urban History* 40:3 (2013), 395-415.

[21] C.L. Grace, *The Book of Shadows* (New York, NY: Minotaur Press, 1996), 1-2

[22] Paul Doherty, *Candle Flame* (Sutton: Severn House Publishers, 2014), is the thirteenth installment in the Brother Athelstan series, in which this setting still prevails.

a hereditary curse, never fully explained, but presented as an accepted part of his otherwise well-ordered, if occasionally precarious world.

At one extreme, then, illness and disability function as medieval scene-setting: we know we are in the Middle Ages precisely because of these things. In Bernard Knight's establishing scene of *The Tainted Relic*, for instance: "Beggars and cripples hunched against walls, and at the gate of the churchyard a leper swung his rattle and hopefully held out his bowl for alms."[23] In depicting the leper's rattle as attracting alms rather than repelling the healthy and fearful, the text aligns with recent scholarship.[24] But most of Knight's section of *The Tainted Relic* uses disease and deformity to create a gothic panoply. A physically impaired clerk is described as "betrayed by a poor body"; he has a hunchback and a lame leg, as well as being small of stature. This is, however, authorial glossing: another perspective on the same plausible reality might emphasize the ways in which the man found a respectable profession suited to his physical capacity.[25] An outlaw has "a nose horribly eroded by some disease"; a tavern's potman lost "one eye and half a foot" as a soldier.[26] Beggars and the leprous are linked as present on the periphery of a hanging, asking for alms.[27] A local "simpleton" is represented as relying on regular charity in food and coin, and another outlaw is described as having "some pustulous disease of his hands and neck."[28] This fantastical scene-setting places us between two of Umberto Eco's models of medievalism: between the medieval as pretext, a colorful background for essentially modern figures, and the medieval as barbaric age, distinguished by its very darkness.[29] A similarly gothic vision of the Middle Ages is found in the opening scene of Roberta Gellis' *A Mortal Bane*, in which a blind woman makes her way through a churchyard,

[23] The Medieval Murderers [here, Bernard Knight,] *The Tainted Relic,* 31.

[24] Luke Demaitre, "The Clapper as vox miselli : New Perspectives on Iconography," in *Leprosy and identity in the Middle Ages: From England to the Mediterranean*, eds. Elma Brenner and François-Olivier Touati (Manchester: Manchester University Press, 2021), 208-65.

[25] Knight, *The Tainted Relic*, 40.

[26] Knight, *The Tainted Relic*, 45, 64.

[27] Knight, *The Tainted Relic*, 87.

[28] Knight, *The Tainted Relic*, 90, 95.

[29] Umberto Eco, "Dreaming of the Middle Ages," in *Travels in Hyperreality*, 68-69. On scholarly imaginings of medieval Europe as a place of disease and disability, see Irina Metzler, *A Social History of Disability in the Middle Ages: Cultural Considerations of Physical Impairment* (London: Routledge, 2013), 1-2.

reflects on the cruelty and prejudice of the clergy, and discovers the body of a murdered man.[30] This character is one of four women with disabilities who work in a brothel under the management of the protagonist. The household's cook is hard of hearing; the three sex workers are respectively blind, mute, and mentally impaired. The hyper-sexuality of the latter is used to clarify the ethics of her sexual consent. Both this and the fact that the mute woman is a "Saracen" who is an expert dancer contribute to the othering of the sexuality of people with disabilities.[31]

Medieval Europe, as imagined here, is a place of discomfort and disease, where deviation from societal norms is punished with quotidian disapproval and not-infrequent violence. Ariana Franklin's *The Serpent's Tale*, published in 2008, reinforces such stereotypes, opening with scenes of a planned assassination, a poisoning, black magic, and a breech birth in rapid succession.[32] Even in less sensational contexts, social suspicion is presented as the norm. In Candace Robb's *A Trust Betrayed*, a man discussing a spy with one leg shorter than the other complains that women are too apt to pity the disabled.[33] In the Apothecary Melchior series, this suspicion is linked to late medieval fear of fraud among those dependent on almsgiving.[34] Less dramatically, colds, coughs, and fevers occur in seven titles, and are almost always successfully cured. An exception is when a young lay brother dies "of a chill," in the assessment of the unhappy almoner, having suffered from symptoms consistent with tuberculosis.[35] The most frequent conditions with which medical

---

30 Roberta Gellis, *A Mortal Bane* (New York, NY: Tor Books, 1999), 1-3.

31 Gellis, *A Mortal Bane*, 14-16; on this othering, see Anna Mollow and Robert McCruer, "Introduction," in *Sex and Disability*, eds. Robert McCruer and Anna Mollow (Durham, NC: Duke University Press, 2012), 1-34.

32 Ariana Franklin, *The Serpent's Tale* (New York, NY: Putnam & Sons, 2008), 1-17.

33 Candace Robb, *A Trust Betrayed* (New York, NY: Mysterious Press, 2002), 156.

34 Indrek Hargla, *Apothecary Melchior and the Mystery of St. Olaf's Church*, trans. Adam Cullen (London: Peter Owens, 2015), 84; Miri Rubin, *Charity and Community in Medieval Cambridge* (Cambridge: Cambridge University Press, 1988), 89-94; Florence Demoulin-Auzary, Pro sustentandis Christi pauperibus: La naissance d'un droit de l'aumône aux xiie et xiiie siècles," in *Der Einfluss der Kanonistik auf die Europäische Rechtskultur: Das Recht der Wirtschaft*, eds. David von Mayenburg, Orazio Condorelli, Franck Roumy, and Mathias Schmoekel (Köln: Böhlau Verlag, 2016), 73-100; Irina Metzler, "Disability in the Middle Ages and Cultural History," *WerkstattGeschichte* 65 (2013), 55-65, esp. 61-63.

35 Indrek Hargla, *Apothecary Melchior and The Ghost of Rataskaevu Street,* trans. Christopher Moseley (London: Peter Owen Publishers, 2016), 109.

practitioners have to contend are those linked to old age. Age itself was viewed as a type of infirmity in the medieval period, and it appears in a dozen titles.[36] Matthew Bartholomew ministers to a man in the early stages of dementia with both sleep aids and companionship; Melchior, similarly, visits an elderly man without declaring this activity to the Council doctor, in order that he may do it more cheaply.[37] Seasonal risks to the health of the elderly are also addressed in several novels.[38] These most common ailments and infirmities, however, are less prevalent in crime fiction's Middle Ages than more dramatic diseases.

François-Olivier Touati once quipped that the Middle Ages, for many modern observers, *is* leprosy.[39] And leprosy is statistically overrepresented in medieval crime fiction, bearing out this claim of its power as a signifier of the medieval. Cadfael's monastery manages a leper hospital, and although it is claimed that the "inmates" are not allowed near Shrewsbury because of a fear of contagion, the hospital is regularly supplied by bread from the abbey bakery, and has privileges of wood-gathering from the Crown.[40] The buildings on the outskirts of medieval Tallinn, too, include a leprosarium dedicated to St. John, described as the place where the "lepers [are] kept."[41] A character in Susanna Gregory's *The Death Toll* observes: "we all know that leprosy is a scourge sent from God to punish the wicked."[42] The widely-traveled sleuth, however, counters that there are multiple forms of leprosy, not all contagious. Even Sharon Kay Penman, widely praised for her fictional evocations of twelfth-century

36 On old age as infirmity, see Joel Agrimi and Chiara Crisciani, "Charity and Aid in Medieval Christian Civilization," in *Western Medical Thought from Antiquity to the Middle Ages*, ed. Mirko D. Grmek (Cambridge, MA: Harvard University Press, 1998), 170-76; Davis, *The Medieval Economy of Salvation*, 208; Shulamith Shahar, *Growing Old in the Middle Ages: 'Winter Clothes Us in Shadow and Pain'* (London: Routledge, 1997), 25, 164-67.

37 Susanna Gregory, *A Plague on Both Your Houses* (New York, NY: St. Martin's Press, 1998), 13-15; Hargla, *The Ghost of Rataskaevu Street*, 164.

38 Susanna Gregory, *The Tainted Relic,* 334; Peters, *Monk's Hood* (New York, NY: Mysterious Press, 1992), 14; Robb, *A Trust Betrayed*, 2-3

39 François-Olivier Touati, *Maladie et Société au Moyen Age: La lèpre, les lépreux et les léproseries dans la province ecclésiastique de Sens jusqu'au milieu du XIVe siècle* (Bruxelles: De Boeck & Larcier, 1998), 19.

40 Peters, *The Devil's Novice* (New York, NY: Mysterious Press, 1983), 288; Peters, *The Pilgrim of Hate* (New York, NY: Mysterious Press, 1997), 11.

41 Hargla, *Ghost of Rataskaevu Street*, 182-83.

42 Gregory, "The Death Toll," in *The Mammoth Book of More Historical Whodunits*, ed. Mike Ashley (New York, NY: Carroll and Graf, 2001), 176.

Europe, depicts medieval lepers as "forsaken by all but God," shunned in life and death, with "every man's hand against them."[43] The same novel repeats the now-discredited theory that a Mass for the dead was routinely said over those diagnosed with leprosy.[44] Michael Jecks' *The Leper's Return* presents both the strict isolation of the leprous and loathing towards them as normative; the novel culminates with an outraged mob attempting to set fire to a *leprosarium* and drive out its inhabitants.[45] In 2011, Jecks wrote in a commentary on the novel: "The life of a leper was so appalling, I still cannot give a talk about them without choking. Naturally, as with most things medieval, the concepts of the treatment were logical for their time – but atrociously cruel in outcome."[46] The assumption that life for those diagnosed with leprosy in medieval Europe was not only appalling, but appallingly cruel, and that this cruelty was a characteristic result of medieval logic, is notable for the ways in which it echoes older medievalisms, rather than recent scholarship.[47] Cadfael, in contrast, echoes popular medieval metaphors in speaking of "leprosies of the heart and ulcers of the soul worse than any of these he poulticed and lanced."[48]

Crime fiction often handles holistic medieval understandings of medicine with accuracy and sensitivity. Humoral theory is explicitly invoked in approximately 20% of the texts under examination, and not always in direct connection to the investigation. Grief, for example, is

---

43 Sharon Kay Penman, *The Queen's Man* (London: Henry Holt, 1996), 11, 78-79.

44 Penman, *The Queen's Man*, 79-80. See Carole Rawcliffe, *Leprosy in Medieval England* (Woodbridge: Boydell and Brewer, 2006), 19-22.

45 Michael Jecks, *The Leper's Return* (London: Headline Books, 1998), 225-29, 305-09.

46 Michael Jecks, Goodreads review, November 16, 2011, www.goodreads.com/review/show/236174512. Last accessed November 23, 2021.

47 E. Jeanselme, "Comment l'Europe, au Moyen Age, se protégea contre la Lèpre," *Bulletin de la Société Française d'Histoire de la Médecine* 25 (1931), 1-12; Anita Homolka, "Die Lebensgewohnheiten der Leprakranken im Spätmittelalter," in:*Aussatz—Lepra—Hansen-Krankheit: ein Menschheitsproblem im Wandel*, ed. Jörn Henning Wolf (Würzburg: Deutsches Aussätzigen-Hilfswerk, 1986), 158; Rawcliffe, *Leprosy in Medieval England,* 13-43. See Krolikoski, "'Have You Come Here to Play Jesus?': The Use and Misuse of Medieval Leprosy," in this volume, for an extended discussion of stereotypes surrounding medieval leprosy.

48 Peters, *The Leper of St. Giles* (New York, NY: Mysterious Press, 1995), 5. Cf. Frederick S. Paxton, "Anointing the Sick and Dying in Christian Antiquity and the Early Medieval West," in *Health, Disease, and Healing in Medieval Culture*, eds. Sheila Campbell, Bert Hall, and David Klausner (New York: St. Martin's Press, 1992), 93-102.

referred to as stirring up morbid humors; anger, too, is presented as dangerous to health.[49] An infirmarian advises his patient to abstain from milk, cream, and bread, fearing a dietary allergy, viz., that his humoral balance might be "hostile to certain foods."[50] Melchior observes that the plague spreads easily in places of "filth" where people do not look after themselves and their streets. He believes that eating clean food and drink and observing healthful practices can help to prevent this dreaded disease. This theory is presented at the conclusion of a debate as to the causes of plague which Melchior holds with two Dominicans; their consensus is that though divine correction may be administered through disease, the disease is not caused by the will of God.[51]

Impairment and disability are more peripheral in historical crime fiction than, in all probability, they were in medieval societies. Those with physical impairments are most often seen as part of marginal groups: of those without resources, employment, or social networks. For named characters, deafness occurs once, epilepsy and unidentified chronic illness twice each, mental disability four times, and lameness five times. Blindness is by far the most frequent sensory impairment, though other forms of impairment also appear approximately half a dozen times. The study of disability in the Middle Ages is a subfield that has seen particularly dramatic growth in the four decades since Brother Cadfael first appeared among his herb beds.[52] Its representation, however, has remained fairly static. In medieval crime fiction, the representation of sickness and, especially, of disability, frequently contributes to the "gothic sensibility" of novels depicting the Middle Ages as distant and exotic.[53] While those with disabilities are sometimes found in historical crime fiction integrated into their societies, they are more frequently on

---

[49] Susanna Gregory, *The Tainted Relic*, 18; Peters, *The Sanctuary Sparrow* (New York, NY: Mysterious Press, 1995), 30.

[50] Grace, *A Maze of Murders*, 128.

[51] Hargla, *St. Olaf's Church*, 100-101.

[52] Cameron Hunt McNabb, "Introduction," *Medieval Disability Sourcebook: Western Europe* (punctum books, 2020), 13-20; Metzler, *A Social History of Disability in the Middle Ages*, 2-7.

[53] Faye Getz, "Black Death and the Silver Lining: Meaning, Continuity, and Revolutionary Change in Histories of Medieval Plague," *Journal of the History of Biology* 24:2 (Summer, 1991) 279.

its edges — and, as in medieval genres of literature, found seeking and receiving miraculous cures.[54]

II. Practitioners

Exceptions to these rules are found in series where practitioner-sleuths are themselves disabled. Owen Archer, for instance, comes to his career as detective-spy after being blinded in one eye. His psychological and physical adjustment to his new identity and social role is prominent in the first novel of the series.[55] This is particularly notable in view of the underrepresentation of disabled protagonists in crime fiction generally. I suggest that the space of the imagined medieval creates possibilities for the representation of impairment as part of protagonists' identity and experience.[56] A number of scholars have hypothesized that social integration was the norm for disabled people in the premodern world.[57] But recovering the experiences of those affected by physical impairment is often challenging; novels can do this imaginatively. While Owen Archer, having suffered a disabling injury in his first career, comes happily to the practice of medicine afterwards, sensory impairment could also pose a threat to professional activity. In Indrek Hargla's series, because the vision – and possibly the acumen – of the Teutonic Order's physician has weakened with age, Melchior uses discretion in following his recipes.[58]

Isaac of Girona, the Jewish doctor of Caroline Roe's series set in fourteenth-century Spain, suffers from degenerative blindness, and has to adjust to this in *Remedy for Treason.* He is shown throughout the series using mobility aids and affected by the anxieties of needing to negotiate unfamiliar spaces. Also, notably, he enjoys a playfully romantic relationship with his wife that is altered, but not interrupted, by his disability. Isaac is, I think, one of the most interesting of medieval

---

[54] Jenni Kuuliala, *Saints, Infirmity, and Community in the Late Middle Ages* (Amsterdam: Amsterdam University Press, 2020), 11-30; Peters, *Pilgrim of Hate*, 51, 163-67.

[55] Candace Robb, *The Apothecary Rose* (New York, NY: St. Martin's Press, 1993), passim

[56] Matthew Shardlake, the protagonist of a mystery series set in 16th-century London, is also disabled. He does not have sensory impairment, but is a hunchback, which is used against him as a term of abuse. See C.J. Sansom, *Dissolution* (New York, NY: Penguin Books, 2003.) The latest in the series was published in 2019.

[57] Metzler, *A Social History of Disability in the Middle Ages,* 72-74, 199-204.

[58] Hargla, *St. Olaf's Church*, 55.

sleuths. The trope of the observant amateur detective is varied by having Isaac's observations made without the faculty of sight. Like any good medieval doctor, he uses his faculties of taste and smell; he is also psychologically acute and emotionally intelligent. His Jewishness, too, makes him sometimes regarded as an outsider: useful or suspect or both. As a practicing urban physician, Isaac is, curiously enough, in the minority of medieval sleuths. Matthew Bartholomew is a university-trained doctor who is writing a treatise on fevers in his spare time. He views the training of physicians as his most important responsibility among many. But Isaac and Matthew, as doctors, are outnumbered by apothecaries, infirmarers, and practitioners of domestic medicine. *The Winter King*, a late installment in Alys Clare's Hawkenlye series, contains, in addition to a respectable apothecary, a "forest woman," one of the main protagonists, who practices mind-reading as well as the provision of basic remedies.[59] Though the nunnery in the book boasts a knowledgeable infirmarian and sub-infirmarian, little medical knowledge is described or used in the plot.

The case of Salerno and its doctors is worth mentioning before we move on to more ordinary practitioners. *Mistress of the Art of Death* introduces Salerno as a place where "men forget their manners and their god in the greater worship of the sick."[60] Throughout the series, Salerno and its school are described as the exception that proves the rule of superstition and narrow-mindedness in determining both who is allowed to be a doctor and how illness is treated. The institutions of the Church, on the other hand, are represented as responsible for the stagnation of medical knowledge, and worse, "every advance necessary for the mental and physical health of mankind."[61] Any form of therapeutic intervention other than the strictly spiritual, in this reading, is viewed by default as suspect, even Satanic.[62] A rather different image of Salernitan medicine is presented in Roberto Tiraboschi's *The Apothecary's Shop*, set in twelfth-century Venice. There, too, a woman doctor is one of the chief protagonists, but she is presented as a brusque eccentric in a world where

---

59 Alys Clare, *The Winter King* (Sutton: Severn House Publishers, 2013), 112-23.
60 Franklin, *Mistress of the Art of Death*, 13.
61 Franklin, *The Serpent's Tale*, 24.
62 Franklin, *Mistress of the Art of Death*, 102.

both medical professionals and medical ideologies are in competition with each other, not as a lone figure of enlightenment.[63]

Medicine as learned and practiced within the household, while it has been the subject of increasing scholarly attention in the past decade, remains peripheral to the medieval mystery novel.[64] In *The Rufus Spy*, the protagonist's aunt helps her with the aftermath of a miscarriage, portraying women's medicine as a still-separate sphere.[65] But where the basic medical knowledge of non-protagonists is represented, it often proves either ineffectual or hazardous.[66] In *The Lady Chapel*, a woman gives her husband a minutely-described medicine, with ingredients including "some barks that [her] mother collected long ago," but it is also proved to contain arsenic.[67] Cadfael provides dried herbs, largely to be used as "preservatives, salts and spices to keep [meat] good and palatable."[68] The elite laywoman who purchases these from him also wants an herbal rub for her son's springtime cough. The protagonist of Candace Robb's Margaret Kerr series has no professional or specialized medical training, but both she and her maidservant are represented as being knowledgeable in domestic medicine, and the opening sequence of the series has them both guarding and washing a corpse.[69] Particularly in

[63] Roberto Tiraboschi, *The Apothecary's Shop: A Novel of Venice 1118 A.D.*, trans. Katherine Gregor (New York, NY: Europa Editions, 2017). This and the other novels in Tiraboschi's Venice trilogy are marketed as literary fiction or, sometimes, noir. They are boldly experimental, with touches of magical realism; for all these reasons, I have not included them as examples of historical crime fiction.

[64] For early examples of such scholarship, see Montserrat Cabré, "Women or Healers? Household Practices and the Categories of Health Care in Late Medieval Iberia," *Bulletin of the History of Medicine* 82:1 (2008), 18-51; and Monica Green, *Making Women's Medicine Masculine: The Rise of Male Authority in Pre-Modern Gynecology* (Oxford: Oxford University Press, 2008.) For a recent example, see Sara Ritchey, *Acts of Care: Recovering Women in Late Medieval Health* (Ithaca, NY: Cornell University Press, 2021.)

[65] Alys Clare, *The Rufus Spy* (London: Severn House, 2018), 31-33, cf. Green, *Making Women's Medicine Masculine*, 29-69. On medicine as practiced within the household, particularly for and by women, see Kristin Uscinski, "For to Cause a Woman to Have Milk: Recipes to Promote Lactation for Medieval and Modern Women," in this volume.

[66] Caroline Roe, *An Antidote for Avarice* (New York, NY: Berkley Publishing, 1999), 28; Robb, *The Lady Chapel*, 42, 50-51; Hargla, *The Mystery of St. Olaf's Church*, 36, 55; Hargla, *The Ghost of Rataskaevu Street*, 109; Gregory, *An Unholy Alliance*, 35-38. Exceptions can be found, as in Peters, *The Virgin in the Ice* (New York: Mysterious Press, 1995), 15-21, 72.

[67] Candace Robb, *The Lady Chapel*, 42, 50-51, 74-75, 99 (quoted at page 99.)

[68] Peters, *Dead Man's Ransom* (New York, NY: Mysterious Press, 1997), 453.

[69] Robb, *A Trust Betrayed*, 1-10.

the first novel of this series, the importance of emotional and spiritual health is highlighted. Corpse-washing is also used in the establishing scene of Laury Silvers' *The Jealous*, where Shatha and Saliha, employed by the Barmakid hospital of Baghdad, are represented as having medical expertise acquired through practice.[70] Through the use of copper basins, and lotus leaves and camphor in their preparations, the apprentice Saliha and the more experienced Shaha are shown uniting practical and theoretical knowledge in their work.[71]

In Silvers' Sufi mysteries, doctors appear as expert consultants.[72] Elsewhere, practitioners of Islamicate medicine, while largely absent from historical crime fiction, are not infrequently referenced. These references are usually linked to orientalist tropes concerning their superior learning and wisdom. In Susanna Gregory's *Plague on Both Your Houses*, protagonist Matthew Bartholomew has received formative education from an Arab doctor in Paris. This doctor has advised him against using leeches, sampling urine, and relying on astrology. This advice serves to bring Bartholomew's practice more into line with modern expectations of medical practitioners, but it deprives him of common and respected medieval tools of diagnosis and treatment. This raises the question of how Bartholomew could establish rapport with his patients without these tools to demonstrate his expertise. The true audience of this expertise, it would seem, is comprised not of the medieval sick but modern readers. In *The Leper of St. Giles*, the leper known as Lazarus receives an early-stage diagnosis from Arab physicians whom he identifies as "wiser than any here."[73] While the influence of Arab medicine on Cadfael's practice is peripheral in the series, it is foregrounded in scholarly analysis of it.[74] Isaac of Girona's use of Arabic-language treatises – and need for an assistant who can read them aloud – is treated matter-of-factly. The medical knowledge of Isaac and his

---

[70] Candace Robb, *A Trust Betrayed*, 1-10; Silvers, *The Jealous*, 18–19.

[71] Silvers, *The Jealous*, 18-22. On the hospital itself, see Michael W. Dols, "The Origins of the Islamic Hospital: Myth and Reality," *Bulletin of the History of Medicine* 61:3 (1987), 383-85.

[72] Silvers, *The Lover*, 15; Silvers, *The Jealous*, 29-31, 49-50.

[73] Peters, *The Leper of St. Giles*, 198.

[74] Lindsay, "The Habit of Detection," 277; Rob Talbot and Robin Whiteman, *Brother Cadfael's Herb Garden: An Illustrated Companion to Medieval Plants and their Uses* (Boston: Bulfinch Press, 1997), 8-9.

daughter, meanwhile, is highly valued by many, but treated as suspect in moments of social and religious tension.[75]

Largely absent from the imagined Middle Ages of crime fiction are fraudulent medical practitioners, although medieval satire shows concern with them.[76] One of Melchior's cases, mentioned in passing, involves poisoning by a man called an "itinerant doctor" by Melchior's wife Keterlyn, and described by Melchior himself as "a thief and a bastard who was peddling all sorts of poisonous rubbish as medicines, which he had stolen."[77] There is a passing reference to fraudulent practitioners in *The Serpent's Tale*, but their danger is represented as more economic than physical; the charlatan of the second Isaac of Girona novel, too, is guilty of nothing more than peddling herbs as a panacea. Only one other novel addresses "false leeches," and even then, the protagonist treats them as mostly harmless.[78] On the other hand, a category of practitioner distinctively found in fiction is those aided by magic powers. *The Winter King*, a late installment in Alys Clare's Hawkenlye series, features pagans who perform mental health interventions through literal mind-reading. In the same novel, in addition to the respectable apothecary, there is a "forest woman," one of the main protagonists, who practices mind-reading as well as the provision of basic remedies; and there is a nunnery with a knowledgeable infirmarian and sub-infirmarian, but little medical knowledge is described or used in the plot. Lassair, the protagonist of the Aelf Fen series set in eleventh-century England, also has magical powers, as well as abundant practical medical knowledge.

A practitioner with a somewhat ambiguous relationship to supernatural as well as natural knowledge is Magda Digby, a recurring character in Candace Robb's Owen Archer series. Magda herself is a semi-legendary figure of historiography: she is a witch-healer, a decidedly and rebelliously non-Christian midwife who lives in a hut on an island,

[75] Roe, *Cure for a Charlatan* (New York, NY: Berkeley Prime Crime, 1999), 51, 58-59; Roe, *Solace for a Sinner* (New York, NY: Berkeley Prime Crime, 2000), 91-92; Joseph Shatzmiller, *Jews, Medicine, and Medieval Society* (Berkeley: University of California Press, 1994), 85-90.

[76] Faith Wallis, ed., *Medieval Medicine: A Reader* (Toronto: University of Toronto Press, 2010), 525-42.

[77] Hargla, *The Ghost of Rataskaevu Street*, 41.

[78] Franklin, *The Serpent's Tale*, 12, contrasts Adelia with "a charlatan who bamboozled his patients with disgusting medicines for high prices." Roe, *Cure for a Charlatan*, 9; Grace, *A Maze of Murders*, 192.

and provides abortifacients and practical wisdom in ways that the other practitioners of the series are less able or willing to do.[79] Tibia (sic), in *Forsaken Soul*, does the same thing "though it is a sin."[80] Meggie, in the Hawkenlye series, fills a similar role, using her emotional intelligence as a healer, though her status as "the bastard child of a forest woman" renders her a social outcast.[81] Magda is the only named midwife I have found, though they are occasionally referenced, and the apothecary Kathryn Swinbrooke is consulted for a challenging birth.[82] Magda is not the only protagonist-practitioner of the Owen Archer series. Both the visually impaired protagonist and his apothecary wife Lucie possess and mediate medical knowledge. The specificity of Lucie's prescriptions makes medieval medical expertise visible to the reader. Series with professional apothecaries as sleuths center ingredients and medicines more than others, showing off the expertise of the sleuths.

Apothecaries are – with the possible exception of Brother Cadfael – decidedly the practitioners who do the most medical practice on the page. The specifics of knowledge and the medical marketplace may be more visible here than elsewhere to compensate for the unfamiliarity of the profession, or perhaps precisely because the demonstrated knowledge of an apothecary functions effectively as medieval exoticism. Sabin, an apothecary in *The Winter King*, fears for her reputation after supplying contraceptives and a soporific to a married woman, and is eventually cleared of suspicion.[83] In Priscilla Royal's series, focusing on a priory, one of the nuns is a former apothecary, giving her convenient medical knowledge.[84] Both Lucie and Owen, in the long-running Owen Archer series, provide remedies and prophylactics even when these are not directly relevant to the plot, establishing their services as integral to the urban life of York. Similarly, Apothecary Melchior, aspiring to his own shop on the town square of late medieval Tallinn, is integrated in his town's lively medical, religious, and civic networks. The therapeutic powers of his most popular specific – a decidedly alcoholic pick-me-up

---

79 See, for example, Candace Robb, *The Lady Chapel*, 84-85.

80 Priscilla Royal, *Forsaken Soul* (Scottsdale, AZ: Poisoned Pen Press, 2008), Chapter 3, timestamp 40:38.

81 Clare, *The Winter King*, 562-63.

82 Peters, *The Virgin in the Ice*, 2; Robb, *The Nun's Tale*, 174; Grace, *A Maze of Murders*, 135; Gregory, *An Unholy Alliance*, 35-38.

83 Clare, *The Winter King*, 71, 141.

84 Royal, *Forsaken Soul.*

– form the basis of an amiable running joke between him and one of his collaborators. Many of the remedies he gives are part of diet regulation and even (acknowledged both by him and the recipients, at least tacitly) placebos for stress. In the character-establishing sequence, his work is characterized as fundamentally social as well as therapeutic, as he provides and receives gossip and news as well as treating "recent illnesses and old pains," mixing up the doctor's medicines to order and selling his own elixirs.[85] Melchior sees his work as a detective as maintaining the moral public health of the city, the health of the collective body.

III. Materials and Knowledge

Medicinal plants are universally treated as central to the practice of medieval medicine – perhaps to a disproportionate degree. The specificity of medieval knowledge, the extent of medieval trade, and the circulation of medical texts are all underrepresented in historical crime fiction. Melchior acquires many of his medicinal herbs at market, from a farmer's wife who is described as having good knowledge of both plants and their properties.[86] In providing medical care as a way of thanking her noble host for hospitality, Kathryn Swinbrooke avails herself of the household's medicine chest, which she expects to find and is gratified to find well-stocked.[87] The establishing scene of *A Morbid Taste for Bones*, Ellis Peters' first Cadfael novel, takes place in the herbalist's garden. Of this the monk is justly proud. The garden is presented as an exceptionally good example of its kind: superior, but not atypical. It is "supplied with herbs both good for spicing meats, and also invaluable as medicine." Cadfael, we are told, has built it up over years, and added to it "many exotic plants" from his experience in the eastern Mediterranean.[88] Similar generalizing descriptions are found in many novels, with the influential Cadfael series remaining unusual in the degree of specificity with which it discusses medicines and *materia medica*. Knowledge of materials was of critical importance to medieval medical practitioners of all kinds, who gained experience from observation and practice, as well as study of medical texts. The honed skills of observation on which practitioner-

[85] Hargla, *St. Olaf's Church*, 15.
[86] Hargla, *The Ghost of Rataskaevu Street*, 51.
[87] Grace, *A Maze of Murders*, 91-92.
[88] Peters, *A Morbid Taste for Bones,* 1-2.

protagonists rely professionally are instrumental in their aptitude for crime-solving. Their medical practice, too, is frequently featured, even when not directly relevant to the resolution of the plot. But the terms in which this practice is imagined are often vague. For most authors, however, indicating the function of medicines is more important than indicating the identity of the substances used to make them. In *The Rufus Spy*, for instance, a hot drink to restore a traveler is made by mixing honey and boiled water with "pinches of this herb and that ground root."[89] Admittedly, the sub-disciplines relevant to examining the uses and understandings of plants in the medieval past are many, and not always in conversation with each other. But the ready accessibility of information about plants' medicinal properties suggests that the very mysteriousness of medical ingredients plays an important role in establishing atmosphere for the writers and readers of historical crime fiction.[90]

Ingredients

Ingredients	Number of Novels Used
Unnamed Herbs	24
Poppy	13
Wine	12
Mint	10
Centaury	6
Betony	5
Camomile	5
Rosemary	5
Cabbage	4
Ginger	4
Sage	4
Willow	4
Mustard	3
Valerian	3
Thyme	2

89 Clare, *The Rufus Spy*, 7.

90 On disciplinary divisions, see Anne Stobart and Susan Francia, "The Fragmentation of Herbal History: The Way Forward," in *Critical Approaches to the History of Western Herbal Medicine,* eds. Stobart and Francia (London: Bloomsbury, 2014), 5-14. On medicinal plants, see for example M. Grieve, *A Modern Herbal*, www.botanical.com/botanical/mgmh/mgmh.html. Last accessed December 7, 2021. See Robin S. Reich, "The Fantasy of Medieval Medicine," in this volume, for a discussion of how the genre of fantasy fiction participates in similar tropes.

Frequency of medical ingredients

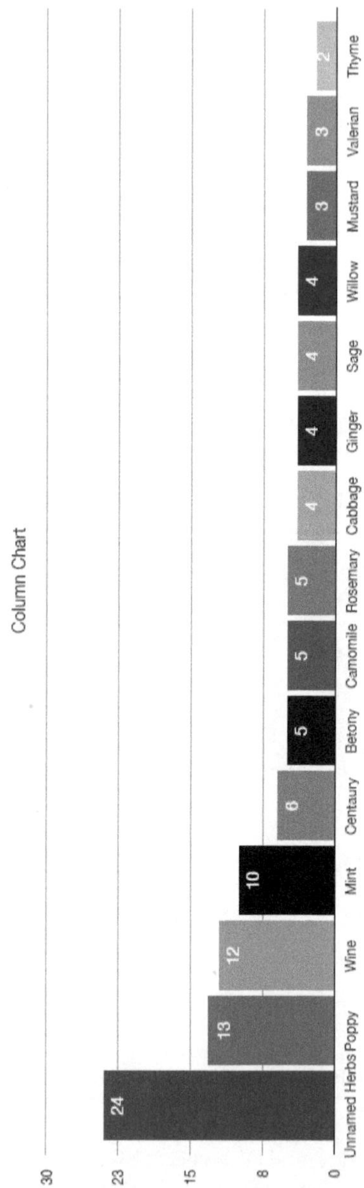

Sometimes not even the function of medicines and *materia medica* is indicated. This is true even in scenes where demonstrating knowledge is important to the plot. In *Mistress of the Art of Death*, in a sequence in which Adelia and her companions establish themselves as trusted practitioners in England, they treat everyday ailments with unspecified ingredients. The exception to this silence is a decoction of willow bark. And while her companions are disheartened by the cold and unfamiliar fen country, Adelia is excited by the abundance of willow trees.[91] This keen awareness of environment and resources would have been a key asset to medieval medical practitioners. But in most medieval mystery novels, this knowledge is presumed rather than demonstrated, and the labor and expertise necessary to collect plants and herbs, for instance, is invisible. The "healthy medicinal herbs" cultivated in the raised beds of a monastery garden in *Wine of Violence* are not identified; "Whispers of the Dead" contains an establishing scene in which a monastic infirmarer grinds leaves in a mortar and pestle, but the reader is not told which leaves he is using, or what he is using them for.[92] Again, the Apothecary Melchior series is exceptional in this regard: the pharmacy kitchen, with its specialized equipment, is described in some detail, possibly as a way of legitimizing the apothecary's craft as a recognizable specialty. Medicines with repulsive ingredients, however, such as "a bitter essence made of marinated wolf's intestines and mummified human remains," Melchior sees as chiefly useful in raising and maintaining his profile as an educated medical practitioner, rather than in practical terms.[93]

The more medieval mystery novels one reads, the more conspicuous the absence of medical specificity becomes. A few ingredients recur regularly, but basil, garlic, and yarrow are far less popular than honey as ingredients in disinfectants. A more surprising favoritism is shown for poppy seeds, not native to any of the regions in which the novels are set. An import from the eastern Mediterranean, poppy seeds are, by far, the most commonly named single ingredient in the medical medievalism of mystery novels. Ginger, while also a popular import, appears far more seldom, and pepper – despite its medicinal uses in drinks to improve circulation – hardly at all. The brandy with ginger and pepper provided

[91] *Mistress of the Art of Death*, 84-85.

[92] Priscilla Royal, *Wine of Violence*, 19; Peter Tremayne, "Whispers of the Dead," 4.

[93] Hargla, *The Ghost of Rataskaevu Street*, 14-15.

by Apothecary Melchior to combat melancholy is exceptional.[94] This is interesting to me as a commentary about how medical plants are imagined: as something that medieval Europe needs to get from elsewhere, and that were always viewed as exotic, rather than (more usually) local plants, carefully observed and collected, with products like ginger and pepper being ordered in substantial quantities by urban hospitals.[95]

The relationship between textual and practical medicine, also of vital importance to medieval medical practitioners, is also underrepresented. Scholars have observed that, often, extant textual sources give us only partial access to medieval medical practice. Increased attention to users' marks in medical manuscripts, too, demonstrates the ways in which oral communication, classical medical texts, and observation of plants and symptoms coexisted as sources of medical expertise.[96] But in crime fiction, elite medicine is largely conspicuous by its absence, and practical medicine is privileged over the textual. Apothecary Melchior, for instance, has many arguments with the Dominican infirmarer in part because the friar is "blindly convinced of what was written in the prescriptive monastic books about the sick." [97] The Matthew Bartholomew series is an exception; Bartholomew, dismayed to find that his university students don't know more about opiates, advises more study of Dioscorides' *De Materia Medica.*[98] Theoretical and practical medicine appear side by side on an afternoon during which Cadfael is overseeing concoctions. While doing so, he is also studying "a copy of Aelfric's list of herbs and trees from the England of a century and a half earlier." This brings him to face the question of whether Aelfric's "dittanders" is identical with the dittany he knows.[99] This dilemma of assessing the changing properties of plants known under similar names is one well known to scholars of medieval medicine. In studying medieval medicine, we are often dealing with the same problems of translation and

---

94 Hargla, *St. Olaf's Church*, 84.

95 Stadtarchiv Mainz 33/1, 33/3.

96 Lucy C. Barnhouse, "Languages of Experience: Translating Medicine in MS Laud Misc. 237," in *New Approaches to Disease, Disability, and Medicine in Medieval Europe,* eds. Erin Connelly and Steffi Künzel (Oxford: Archaeopress, 2018), 94-108.

97 Hargla, *The Ghost of Rataskaevu Street*, 53.

98 Susanna Gregory, *An Unholy Alliance*, 39-43.

99 Peters, *The Devil's Novice*, 188-189.

problems of time that Brother Cadfael is when reading Aelfric on a rainy day.

Dorothy L. Sayers once had her Lord Peter Wimsey quip that in detective novels, "virtue is always triumphant," and this classic formulation holds true for series set in the Middle Ages.[100] Unsolved crimes and morally ambivalent sleuths are less common than in much contemporary detective fiction. For all the violence that is present in the medieval worlds of historical crime fiction, and for all the suffering with which characters may have to contend, clear and complete resolution is the norm. The protagonists are motivated by a spirit of inquiry and compassion, linked to their callings as medical practitioners, and these humane characteristics help them find holistic solutions to the problems confronting them. Sherlock Holmes once defined the essence of his calling as bringing peace to troubled souls; medieval sleuths might well do the same.[101] Compassion is often more crucial than medical expertise to their crime-solving. Medieval medical knowledge and practice are far more often invoked and assumed than described. Despite the ways in which it is treated as anticipating or analogous to modern scientific knowledge, the logic of medieval medicine is still made largely inaccessible to readers. While practitioners are almost invariably successful in providing cures as well as solving crimes, the medicine they practice remains fundamentally mysterious and even quasi-mystical. This persistent othering of medieval medicine forms part of the othering of the Middle Ages themselves. Still, some of the boldest and most successful novels under discussion here examine ways in which medieval desires, fears, and intolerances resemble those of our contemporary world.

---

[100] Dorothy L. Sayers, *Strong Poison* (New York, NY: Avon Books, 1967), 99.

[101] Arthur Conan Doyle, "The Yellow Face," in *The New Annotated Sherlock Holmes*, vol. 1, ed. Leslie S. Klinger (New York, NY: Norton and Company, 2005), 454.

SECTION III

Women's Medicine, Medieval and Modern

HOW TO TREAT A WOMAN'S COLD AND POROUS BODY: MUGWORT FUMIGATION FOR FERTILITY IN MEDIEVAL AND MODERN FOLK MEDICINE OF WESTERN AND ASIAN CULTURES

MINJI LEE*

In the history of gynecology and obstetrics, many medical interventions – direct and indirect – have been suggested to aid women's fertility. Even when women's sexual and reproductive organs were not visible to or easily treatable by the medical practitioner, premodern medicine tried to provide women with the right diagnoses and treatments. Fertility affects not only whether women can have children but also whether women can survive birth procedures. Today, ultrasounds and other tests are vital and standard diagnostic tools in gynecology. But the absence of these medical technologies did not mean that medieval medicine lacked methods to aid women in agony, either by urgent direct interventions or gradual health management. While medieval people did check the uterus or vagina, their diagnoses and treatments were often interconnected with beliefs about and representations of the body, which can sometimes still be seen in modern popular beliefs and alternative medical practices.

Learned medicine in premodern Europe was influenced by both Aristotelian elemental theory and Galenic humoralism. Galenic

* Department of Religion and Medical Humanities Program, Montclair State University.

humoralism was based on Aristotle's theory that the whole cosmos is composed of four different elements: fire, earth, water, and air. These elements were mirrored by the humors in the human body: yellow bile, black bile, phlegm, and blood. The four elements and humors were defined by the combination of the qualities heat, cold, dryness, and wetness. Individuals had different combinations of humors, producing different temperaments, and personal health was guaranteed by keeping the right balance among these humors. Gender was a key factor in determining how this balance was understood in an individual. According to Galenic medicine, men were hotter and drier than women, whose bodies were naturally inclined to be cold and wet.[1] Even though women's ideal balance of humors or qualities was colder than men's, heat was required for reproduction. Having the right measure or balance of heat was essential to everyone's health; it was believed that heat was required for conception and other reproductive processes like menstruation, pregnancy, and childbirth. Barrenness and impediments to reproduction were thus associated with an excess of cold humors in women.[2]

Since heat and moisture were believed to be essential to keep one fertile, mugwort fumigation often functioned as a useful way to supply heat. Treatments with mugwort (several plants in the genus *Artemisia*) were believed in several premodern cultures, European and Asian, to heat a woman's body. If a woman was perceived as not generating enough heat to ensure reproduction and fertility on her own, she could use medicines that, like mugwort, were classified as having a hot nature. Moreover, fumigation could be the best way to insert what was needed in the uterus, so what was used to make the smoke also mattered.

Mugwort fumigation is a gynecological treatment found in many cultures. Comparing mugwort fumigation in premodern European and Asian texts and practices can shed light on understandings of women's general health and bodies. This analysis reveals shared cultural

[1] Helen King, "The Mathematics of Sex: One to Two, or Two to One?," *Studies in Medieval and Renaissance History: Sexuality and Culture in Medieval and Renaissance Europe* 2, no. 3 (2005), 47.

[2] The lack of heat was applied to both sexes' infertility, but women were more often used to explain infertility. Catherine Rider, "Gender, Old Age, and the Infertile Body in Medieval Medicine," in *Gender, Health, and Healing, 1250-1550*, ed. Sara Ritchey and Sharon Strocchia (Amsterdam: Amsterdam University Press, 2020), 270.

assumptions about women's bodies: they are cold in nature, lacking both heat and the ability to absorb heat as needed. Moreover, the usage of mugwort in modern Korean medicine can provide insights into how medieval medical practitioners might have used mugwort and understood its effects on gynecological issues. Mugwort could be used as a medicine to supply heat to women, correcting humoral imbalances. This herb and its applications illustrate medical, cosmological, theological, and popular understandings of women's bodies. More specifically, these medical traditions suggest that a woman's body, particularly the uterus and vagina, was believed to lack its own heat but was porous enough to receive heat from herbs with a hot nature, including mugwort.

Premodern medical or gynecological texts from West and East alike provide sick women with treatments for heating them through fumigation with mugwort, or other materials of a hot nature. This evidence includes descriptions from medieval European medical books composed partially or entirely by women, such as the *Trotula*,[3] a compilation of texts on women's medicine created in Salerno, Italy, and Hildegard of Bingen's medical writings in twelfth-century Germany. Both texts present mugwort as a major ingredient, powdered or fumigated, for provoking menstruation in women with irregular periods by supplying necessary heat. Asian medicine presents mugwort fumigation as an important way to boost a woman's fertility and general health. Korean women's use of mugwort today shows how this treatment is still exercised daily and expected by women.[4] While women can receive prescriptions for the complicated medication containing mugwort from traditional doctors, they also drink, eat, insert, and fumigate with mugwort based on folk medical traditions without a doctor's prescription. These examples, despite the substantive temporal and geographical gap between them, share a common foundation: the belief that smoke or

[3] The *Trotula* consists of three books, "Book on the Conditions of Women (*Liber de sinthomatibus mulierum*)," "Treatments for Women (*De curis mulierum*)," and "Women's Cosmetics (*De ornatu mulierum*)." While the authors are not known, it is possible that "Treatments for Women (*De curis mulierum*)" was written by women at least partially. For more information, see Monica Green "Who/What is "Trotula"?," last updated January 6, 2020, www.academia.edu/41537366/WHO_WHAT_IS_TROTULA_2020.

[4] Saunjoo L. Yoon, and Jeong-Hee Kim. "Factors Contributing to the Use of Complementary and Alternative Medicine in Rural Older Women with Chronic Pain in South Korea." *Applied Nursing Research* 26, no. 4 (2013), 186.

steam from mugwort can treat women's issues, including irregular menstruation.

I. Understanding the Porous Body of a Woman: Dangers and Possibilities

Fumigation was believed to work due to the supposed permeability of the body: the idea that human beings and their bodies could exchange properties and materials with the outer world. Although this permeability was shared by women and men, a woman's body was perceived as more permeable due to the opening of her reproductive organs. The permeability of the human body is linked to humoralism in Galenic medicine. If anyone had health issues due to a deficient or excessive humor, appropriate treatment would provide what is lacking or, alternatively, get rid of something in the body. In case of immoderate heat or coldness, or even humidity or dryness, the opposite humor or elements should be provided to treat the symptoms and balance the elemental qualities. The *Trotula*, a twelfth-century compilation of at least three books on women's health, in describing the treatments for diseases or symptoms which were believed to be caused by the lack of heat, or from excessive cold, asserted: "[C]ontraries are cured by contraries."[5]

If an excess of a humor or elemental quality caused any diseases or symptoms, the contrary humor or elements needed to be supplied to keep the right balance. But how could medieval people supply what was needed? Medieval *materia medica*, or "healing substances," indicated treatments using parts of various herbs to modify the humors. Different cultures have their own rich traditions of *materia medica*, including how to understand the human body, improve health, diagnose, treat, and prevent certain diseases, and make remedies. At the same time, different knowledge about and substances of *materia medica* were imported and exported from an early period in the history of medicine.

While medieval medicine represented both male and female as open and permeable for receiving medicines and the elements, there were gendered differences in the degree to which bodies could be opened.

[5] Monica H. Green, ed. and trans., *The Trotula: A Medieval Compendium of Women's Medicine* (Philadelphia: University of Pennsylvania Press, 2001), 117.

In other words, even when the human body was believed to exchange elements with the cosmos, a woman's body was thought to be weaker and thus more open to external entities, an idea which could be traced back to ancient medicine.[6] While this open nature of women's bodies was usually a vulnerability, it also made specific treatments of subtle intervention possible when more direct intervention was not physically available or recommended. In particular, a mother's body was understood to be more physically open as it needed to exchange elements and soul with the fetus.[7]

A woman's pregnant body was not just exchanging humors and substances with the fetus. It also received elements and humors from the surrounding world and sent them back out again. According to some medieval Western authors, like Hildegard of Bingen, women's porosity can be traced back to the Biblical story of creation. The body of Eve, perfect before the Fall, became porous after her transgression of swallowing the forbidden fruit. Women, Eve's descendants, inherited the consequences of Eve's first sin and punishment: pain in menstruation and childbirth.[8]

II. Heat for Health and Reproduction

Menstruation was related to the possibility of pregnancy and childbirth. In medieval medicine, menstruation was also believed to be a purgation due to women's inferiority and inability to consume bodily residues. Following Galenic humoralism, medieval medical authors claimed that a woman's body lacked the heat and dryness essential to burn off superfluities. According to the "Book on the Conditions of Women" in *The Trotula*: "Because there is not enough heat in women to dry up the bad and superfluous humors, nor is their weakness able to tolerate sufficient labor so that Nature might expel [the excess] to the outside

[6] Laura Josc, "Monstrous Conceptions: Sex, Madness and Gender in Medieval Medical Texts," *Comparative Critical Studies* 5, no. 2 (2008), 157.

[7] Barbara Newman, *The Permeable Self: Five Medieval Relationships* (Philadelphia: University of Pennsylvania Press, 2021), 156-208

[8] This understanding of the gendered body after Original Sin is seen in many Christian writers, including Hildegard of Bingen. In her *Scivias* and *Cause et cure*, Hildegard explains woman's porosity as flows entering Eve's body after transgression. On the other hand, the Virgin Mary's body was often described as sealed and kept intact: Miri Rubin, *Mother of God: A History of the Virgin Mary* (New Haven: Yale University Press, 2009), 27.

through sweat as [it does] in men, Nature established a certain purgation especially for women, that is, the menses, to temper their property of heat."[9]

Granted that medieval medicine did not depend on one single theory, it was widely believed that women and men were distinguished by different degrees of heat and dryness. Many sex differences, including internal organs and external appearances, were explained by the varying degrees of these qualities. In Aristotelian theory, which medieval medicine also highly depended on, coldness and wetness were used to define inferior bodies.[10] The man's larger body and quick digestion were explained by greater heat.[11] With this heat, men could make the highest form of humors, semen. In Hildegard's *Cause et cure*, men are described as having more hair and sweat due to their hot nature,[12] defining heat as a primary cause of physical differences.[13]

Not just that. In medieval Christian thought, woman also had an inferior body because Eve was made of Adam's flesh while Adam was made of earth and God's breath. The woman's body was colder and wetter, which was believed to cause sex differences. Women were believed to have had other ways to cleanse impurities because their bodies lacked heat and dryness, which were essential to burn the residues of humors and other bodily fluids to keep themselves healthy. They were unable to refine the secretion inward because this refinement required sufficient heat which was lacking in the woman's body. While men were hot and dry enough to burn off and eliminate the bodily residues by making semen out of blood, women needed menstruation to perform the same function. While menstruation was described as a solution to cleanse the female body which lacks the required heat, menstruation itself also required heat. So, if a woman's body is too cold, it could not expel

---

[9] Green, *The Trotula*, 66.

[10] Joan Cadden, *Meanings of Sex Difference in the Middle Ages: Medicine, Science, and Culture* (New York: Cambridge University Press, 1993), 23.

[11] James A. Brundage, *Law, Sex, and Christian Society in Medieval Europe* (Chicago: University of Chicago Press, 1987), 426.

[12] Hildegard of Bingen, *Causes and Cures*, trans. Priscilla Throop (Charlotte, VT: MedievalMS, 2006), 28.

[13] Hildegard of Bingen is unique in seeing the woman's sexual delectation as weaker due to lesser heat and smaller body contrasting to the man's fiery nature and bigger body. Hildegard of Bingen, *Causes and cures*, trans. Throop, 63-64.

menstrual blood. Hildegard of Bingen explains that heat can open the blood vessels and make the blood flow.[14]

Heat was also responsible for making the body fertile and aroused.[15] Heat was related to reproduction and was used to explain why the too young or elderly do not have children: "[t]he young and old of both sexes lacked the necessary physical capabilities to make healthy seed, or had cold and dry humors."[16] It was important that both women and men had enough – and not too much – heat for fertility.[17] People who wanted to have children could manage their diet and activities with a view to maintaining or obtaining this desired heat. Similarly, people avoided heat when they did not want to have sexual arousal or fertility. Monks, who vowed to keep a celibate life, were advised not to eat too much hot food, such as wine or meat, since it was believed to arouse lust.[18]

A woman's reproductive body needed sufficient heat: first, of course, to remain healthy, but second to avoid womanly disorders, and third to succeed in conception, pregnancy, and childbirth. The declining heat associated with old age, for example, was understood as a cause of post-menopausal women's infertility.[19] Hildegard of Bingen also related heat to procreation. A woman could conceive if she had "the fluid of fertility with heat." Otherwise, "she would remain fruitless like dry ground, which does not yield itself to any fruitful use."[20] This heat was required not just for conception, but also for menstruation even before coitus. Medieval people believed that regular menstruation was needed for successful reproduction. Therefore, it was important to use medical interventions if a woman did not menstruate regularly. "The Book on

---

[14] Hildegard of Bingen, *Causes and Cures*, trans. Throop, 146

[15] Dianne M. Bazell, "Strife among the Table-Fellows: Conflicting Attitudes of Early and Medieval Christians toward the Eating of Meat," *Journal of the American Academy of Religion* 65, no. 1 (1997), 77. Sexual arousal, which was believed to be necessary for conception, was also understood as dependent on heat, and for successful conception, women required a certain level of heat. Brundage, *Law, Sex, and Christian Society in Medieval Europe*, 451.

[16] Rider, "Gender, Old Age, and the Infertile Body in Medieval Medicine," 276.

[17] Rider, "Gender, Old Age, and the Infertile Body in Medieval Medicine," 270.

[18] Bazell, "Strife among the Table-Fellows," 77.

[19] The lack of heat was applied to both sexes' infertility, although women were more often used to explain infertility: Rider, "Gender, Old Age, and the Infertile Body in Medieval Medicine," 270.

[20] Hildegard of Bingen, *Scivias*, trans. Columba Hart, Jane Bishop (New York: Paulist Press, 1990), 177.

the Conditions of Women" in *The Trotula* explains why women could have irregular menstruation: "Sometimes there is diarrhea on account of excessive coldness of the womb, or because its veins are too slender, as in emaciated women, because then thick and superfluous humors do not have a free passage by which they might break free."[21]

While, as this passage illustrates, there might be many reasons for menstrual retention, lack of heat was understood as one of the major causes of this condition. Hildegard of Bingen, like *The Trotula*, presented a lack of heat and lack of fertility as linked.[22] Heat, Hildegard explained, could open the blood vessels and make blood flow.[23] For successful reproductive sex, she prescribed lard, meat, and fat, which were believed to contain heat and add it to the woman who ate them. She even recommended taking the bodily fluids from animals' or other women's reproductive parts, showing the belief that other females' fluids would stimulate menstruation.

As lack of menstruation was linked to a lack of heat, excessive menstruation was linked to excessive heat. If women experienced heavy menstruation due to strong heat, this heat should be mitigated by ingredients with a cold nature. Hildegard instructed women to wet a linen cloth with cold water and wrap their thighs with it. Heated celery also worked to hasten the heavy flow because its cold nature "resists the contrary flow."[24]

Heat was necessary for a woman's health. If a woman's body failed to secure a certain amount of heat, she might experience issues with her health. The tricky part, however, is that the woman's body is by nature cold, requiring even more heat to have children since reproduction needs a greater level of heat. The examples above from premodern European sources suggest that women could have issues in fertility, especially when they lacked heat. What treatments might they choose to address these issues?

---

[21] Green, *The Trotula*, 73.

[22] Hildegard of Bingen, *Causes and Cures*, trans. Throop, 146.

[23] Hildegard of Bingen, *Causes and Cures*, trans. Throop, 149-150.

[24] Hildegard of Bingen, *Causes and Cures*, trans. Throop, 150.

III. Mugwort

Mugwort, in many medieval medical texts, is a common name for several herbs in the genus *Artemisia*,[25] especially *Artemisia vulgaris*,[26] or it is used for a loose category of different herbs.[27] Mugwort was popularly used in both Europe and Asia[28] and was widely used both for gynecological reasons and for general treatments. Mugwort is still one of the most popular herbs in East Asian countries such as China, Japan, and Korea. According to many traditions of medicine, mugwort was a powerful herb for curing women's reproductive issues. While mugwort is used in various ways, this essay focuses on mugwort treatments related to heat. Across European and Asian medical traditions, mugwort is presented as a provider of heat. This is crucial to understanding why mugwort fumigation was believed to be effective for managing women's health, and what this treatment tells us about how women's bodies were represented and taken care of.

Mugwort was one of the most popular herbs in premodern European medicine as well and was known as "the mother of all herbs." It "succors mothers with assistance as a friend," as described in Henry of Huntingdon's *Anglicanus ortus*.[29] The medieval gynecological understanding of the therapeutic uses of mugwort shows both a religious and medical understanding of women who failed to sustain enough bodily heat. If women lost heat even more, given that they are colder than men already, they would develop physical symptoms according to contemporary medical beliefs; in particular, those symptoms happen in the reproductive organs that need a certain heat to receive semen and to conceive.

---

[25] Ekiert Halina et al., "Significance of *Artemisia Vulgaris* L. (Common Mugwort) in the History of Medicine and Its Possible Contemporary Applications Substantiated by Phytochemical and Pharmacological Studies," *Molecules* 25, no. 19 (2020), 4415.

[26] W. Greuter, "Compositae (pro parte majore)," Compositae. *Euro+Med Plantbase - The Information Resource for Euro-Mediterranean Plant Diversity*, ed. W. Greuter and E. von Raab-Straube, Accessed May 13 2022, http://ww2.bgbm.org/euroPlusMed/PTaxon Detail.asp?UUID=30F7AED4-1BAC-4C46-A86D-ECC7A13DF924.

[27] "The Artemisia genus belongs to subtribe Artemisiinae of tribe Anthemidae from Asteraceae family and comprises more than 500 species," Halina et al., "Significance of *Artemisia Vulgaris*," 4415.

[28] Linda L. Barnes, *Needles, Herbs, Gods, and Ghosts: China, Healing and the West to 1848*: (Cambridge, MA: Harvard University Press, 2009), 23-24.

[29] Henry Huntingdon, *Anglicanus ortus: A Verse Herbal of the Twelfth Century*, ed. and trans. Winston Black (Toronto: Pontifical Institute of Mediaeval Studies, 2012), 79-81.

Therefore, ingredients that brought heat to a woman's body could restore women with gynecological issues including menstrual retention, as discussed above. Mugwort was thus suitable for this heating treatment.

Hildegard of Bingen explains mugwort as possessing a hot nature in her book on natural philosophy, the *Physica*:

> Mugwort (*biboz*) is very hot, and its juice is of very great value. If it is cooked and eaten as a puree, it heals ailing intestines and warms a cold stomach. But, if someone eats or drinks something which has given *them* pain, then *they* should cook and eat warmed mugwort with meat or lard, or as a puree, or with any other condiment. It will attract the rotten matter which was in the previously ingested food or drink, and chase it away. If bad humors gather in some part of the body, flowing out from broken skin where there is no poisoned wound, the person should take mugwort and express the juice. To the juice he should add a smaller amount of honey. *They* should spread this on the afflicted area, then cover it with egg white, and tie it with a cloth. *They* should do this until he is better.[30]

In this passage, mugwort is described as hot in nature and beneficial in general. Primarily, its hot nature and effect of warming a cold stomach are highlighted. Mugwort's characteristic of having a "very warm" nature is an integral part of its efficacy.

Throughout the *Physica*, mugwort frequently appears as a major ingredient. It is often heated on its own or used in a steam bath and is often accompanied by other herbs or ingredients to treat serious diseases such as cancer and strangury (a condition caused by blockage or irritation at the base of the bladder). According to Hildegard, mugwort is beneficial to both men and women. It is used consistently in heating treatments. Here, mugwort is presented as one of the significant herbs to fix reproductive health issues. According to *The Trotula*, claiming Galen as an authority, mugwort effectively regulates the menstrual cycle.[31]

---

[30] Modified from Hildegard of Bingen, *Physica: The Complete English Translation of Her Classic Work on Health and Healing*, trans. Priscilla Throop (Rochester: Healing Arts Press, 1998), 56; italics mine.
[31] Green, *The Trotula*, 77.

More particularly, mugwort in *The Trotula* seems to function in the following ways: providing heat or lessening an immoderately cold condition (especially for women), reducing pain, and stopping severe bleeding after birth. This mixed usage of mugwort is also something found in Asian culture, which will be discussed below. Mugwort is regarded as generally beneficial to health, particularly women's reproductive health. For example, mugwort can benefit women who are experiencing irregular menstruation. It appears among many ingredients used to cure "the paucity of the menses" in *The Trotula*. The authors suggest several ways of using mugwort to draw out menstruation. Women could ingest mugwort with wine after it is heated, and this medication could be traced back to Galen, according to *The Trotula*. Mugwort could be used alone or with any combination of other herbs such as sage, oregano, cumin, and pennyroyal, with their similar warming qualities or emmenagogic virtues. At the same time, women could absorb mugwort or its power in other ways than ingesting it directly. The other treatment consisted of applying powdered mugwort on the belly, probably expecting the woman's womb to receive its properties through her navel or skin. Similarly, mugwort could be dipped in heated bathwater, placed near the navel, or placed in a sack after being heated.[32]

When the authors of *The Trotula* suggest these treatments, there is a warning presented which supports the warming power of mugwort: "But for the woman who frequently makes applications of this kind, it is necessary that she anoints her vagina inside with cold unguents lest she becomes excessively heated."[33] This warning suggests that these herbs and foods and the treatment methods were intended to bring heat to the woman's body, but that excessive heat is also not healthy for women. The key to keeping healthy is finding the right balance between heat and cold and moisture and dryness. Repeatedly, mugwort is listed with other herbs that provoke menstruation in the sections of *The Trotula* "On Retention of the Menses"[34] and "On Paucity of the Menses."[35]

In *The Trotula,* mugwort and its heat were helpful in solving retention of menses caused by lack of heat or excess of cold. Also, mugwort aided difficult births when the birth was delayed or the fetus was dead and

[32] Green, *The Trotula*, 67-68.
[33] Green, *The Trotula*, 69.
[34] Green, *The Trotula*, 77.
[35] Green, *The Trotula*, 79.

remained inside the mother's body. Just as it could provoke menstruation, mugwort was believed to provoke childbirth or delivery of the dead fetus.[36] In other parts of *The Trotula* regarding difficulties of birth, mugwort is prescribed in wine or lupin broth in the case of the dead fetus.[37] These treatments using mugwort all focused on releasing something stuck in the woman's body, whether it is the menses, a living baby, or dead fetus. In this sense, the hot nature of mugwort is beneficial for bringing forth fluids or a fetus which would harm the woman's life if retained. Also, mugwort is mentioned as an ingredient to be taken by the mother-to-be after being heated in wine with other herbs for an easy delivery.[38] It can be ground and mixed with oil and sugar to be placed on the skin near the womb to quicken the delivery of a baby.[39] Most treatments assume that mugwort is hot by nature.

Other than facilitating menstruation and delivery, mugwort could be used on other occasions to help women with pregnancy symptoms, such as lessening the pain after birth. Mugwort was recommended with other herbs, in musk oil or pennyroyal oil, or warmed in a pot, wrapped in a cloth, and inserted as a suppository.[40] Mugwort juice was also recommended with other herbs to stop an immoderate flow of blood.[41] Another usage of mugwort was for impediments to conception. The authors explain that in some cases women cannot conceive due to immoderate heat and dryness, which likely burns up the semen. In such cases, mugwort can be used with cooling substances such as marshmallow, which is known to have a cold nature.[42] The mugwort, then, prevents the woman's body from being cooled too much by the marshmallow treatment because her body still needs a certain level of heat for reproduction. Although *The Trotula* shows somewhat inconsistent usage of mugwort, it seems that its main function is to provide heat to the woman's naturally cold body.[43]

---

[36] Green, *The Trotula*, 82.
[37] Green, *The Trotula*, 101.
[38] Green, *The Trotula*, 105.
[39] Green, *The Trotula*, 103.
[40] Green, *The Trotula*, 161.
[41] Green, *The Trotula*, 125.
[42] Green, "Introduction," in *The Trotula*, 38.
[43] It is noteworthy that mugwort is also referred to as an abortifacient, although this paper does not discuss this aspect. See Elizabeth Ann Conover, "Herbal Agents and over-the-

IV. Fumigation

How can mugwort be used and enter the woman's body, especially the uterus or vagina, if the woman suffers from reproductive issues? In many cultures, fumigation and suppositories are popular methods of delivering mugwort's virtues.[44] Fumigation especially is recommended to bring the uterus back to its original place in the *Gynaikeia*, or "Diseases of Women," part of the *Hippocratic Corpus*[45] when it was believed in ancient tradition and medieval southern Italian medicine that the womb could wander in the woman's body and cause gynecological issues.[46]

Fumigation could be used in many ways, but for gynecological reasons its use was supported by the belief that the fumes could be delivered to the genitals, the place where the patient was suffering. Fumigation was understood as a strong, efficient method of medical intervention by letting the healing materials enter the body and be absorbed. The author of the *Gynaikeia* suggests that women could receive benefits by receiving mugwort smoke directly into their wombs. *The Trotula* explains the procedure: "let it be cooked in a pot and let the woman set a perforated chair over it and let her sit there covered all over and let the smoke come out through a reed, so that the smoke is received

---

Counter Medications in Pregnancy," *Best Practice & Research Clinical Endocrinology & Metabolism* 17, no. 2 (2003), 237-51. The tricky part of this remedy is that often mugwort fumigation appears to provide the patients with coldness. It is also noted that fumigation is recommended for women who cannot conceive due to too much heat, which would burn the semen. Then, the remedy is this: "If she is young and the disease is not chronic, you should aid her in this way: take marsh mallow and mugwort, and cook them in water, and with such a decoction you should fumigate the patient three or four times." The authors recommend this explaining "from the many fumigations the womb receives some strength, smoothness, and softness, and from the benefit of this suppository and these fumigations it will be dried out, and from this medicine should receive some strength. Green, *The Trotula*, 85-86.

44 Eleni Voultsiadou, "Therapeutic Properties and Uses of Marine Invertebrates in the Ancient Greek World and Early Byzantium." *Journal of Ethnopharmacology* 130, no. 2 (2010), 246; for more information on suppositories, see William John Stewart McKay, *The History of Ancient Gynæcology* (London: Baillière, Tindall and Cox, 1901), 281-82.

45 For a detailed explanation of fumigation, see Helen King, "Once upon a Text: Hysteria from Hippocrates," in *Hysteria Beyond Freud*, ed. Helen King, Sander L. Gilman, Roy Porter, G. S. Rousseau, and Elaine Showalter (Berkeley: University of California Press, 2020), 21.

46 Green, "Introduction," in *Trotula*, 26.

inside penetrating through the reed up to the womb."[47] Fumigation made it possible for male doctors to avoid applying ointments directly to the woman's reproductive organs. The patients themselves, or their husbands or friends could conduct this treatment with or without the guidance of doctors.[48]

V. Asian Methods of Using Mugwort

Like medieval European medicine, Korean traditional medicine assumes that mugwort can supply heat to women who are experiencing reproductive issues due to a lack of heat. In Korean traditional medicine, as in medieval Europe, mugwort is believed to have a hot nature, which women lack in general. In traditional East Asian medical theory, women are closer to *yin*, the weaker, wet, dark, and cold nature, while men take more from *yang*, the stronger, drier, bright, and hot nature. The category of *yin* was thought of as inferior to *yang*. As in medieval European medical theory, which can be traced back to Aristotle and Galen, the woman's body was thought of as colder and wetter than the man's. Women's cold and moist nature, too, is understood as inferior to men's generally hot and dry nature.

In Korea, the most popular mode of using mugwort is via ingestion. Korean medicine has several methods for eating and consuming mugwort with food, such as in rice cakes. Mugwort is also heated, dried, and ground into a green powder. It is also used in moxibustion. Moxibustion is a medical practice of burning *moxa*, a dried sponge made of mugwort, on or above the skin, a procedure which is believed to deliver heat and drive away cold, boosting *qi* (or *chi*, "energy") and lessening pain.[49] Mugwort can be taken in various ways, although moxibustion and fumigation are uniquely used for this herb. While the benefits of taking it are varied, it is specifically recommended for women's reproductive health. Moreover, mugwort is spiritually important in East Asian culture. For example, it is believed to have a protective power that can drive away harmful insects or spirits which

---

[47] Green, *The Trotula*, 67.

[48] Jennifer Evans, "Female Barrenness, Bodily Access and Aromatic Treatments in Seventeenth-century England." *Historical Research* 87, no. 237 (2014), 426-27.

[49] Y. Run-Ming, "The Origin and Development of Chinese Acupuncture and Moxibustion." *Ancient Science of Life* 4, no. 4 (1985), 227.

might cause diseases in people.[50] Mugwort also appears in the founding myth of Korea, in which a bear is transformed into a woman after eating garlic and mugwort for a hundred days in a cave, which leads to her marriage to the founder of Korea.[51]

As illustrated in this mythical origin story, mugwort's significance in Korean medicine is of long standing. Let us briefly examine mugwort in the textual tradition of Korea. While Korean traditional medicine was highly indebted to Chinese medicine from the tenth century CE, Korean medicine also developed a distinctive tradition of documents and practices.[52] One of the most popular and well-known premodern medical books is the *Donguibogam* (동의보감, 東醫寶鑑) composed by Heo Jun, a court physician, in 1613.[53] The *Donguibogam* contains general medical information for diagnosing and treating patients, including gynecological topics, while focusing on *qi* and spirits as essential parts of physical health. It introduces various bodily symptoms, preventative methods, and treatments, including specific recipes and medications. As in Galenic humoralism, Heo Jun presents the right balance of hot, cold, dry, and humid properties to be maintained for health. This book was widely circulated and is still popularly used by traditional Korean doctors.[54] In fact, this book was also used by women in the royal courts

[50] Zaehi Kim, "Reinterpretation of Ungnyeo through Eurasian Bear Worship and Mugwort and Garlic from Dangun Myth," *The Korean Folklore* 67 (2018), 44.

[51] Choon H. Do, "Progress of Chemistry in South Korea," *Chemistry International* 37, no. 5-6 (2015), 4-11. This story originated in *Samguk yusa* (*Memorabilia of the Three Kingdoms*), thirteenth-century historical documents. The reason why mugwort and garlic had to be consumed is not clear, but they had been used for medicine, supplying heat to people who ate them. There is another explanation: for a bear to rely on mugwort and garlic is to go through hardship so that it can transform into a human being, which is a higher state than animals. Gunhyuk Park, "Oxidative Damage in Korean Medicine," *Antioxidants* 11, no. 3 (2022), 600.

[52] See Wung-Seok Cha, Jun-Ho Oh, Hi-Joon Park, Sang-Woo Ahn, Se-Young Hong, and Nam-Il Kim, "Historical Difference between Traditional Korean Medicine and Traditional Chinese Medicine," *Neurological Research* 29, no. 1 (2007), 5-9. See also Ng, "The Art of Giving Birth in China," in this volume, on reproductive practices in Middle Kingdom China, and on continuities between the premodern past and the present.

[53] In the Korean naming system, the last name comes first followed by given name; therefore, I keep this system to refer the physician: Heo is his last name and Jun is given name. For more information on this book, see Bong-Keun Song, Jin-Hee Won, and Sungchul Kim, "Historical Medical Value of *Donguibogam*," *Journal of Pharmacopuncture* 19, no. 1 (2016), 16.

[54] Song, Won, and Kim, "Historical Medical Value of *Donguibogam*," 17.

who must have had more limitations than non-elite women in seeing and being examined by male doctors.[55]

The *Donguibogam* sees lack of heat as a major cause of irregular menstruation. As to timing, the *Donguibogam* says that if a woman has a period earlier or more often than her normal cycle, it means that she might have too much heat (13.9.4).[56] Or if she does not menstruate on time, it might mean that she lacks *qi* (13.10). Among many reasons, heat seems a major explanation for irregular menstruation because it interrupts blood flow: "the shift of heat from the small intestine to the large intestine forms abdominal mass and eventually amenorrhea." An annotation states that if the blood is too thick to flow freely, it can also lead to blocked menstruation (13.10.2).[57]

Here Heo Jun says that irregular menstruation can be a symptom of or reason for a complicated pregnancy. Since the woman's body was understood as already cold, if her womb were cold beyond measure, she could not conceive. The treatment is to heat the woman's womb. For this, mugwort is recommended. According to the *Donguibogam*, the treatment would be to make the medication *Mookboohwan* (묵부환, 墨附丸) which contains mugwort as a major ingredient:

> It regulates the menstrual cycle and treats infertility from a cold uterus. Cyperi Rhizoma (香附子) 1 geun (divide into 2 bags and soak in children's urine and rice vinegar for 9 days and after refining, evenly mix with 4 nyang of old mugwort. Prepare by putting the mixture into a porcelain china bowl along with 5 bowls of vinegar and boiling down until it is dry), 2 nyang each of Cnidii Rhizoma (川芎), Angelica Gigantis Radix (當歸), Paeoniae Radix Alba (白芍藥), Rehmanniae Radix Preparata (熟地黃), Rehmanniae Radix

55 e 조선궁중여성. Accessed December 1, 2021. https://terms.naver.com/.

56 "A shorter menstrual cycle means heat in both the qi and blood for which a Four Substances Clear Channels Decoction can be used. A Four Substances Decoction with Bupleuri Radix (**柴胡**), Scutellariae Radix (**黃芩**), and Coptidis Rhizoma (**黃連**) can also be used." Heo Jun, "Donguibogam," 한의학고전 DB, https://www.mediclassics.kr/books/8/volume/3/#content_1130.

57 Heo Jun, "Donguibogam," 한의학고전 DB https://www.mediclassics.kr/books/8/volume/3/#content_1169.

> (生乾地黃), and Myrrha (沒藥), 1 nyang of Succinum (琥珀). Grind up these herbs and knead with vinegar added paste. Form pills as big as the seed of a royal foxglove tree and take 100 pills with a Zingiberis Rhizoma Crudus (生薑) and mugwort decoction on an empty stomach (13.9.6.1).[58]

Even when people are using a variety of herbs and ingredients for improving fertility, the goal of the treatments is to provide women with heat to provoke menstruation using medications mixed with mugwort like Chokyungsan (조경산, 調經散), or "medicine to regulate menstruation" in English.[59]

In a different section, the author introduces treatments for unmarried women who are having uneven menstrual periods, such as *Samsinhwan* (삼신환, 三神丸):

> It treats irregular menstruation and stomachaches in unmarried women. 2 nyang of Citrus Unshius Exocarpium (橘紅), 1 nyang each of Corydalis Tuber (玄胡索) (processed with vinegar), and Angelica Gigantis Radix (當歸) (moistened with wine and stir-fried). Grind up these herbs and knead with wine-added paste to form pills as big as the seed of a royal foxglove tree. Take 100 pills at a time along with a mugwort and vinegar decoction. (13.12.1)[60]

Here, along with other herbs, mugwort is an important ingredient in this recipe. At the same time, it is recommended to take it with wine or vinegar, heated. Since vinegar and wine are also treated as heating, the heating action of mugwort would work even better.

While mugwort fumigation is not explicitly recommended here, mugwort is commonly used to treat menstrual retention, and fumigation facilitates blood and *qi* circulation, or removal of something stuck in the

---

58 Heo Jun, "Donguibogam," 한의학고전 DB https://www.mediclassics.kr/books/8/volume/3/#content_1146.

59 Heo Jun, "Donguibogam," 한의학고전 DB www.mediclassics.kr/books/8/volume/3/#content_1133.

60 Heo Jun, "Donguibogam," 한의학고전 DB https://www.mediclassics.kr/books/8/volume/3/#content_1217.

body such as feces or a blockage of the throat, benefiting longevity because it provides heat.[61] It should be noted that the Korean understanding of fumigation is more complicated than the European practice explained above. It is not simply treating specific organs, such as the womb in the matter of menstrual retention, but it aims to enhance the general physical condition of the patient. If any medication including mugwort ignores the overall condition of the body, it might fail to help the patient.

How are women making use of this premodern textual knowledge now? An interesting use of mugwort today is in fumigatory treatment, which has many similarities with the treatment described in the *Trotula*. 쑥훈증(燻蒸), "mugwort fumigation" in English, is popular in Korean traditional medicine. Even though doctors examine patients and perform mugwort fumigations on them, women can use a simplified method without visiting a doctor. Women can have their own personal facilities for fumigation at home, or they can receive treatments in a public sauna. According to popular belief, mugwort is thought to have a hot nature without serious side effects, which makes it easy for patients to use.[62] While there are different kinds of mugwort, *Artemisia vulgaris* is believed to work best for women's diseases.

The most apparent and desired effect of mugwort fumigation is to return menstruation to a normal cycle. However, mugwort is believed to help solve many female diseases and symptoms. According to a 2008

[61] Alternatively, there is one fumigation treatment to stop their wives from having intercourse with ghosts in their dream: "It [Benzoinum] cures women having sexual intercourse with ghosts in their dreams. Mix with Realgar (雄黃) and make pills. Burn it and fumigate on the pubic area, and she will not have such dreams. 《本草》" https://www.mediclassics.kr/books/8/volume/2/#content_505; "Therefore, warming the navel to strengthen the stem is like a plant growing spontaneously after being supplied with water and earth. When the person always warms the navel in the right way, defense and nutrients become harmonized, and the corporeal and ethereal souls become stable. Therefore, the heat or cold cannot invade the person, and the body becomes light and strong and thus wondrous inside, https://www.mediclassics.kr/books/8/volume /7/#content_837.

[62] Kwang-Ok Lee, Sun-Bok Jang, and Ji-Soo Yoo, "Content Analysis of Wormwood Smoke (Ssukjahun) Experiences in Women," *Journal of East-West Nursing Research* 14, no. 1 (2008), 74.

Korean study, "Content Analysis of Wormwood[63] Smoke (Ssukjahun) Experience in Women," fifteen women beyond their twenties reported that they expected various effects from fumigation including curing vaginitis, cramps, insomnia, leukorrhea, and other diseases; preventing miscarriages; and enhancing blood circulation. Their reported experiences during the treatment included sweating, cleaning, mind settling, disinfection, and heat. After the treatment, the women reported that they experienced good skin, reduced leukorrhea, muscle relaxation, weight loss, increased energy, and better sleep. Although they had side effects such as blisters, pains, headaches, or pimples, most women understood these as part of the health effects[64] as Korean traditional medicine assumes that recovery is accompanied by *Myunghyun Symptom* (瞑眩現狀), the discharging of negative energies or humors out of one's body.[65]

Women experiencing menstrual retention might have an even greater lack of heat; therefore, their bodies lose the balance of the cold and became wetter. Therefore, Korean folk medicine, with Chinese medicine as its basis, focused on supplying the needed heat to troubled women to restart menstruation, which in turn was understood as inducing a healthy state for reproduction. According to Korean traditional medicine, mugwort is believed to contain heat which is necessary for fertility and fumigation is seen as an effective way to deliver its heat to the womb so that women can have regular menstruation and safe child delivery.

VI. Conclusion

In both European and Asian medical traditions, mugwort was believed to supply heat that was already lacking in healthy women and even was

---

[63] In Korea, different herbs in the genus *Artemisia* are used interchangeably and historically recognized as one herb "Ssuk 쑥" not distinguished by its different kinds. Kim, "Reinterpretation of Ungnyeo through Eurasian Bear Worship and Mugwort and Garlic from Dangun Myth," 43-45; the most common herbs are *Artemisia vulgaris* (mugwort) and *Artemisia montana Pampan* or *princeps* (wormwood).

[64] Lee, Jang, and Yoo, "Content Analysis of Wormwood Smoke (Ssukjahun) Experiences in Women," 68-77.

[65] Yong-Jae Jeong, "A Sasang Constitutional Study on the Myunghyun Symptom," *Journal of Sasang Constitutional Medicine* 21, no. 1 (2009), 20-27.

more insufficient in women during menstruation. Fumigation with mugwort was a particularly popular treatment, believed to deliver the needed element or energy of heat deep inside the body. The assumption that the fumes of mugwort can enter through the vagina, reach the womb, and bring the herb's elemental heat to the woman's body also shows that the woman's body was reckoned as more permeable or weaker than a man's. Mugwort fumigation treatment can help us rethink how a woman's sexual or reproductive body was understood in medieval medicine and cosmology. Lastly, I suggest that comparing this herbal treatment in two different cultures can help fill in the gaps between Western Europe and East Asia. Recent studies have shed light on the medieval transmission of medical knowledge across Eurasia, as exemplified in the Dunhuang manuscripts or in Malay humoralism.[66] Also, the documents from the al-Sham region (part of modern Syria) list plants from East Asia in their *materia medica* during the Middle Ages and Ottoman period, showing the active transportation of pharmaceutical ideas, practices, and materials.[67] The circulation of mugwort and beliefs concerning it in the medieval world should be researched further.

As this essay has shown, parallels and resonances can be found between uses and understandings of mugwort in medieval European treatments and modern Korean medicine. While mugwort is used for various reasons, its major effect is to provide heat to female patients suffering from lack of it. While some European medicine assumed that mugwort works as an emmenagogue or abortifacient as it could bring menstruation back with its hot nature, so even modern mugwort supplements warn women not to take it during pregnancy to avoid miscarriages, which supports the heating power of mugwort. In Western

[66] Ronit Yoeli-Tlalim examines the Central Asian and Tibetan traditions to uncover the medical theories and practices transmitted between Europe and Asia, mainly based on the Judeo-Arabic manuscripts discovered in the Dunhuang library cave. The author argues for the common topos of medicine encompassing Persian, Greek, Syrian, and Arabic in the premodern world. See Ronit Yoeli-Tlalim, *ReOrienting Histories of Medicine: Encounters along the Silk Roads* (New York: Bloomsbury Publishing, 2021), 29-30. Carol Laderman introduces the Malay pregnancy-related rituals and beliefs combined with Chinese, Ayurvedic, and Islamic premodern medicine, representing direct interactions between different cultures. Carol Laderman, "A Welcoming Soil: Islamic Humoralism on the Malay Peninsula," in *Paths to Asian Medical Knowledge*, ed. Charles Leslie and Allan Young (Berkeley: University of California Press, 1992), 272-290.

[67] Efraim Lev, "Reconstructed *Materia Medica* of the Medieval and Ottoman al-Sham," *Journal of Ethnopharmacology* 80, no. 2-3 (2002), 176.

medieval medicine, the hot properties of mugwort encourage blood flow in women, which is to be avoided when their womb needs to keep the fetus. Korean traditional medicine has different recommendations for mugwort, sometimes encouraging the mother-to-be to take it, saying that it will prevent miscarriages, and sometimes discouraging its use, which shows the more general beliefs that mugwort can prevent excessive bleeding and treat women's diseases in general.[68]

This chapter is not advocating for the efficacy of mugwort fumigation. Instead, it has examined both how women's bodies were understood and defined, and how women took care of their bodies, in medieval European and Asian cultures. When a woman's body was understood as having reproductive issues due to a lack of heat, there were ways of providing the needed heat to the woman's sexual organs. As seen in the mugwort recipes and fumigation described above, this herb has been popularly used in Western and Eastern medicine as a way of delivering heat to the deepest parts of the woman's body to secure its reproductive functions.

While the woman's body was already understood to be colder than the man's in European and Asian premodern medicine, women could have difficulties having children, even suffering life-threatening events, such as serious delays in delivery or a dead fetus retained in the womb, due to immoderate coldness in their body. According to *The Trotula* from premodern European gynecology and the *Donguibogam* from premodern Asian medicine, these issues associated with the coldness of the woman's body could be resolved by mugwort with its warming nature. Women in both cultures used mugwort through fumigation, ingestion, moxibustion, cooked with wine, soaked in a bath, placed near the womb, and mixed with other ingredients, showing its highly variable applications. Granted that there are differences in the range of uses, the two medical traditions suggest that mugwort was considered throughout premodern Eurasia as a warming ingredient, particularly helpful to women, whose naturally cold bodies needed sufficient heat for safe reproduction. While mugwort in European medicine is no longer a major medicinal herb, it has survived and is still widely used in East Asia as a traditional remedy or in a modern form as a medical supplement, continuing to help women with a range of health issues.

68 Su-Noh Ryu and Sam Sik Kang, "Analysis of Available Component in Artemisiae Herba," *Korean Journal of Crop Science* 49 (2004), 174.

FOR TO CAUSE A WOMAN TO HAVE MILK: RECIPES TO PROMOTE LACTATION FOR MEDIEVAL AND MODERN WOMEN

KRISTIN USCINSKI*

For to cause a woman to have milk.
Take vervain and drink it with wine
or fennel and eat lettuce
and butter and drink wine with fennel seed.
Or take (a) crystal and break it and
make powder thereof and
drink it with milk.

– 15th-century English medical recipe from Bodleian Library,
Ashmole 1447, fol. 99 (authorial translation)

I. Introduction

This recipe, designed to provoke lactation in medieval women, raises many questions in under fifty words. How common was the complaint it purports to address? Why would medieval women seek recipes meant to increase lactation? Why fennel, why lettuce, why vervain? What was the significance of these ingredients to the recipe user? How accessible would they have been to an English woman in the fifteenth century when

* Department of History, SUNY Purchase College.

this recipe manuscript was compiled? And finally, what do we do with these remnants of medieval medical practice today when so many negative medievalisms surround medieval medical theory and practice, and when testing for clinical efficacy in medieval recipes is difficult at best?

Women can be remarkably difficult to see in medieval sources, particularly in the world of scholastic and professional medical care, but recipes provide significant insight into the relationship between this elite medical tradition and the uncredited home practitioner. As Sara Ritchey has pointed out, we need to "heed the trace" of women's participation in medical practice, even if we cannot see women directly in the source material.[1] Prefaces to medieval recipe collections, and references in the recipes themselves, point to women's presence in treatments for obstetrical and gynecological conditions, as well as those that deal with female anatomy – women's medicine.[2] Some of these may have been products of literary tropes, aimed at legitimizing men's authority over women's intimate conditions.[3] But there are still many clues that indicate the likelihood of female involvement.

---

[1] Sara Ritchey, *Acts of Care: Recovering Women in Late Medieval Health* (Ithaca: Cornell University Press, 2021), 1-24.

[2] For examples of medical texts known to be owned by individual medieval women and medical texts commissioned by and/or addressed to women, see Richard Aspin, "Queen Isabella's Regimen of Health," *The Wellcome Library,* 17 June 2022, http://blog.wellcome library.org/2017/01/queen-isabellas-regimen-of-health/; Green, "The Possibilities of Literacy and the Limits of Reading: Women and the Gendering of Medieval Literacy," in *Women's Healthcare in the Medieval West: Texts and Contexts* (Aldershot: Ashgate, 2000), 1-76, at 49-57, 62-69. For discussion on female and male users of the text *The Sickness of Women* and a discussion on the text as intended for direct use by women due to its content, its circulation in small codices in the vernacular, which were the type of medical manuscript most often known to have been owned by women, see Monica H. Green and Linne R. Mooney, "The Sickness of Women," in *Sex, Aging, and Death in a Medieval Medical Compendium: Trinity College Cambridge MS R.14.52, Its Texts, Language, and Scribe,* ed. M. Teresa Tavormina (Tempe, AZ: Arizona Center for Medieval and Renaissance Studies, 2003), 455-568, at 463, 473-74; Monica Green, "Obstetrical and Gynecological Texts in Middle English," *Studies in the Age of Chaucer,* 14 (1992): 53-88. Green and Mooney take care to point out that there are no "marks to confirm female ownership" on either of these two manuscripts (BL Sloane 249 and Royal College of Surgeons MS 129) but nevertheless seem confident that the possibility that women used them was very real.

[3] Monica Green, *Making Women's Medicine Masculine: The Rise of Male Authority in Pre-Modern Gynaecology* (New York: Oxford University Press, 2008), 220-25.

The predominantly botanical nature of medieval recipe ingredients means that some ingredients could be found in the domestic garden and others were available for purchase.[4] Once these ingredients were gathered, the methods and equipment required for women's recipes indicate that they were easy to make and drew on skills and utensils that overlapped with those of the ordinary medieval kitchen.[5] The chopping, mixing, heating and pounding called for in medical recipes were also the tasks of medieval kitchens. And the most logical person to proficiently wield these skills was the one most likely to be in the kitchen: a woman. No special equipment is specified in Ashmole 1447 – and many medical recipe collections like it – because the recipe user was assumed to be already familiar with these tasks and could use their own judgment to get it done. The same social expectations that placed women in the home as domestic caretakers also positioned them squarely in the kitchen, the most sensible location for the production of medical recipes.[6]

Taken together, all these recipe elements – ingredients, methods, production locations, and modes of access – impart a clearer picture of women's involvement in matters of health. Women's practice of domestic medicine using medical texts was increasingly likely by the later Middle Ages, when the general consumption of medical literature had grown, as had the likelihood of its presence in a wider variety of medieval

[4] Jerry Stannard, "Alimentary and Medicinal Uses of Plants," in *Medieval Gardens,* ed. Elisabeth B. MacDougall (Washington, DC: Dumbarton Oaks, 1986), 69-92; Stannard, *Herbs and Herbalism in the Middle Ages and Renaissance* (London: Routledge, 1999); see also Stannard, "STANBIS (STannard's ANnotated Bibliographical Information System)" (University of Kansas Libraries, Spencer Research Library, 1952-1988), accessed 30 May 2022, https://archives.lib.ku.edu/repositories/3/resources/3443.

[5] The equipment, skills, and personnel of the medieval kitchen have been illuminated by Peter Brears, *Cooking and Dining in Medieval England* (Devon: Prospect Books, 2008); C. M. Woolgar, *The Culture of Food in Medieval England, 1200-1500* (New Haven: Yale University Press, 2016); Terence Scully, *The Art of Cookery in the Middle Ages* (Rochester: The Boydell Press, 1995).

[6] Jennifer Ward, *Women in Medieval Europe, 1200-1500* (New York: Routledge, 2016), 19, 74. Medieval women's connections to food and cooking have been part of the dialogue on gender and authority since Carolyn Walker Bynum first argued that women's role in the production of food was one of their primary expressions of control: Carolyn Walker Bynum, *Holy Feast, Holy Fast: The Religious Significance of Food to Medieval Women* (Berkeley: University of California Press, 1987).

households and in the vernacular.[7] Recipe users need not necessarily have been only lettered individuals; and women were not invariably illiterate. Medieval literacy went beyond the ability to put pen to paper and included more than just reading and writing.[8] The pursuit of recipe collecting in the early modern period, associated most with women, has firm roots in medieval England, where women were involved in both the supply and demand of medical recipes.[9] Women who were exposed to the content of recipe collections were predisposed to making those recipes, most especially the ones which affected them directly.

Even the most detailed medieval medical recipes are usually too vague to enable either replication or determination of efficacy. How fine should that crystal be powdered? How many fennel seeds? How much wine? Similarly, one woman's lettuce may be another woman's spinach. Even if medieval recipes meant lettuce when they wrote lettuce, the plants of fifteenth-century England are not the same as those that grew in the twelfth-century medical center at Salerno, nor are they the same as those growing today, making choosing a chemically identical plant impossible,

---

[7] Elizabeth Dearnley, "'Women of Oure Tunge Cunne Bettir Reede and Vnderstonde This Language': Women and Vernacular Translation in Medieval England," in *Multilingualism in Medieval Britain (c.1066-1520)*, eds. Judith A. Jefferson and Ad Putter (Turnhout: Brepols, 2013), 259-72. For the increase in vernacularization of medical and scientific texts, see Päivi Pahta and Irma Taavitsainen, "Vernacularisation of Scientific and Medical Writing in Its Sociohistoric Context," in *Medical and Scientific Writing in Late Medieval English*, eds. Irma Taavitsainen and Päivi Pahta (Cambridge: Cambridge University Press, 2004), 1-22.

[8] Joyce Coleman, "Aural Illumination: Books and Aurality in the Frontispieces to Bishop Chevrot's *Cité de Dieu*," in *Orality and Literacy in the Middle Ages: Essays on a Conjunction and its Consequences in Honour of D. H. Green* (Turnhout: Brepols, 2005), 223-252, at 223; Coleman, *Public Reading and the Reading Public in Late Medieval England and France* (New York: Cambridge University Press, 1996), 34-51; Ruth Crosby, "Oral Delivery in the Middle Ages," *Speculum* 11 (1936): 88-110, at 88; Cheryl Glenn, "Medieval Literacy Outside the Academy: Popular Practice and Individual Technique," *College Composition and Communication* 44, no. 4 (1993): 497-508, at 498; Rosamund McKitterick, *The Uses of Literacy in Early Medieval Europe* (New York: Cambridge University Press, 1990), 2-3; Brian Stock, *The Implications of Literacy: Written Language and Models of Interpretation in the Eleventh and Twelfth Centuries* (Princeton: Princeton University Press, 1983), 7.

[9] Monica Green, "The Possibilities of Literacy and the Limits of Reading: Women and the Gendering of Medieval Literacy," in *Women's Healthcare in the Medieval West,* 46; see also Elaine Leong, "Collecting Knowledge for the Family: Recipes, Gender and Practical Knowledge in the Early Modern English Household," *Centaurus* 55, no. 2 (2013), 81-103.

to say nothing of amounts used or precise methods followed.[10] Trying to match modern diagnoses with medieval ones also has its problems.[11] A recipe to help with sore breasts might have been used to address a variety of health complaints. And of course, finding a recipe written out does not tell us whether it was used, if it functioned as its author claimed it could, or what other recipes existed that never got written down.

These questions may never be fully answered, but they remain productive to ask. Medieval authors considered a range of factors when deciding which recipes to place in collections: pharmacological efficacy, the effect a person's emotions and diet could have on the body, ritual tradition, as well as ease of transmission and execution. It is feasible to consider these as therapeutic possibilities without imposing modern scientific standards on the indefinite elements of medieval recipes – while remembering that some modern and medieval cures bear a close resemblance.

Many of the same ingredients from the Ashmole 1447 recipe appear in modern galactagogues, remedies designed to promote lactation. What we now know about their chemical composition, moreover, confirms their positive effects on breastfeeding. As will be discussed below, fennel, and to a lesser extent vervain, are ingredients in modern remedies designed to help women with lactation. Eating a balanced diet, abounding in leafy greens, is frequent advice in online medical forums like La Leche League and Healthline, not to mention in the many (many) "mommy blogs" and communities to be found on the internet.[12] Even

[10] Helen King, "Why I Wasn't Excited About the Medieval Remedy That Works Against MRSA," *The Conversation*, 9 April 2015, accessed 30 May 2022, https://theconversation.com/why-i-wasnt-excited-about-the-medieval-remedy-that-works-against-mrsa-39719.

[11] Monica Green has rightly noted that recent generations of historians are averse to using modern scientific categories of disease and have largely avoided "retrospective diagnosis." Monica Green, "Editor's Introduction to *Pandemic Disease in the Medieval World: Rethinking the Black Death,*" in *Pandemic Disease in the Medieval World: Rethinking the Black Death,* ed. Monica Green (Kalamazoo: ARC Medieval Press, 2015), 9-26, at 15.

[12] Diana Cassar-Uhl, "Feeding the New Mother," *La Leche League International,* accessed 20 May 2022, www.llli.org/feeding-the-new-mother/; Natalie Gingerich Mackenzie, "How to Eat a Healthy Breastfeeding Diet," *The Bump,* accessed 20 May 2022, www.thebump.com/a/breastfeeding-diet; Jessica Timmons, "Galactagogues: 23 Foods That Increase Breast Milk," medically reviewed by Valinda Riggins Nwadike, MD, Ph.D., *Healthline,* accessed 2 February 2021, www.healthline.com/health/parenting/galact

crystals have their supporters, and the placebo effect does have recognized clinical value.

Medieval lithotherapy was often a serious affair in the scientific and medical community, which stemmed from classical tradition and incorporated much of the same medical theory as herbal cures.[13] The inclusion of crystals in a medieval recipe does, however, tend to trigger the sort of incredulity that haunts the history of medicine. It is certainly true that occasionally medieval recipe users were instructed to say a string of thaumaturgic nonsense syllables that may or may not resemble liturgical Latin, perhaps eat the item it was written on, or wear animal parts as talismans.[14] A quick Google search for medieval medicine yields no shortage of articles, ever-fond of the itemized list, hyping "weird," "crazy," and "horrifying" medieval treatments "that will make your stomach turn" – things like owls burnt to a powder and animal dung being used as topical treatments and hot irons applied to hemorrhoids,[15]

---

agogues#Your-breastfeeding-diet; "10 Foods to Nourish Breastfeeding Moms," *Mom365,* accessed 20 May 2022, www.mom365.com/baby/breastfeeding/10-foods-to-nourish-breastfeeding-moms.

[13] John Riddle, "Lithotherapy in the Middle Ages: Lapidaries Considered as Medical Texts," *Pharmacy in History* 12, no. 2 (1970), 39-50.

[14] A recipe for a woman whose child is dead in the womb: "[L]et these names be written on cheese or butter: '+ sa. e. op. ab. z. po. c. zy. e pe . pa. pu. c. ac. sator arepo tenet os pera rotas,' and let them be given to eat." Monica H. Green, ed. and trans., *The Trotula: An English Translation of the Medieval Compendium of Women's Medicine* (Philadelphia: University of Pennsylvania Press, 2001), 80. A recipe for contraception: "also take pyones seed w(i)t the heert of the mulys ere & medyl hem to gyd(er) & put hem in a gyrdyl a but it & sche schall nat conseyve as long as sche berythe hit upon her;" [Also take peony seeds with the heart of the mule's ear and muddle them together and put them in a girdle about it and she shall not conceive as long as she wears it.] Royal College of Physicians, MS 411, fol. 94v.

[15] "Crazy Potions and Nasty Nostrums: Six Bizarre Medieval Medicines," *History on the Net,* accessed 17 June 2022, www.historyonthenet.com/crazy-potions-and-nasty-nostrums-six-bizarre-medieval-medicines; Esh, "9 Horrifying & Weird Medieval Medical Practices," *Medium.com*, 16 January 2021, accessed 17 June 2022, https://medium.com/lessons-from-history/9-horrifying-weird-medieval-medical-practices-8188901ae45; Stephanie Schoppert, "8 Medical Practices from Medieval Times That Will Turn Your Stomach," *History Collection,* 16 March 2017, accessed 30 May 2022, https://historycollection.com/medieval-medical-practices-sure-turn-stomach/; Adam Wenger, "11 Old Medical Treatments That Will Make Your Stomach Turn. Including Heroin for Kids!" *Healthline*, 1 September 2017, accessed 30 May 2022, www.healthline.com/health/old-medical-treatments-make-your-stomach-turn. For medieval medicine as presented in the

or perhaps ingesting powdered crystals to promote lactation. People like to be horrified at the past, to feel better about their present. These sites tend not to explain medieval rationales and do not emphasize the more relatable aspects of medical practice, which make up the bulk of the evidence.

Medieval medical recipes have extraordinary potential to reveal the practice of medicine and medieval perceptions of the body and disease. In this chapter, I use recipes for lactation to highlight the commonality between medieval and modern women and to demonstrate the fragility of these negative medievalisms. The following discussion draws on my database of 1960 recipes for women's healthcare in medieval England, compiled as a representative sample of recipes for women's health from over fifty recipe collections, written in Latin, Middle English, and Anglo-Norman, and disseminated in England from the twelfth through the early sixteenth centuries. For the first time in one place, there are hundreds of recipes that show us a larger picture of women's healthcare. My **M**edieval **E**nglish **R**ecipes for **W**omen's **H**ealthcare database (abbreviated hereafter as MERWH) draws on unedited manuscripts currently in England at the British, Bodleian, and Wellcome Libraries, as well as those in the collections of Trinity College, Cambridge, and Magdalene College, Cambridge, and the Royal College of Physicians in London. Also included are recipes from three well-known edited collections—the *Trotula* Ensemble, *The Sickness of Women*, and *The Knowing of Woman's Kind in Childing*—which provide a comparative framework for other texts such as *Agnus Castus, Macer Floridus de Viribus Herbarum, The Alphabet of Galen*, and Hildegard of Bingen's *Physica* which discuss specific properties of the ingredients themselves. [16] Analyzing recipes from women's recipe collections, herbal texts, and from anonymous, general recipe collections using a quantitative database is a new methodology for examining the genre of medical recipes. Such an approach considerably augments our understanding of medieval health and medicine by categorizing the

fictional world, see Robin S. Reich, "The Fantasy of Medieval Medicine: Orientalizing Experiential and textual Traditions in the Imagined Medieval Past" and for popular perceptions compared to the archaeological record of medieval surgery, see Claire Burridge, "Early Medieval Surgery: Challenging Popular Stereotypes with Archaeological Evidence," in this volume.

[16] Kristin Uscinski, "Recipes for Women's Healthcare in Medieval England," PhD diss., (Fordham University, 2017), Appendix D.

conditions, applications, and ingredients in recipes for women's health. This also makes it possible to see what conditions received the most attention, what ingredients were popular, what cures were considered efficacious, and how these cures were made. Overall, botanical ingredients account for almost half of MERWH recipes, and fennel, vervain, and lettuce make frequent appearances across all women's recipes.[17] Crystals are there too, but only rarely, and in the case of the Ashmole 1447 recipe, they are offered as an alternative.[18] These recipes for lactation were potentially accessible to a meaningful portion of the medieval English population – and there was great need for them.

II. Modern Lactation and the Efficacy of Medieval Remedies

Today, we understand that many factors may be responsible for an insufficient milk supply, from thyroid conditions to heart disease, to even a cleft palate – but insufficient nutrients could certainly be to blame.[19] Modern medicine has shown that the mother's diet does, in fact, have an effect on breastmilk production and composition.[20] Breastmilk production relies on glucose, amino and fatty acids and folates, minerals, and a range of vitamins, all of which flow from the mother's blood into cells of the mammary glands and to the infant.[21] Zinc, copper, and iron play important roles in growth, metabolic and neurological function, sexual development, and the health of the blood , and are best passed via breastmilk to an infant through the mother's

[17] Fennel appears in 80 recipes, vervain 51, and lettuce 25; Uscinski, "Recipes for Women's Healthcare in Medieval England," Appendix D.

[18] Crystals appear in 15 recipes; Uscinski, "Recipes for Women's Healthcare in Medieval England," Appendix D.

[19] Jacqueline C. Kent, Daneille K. Prime, and Catherine P. Garbin, "Principles for Maintaining or Increasing Breast Milk Production," *The Association of Women's Health, Obstetric, and Neonatal Nurses,* 41 (2012), 114-21, at 116; Ruth Lawrence and Robert Lawrence, *Breastfeeding: A Guide for the Medical Profession,* 7th edition (Maryland Heights, MO: Elsevier, 2011), 114-121, at 116.

[20] Jacqueline C. Kent, "How Breastfeeding Works," *The American College of Nurse-Midwives,* 52: 6 (2007), 564-570, at 564.

[21] Kent, "How Breastfeeding Works," 564; see also A. M. Smith, M. F. Picciano, and R. H. Deering, "Folate Supplementation During Lactation: Maternal Folate Status, Human Milk Folate Content, and Their Relationship to Infant Folate Status," *Journal of Pediatric Gastroenterol Nutrition* 2, no. 4 (1983), 622.

dietary intake.[22] Lactating women require more potassium – an electrolyte that works to maintain osmotic pressure, neural impulse transmission, muscle contractions, cardiovascular function, and regulates blood pressure – than non-lactating individuals because this mineral is secreted through the breastmilk.[23] Without adequate potassium – or indeed any of these vitamins and minerals – the mother's body is compromised.

Medieval recipes for lactation often call for ingredients we now know to be rich in the above minerals and vitamins, which points to the possibility of an awareness of health benefits, even without the same understandings of the biomechanics behind them. The humoral theories of Hippocrates and Galen dominated the medieval scholastic medical tradition, which in turn informed dietary considerations and medicinal cures. Most ancient authors, from Aristotle on, believed lactation to be a byproduct of pregnancy, a transformation of menstrual blood into breastmilk.[24]

Care of the whole person had to be considered, and this theoretical approach to medicine was manifested in everyday life, such as in choice of food, drink, and exercise. Soranus' *Gynecology* recommends that, if disease was not the cause of an unsatisfactory milk supply, the lactating woman should do things that exercised the upper half of her body, take baths, and eat "food which has wholesome juices."[25] The Cleveland Clinic agrees: "a healthy, well-balanced diet is key" to successful breastfeeding.[26] Galen's *On the Power of Food* includes fennel in a list of bitter herbs that can be found in culinary books, as it has properties useful to both physicians and cooks. Lettuce, he writes, is considered a

---

[22] Yun Kyung Choi, et al., "Association of Maternal Diet with Zinc, Copper, and Iron Concentrations in Transitional Human Milk Produced by Korean Mothers," *Clinical Nutritional Research* 5, no. 1 (2016), 15-25.

[23] Daniela Storm, et al., "Revised Reference Values for Potassium Intake," *Annals of Nutrition and Metabolism* 71, no.1-2 (2017), 118-124.

[24] Belle Tuten, "Lactation and the Breast in Antiquity: Medical Authorities on Breast Health and Treatment," *Quaestiones Medii Aevi Novae* 19 (2014): 159-186, a 164-169.

[25] Soranus, *Soranus' Gynecology*, trans. Owsei Temkin (Baltimore: The Johns Hopkins University Press, 1956), 102.

[26] "Foods to Eat While Breastfeeding: A Healthy, Well-Balanced Diet is Key," *The Cleveland Clinic*, 11 October 2021, accessed 1 June 2022, https://health.cleveland clinic.org/breastfeeding-diet/.

vegetable "superior to all others" by physicians. It has the best juices and produces a lot of blood without affecting the other humors.[27]

Humoral theory was the principal governing medical theory in medieval Europe, persisting into the early modern and modern eras, in both gynecological and obstetric medicine.[28] Understood in terms of their humoral pathology, remedies operated in opposition to the illnesses they aimed to treat and according to the baseline of the individual's humoral complexion.[29] The remedies medieval breastfeeding women sought are largely comprised of rather ordinary, readily accessible herbs and foods such as fennel, vervain, lettuce, butter, and wine in the recipe from Ashmole 1447. A version of this recipe appears fifteen times in MERWH.[30] Many anonymous medieval English recipe collections are bare-bones, and they do not often explain the reasoning behind each ingredient. Because of this, other medieval medical texts such as *The Alphabet of Galen, Macer Floridus, Agnus Castus,* Hildegard of Bingen's *Physica,* and *The Trotula* – all of which apply classical medical theory in some way – help to clarify the thinking behind these ingredient choices.

Fennel (*Foeniculum vulgare*) is a plant from the carrot family. Indigenous to the Mediterranean basin and India, it has been naturalized in many parts of the world, including Northwestern Europe, where it grows wild.[31] *The Alphabet of Galen*, a seventh-century pharmacological

[27] Mark Grant, "On the Powers of Foods: Book 2," in *Galen on Food and Diet* (New York: Routledge, 2000), 109-153, at 138, 144.

[28] Frederick W. Gibbs, *Poison, Medicine, and Disease in Late Medieval and Early Modern Europe* (New York: Routledge, 2019), 1-38; Nichola E. Harris, "Loadstones are a Girl's Best Friend: Lapidary Cures, Midwives, and Manuals of Popular Healing in Medieval and Early Modern England," in *The Sacred and the Secular in Medieval Healing: Sites, Objects, and Texts,* ed. Barbara S. Bowers and Linda Migl Keyser (New York: Routledge, 2016), 182-218, at 182-83; Etienne van de Walle, "Flowers and Fruits: Two Thousand Years of Menstrual Regulation," *Journal of Interdisciplinary History* 28, no. 2 (1997), 183-203, at 186; Stanley W. Jackson, *Melancholia and Depression: From Hippocratic Times to Modern Times* (New Haven: Yale University Press, 1986), 116-246.

[29] Thomas F. Glick, "Communication," in *Medieval Science, Technology, and Medicine: An Encyclopedia*, eds. Thomas Glick, Steven J. Livesey, and Faith Wallis (New York: Routledge, 2005), 135-39, at 137.

[30] Occasionally, this recipes appears with the addition of celandine, which could be either Greater or Lesser Celandine, plants that are not botanically related; "celandine, n.," *OED Online* (Oxford University Press, 2022), accessed 1 June 2022, https://www-oed-com.avoserv2.library.fordham.edu/view/Entry/29399?redirectedFrom=celandine.

[31] Maud Grieve, *A Modern Herbal, Volume I A-H* (New York: Dover Publications, 1971), 293-297, at 293.

text that went on to have a long medieval life, claims that fennel was common and quite useful in many medicines.[32] Hildegard of Bingen, the twelfth-century visionary nun and philosopher, claimed that fennel had many health benefits, from improving digestion to helping a person sleep.[33] Neither *The Alphabet* nor Hildegard make any mention of fennel's effect on lactation, but "The Book on the Conditions of Women" from the *Trotula* ensemble does recommend porridges made of bean flour, rice, or wheat bread with milk, sugar, and a little fennel seed.[34] Macer Floridus's *De Viribus Herbarum* and *Agnus Castus,* both popular herbal texts in medieval England, recommend fennel as a treatment for stomach, ear and eye complaints, as well as a galactagogue.[35] In North American folk medicine, fennel is perceived to increase a woman's milk supply.[36] Fennel, along with dill and ginger, is a common ingredient in modern "gripe water," which is designed to calm infant digestion.[37] In MERWH, fennel appears in 80 recipes, in conditions that echo all these complaints, making it one of the most popular medieval ingredients.[38]

Vervain, or verbena, (*Verbena officinalis*) is another widely distributed plant. In England, it grows along roadsides and in pastures and has been around since at least the early Middle Ages.[39] *The Alphabet of Galen,* Macer Floridus, and Hildegard likewise tout the healing powers of vervain, but

---

[32] *The Alphabet of Galen: A Critical Edition of the Latin Text with English Translation and Commentary,* ed. and trans. Nicholas Everett (Toronto: University of Toronto Press, 2012), 230-231. This text exists in manuscripts dating from the seventh through the eleventh centuries, and the text appears to be based on ancient Greek medicine, rather than medieval; *The Alphabet of Galen,* trans. Everett, 5-6.

[33] Hildegard of Bingen, *Hildegard von Bingen's Physica: The Complete English Translation of Her Classic Work on Health and Healing,* trans. Priscilla Throop (Rochester, VT: Healing Arts Press, 1998), 39-41.

[34] Green, ed. and trans., *The* Trotula, 85.

[35] Gösta Frisk, *A Middle English Translation of* Macer Floridus de Viribus Herbarum (Lundequistka: University of Bokhandein, 1949), 88; Gösta Brodin, *Agnus Castus: A Middle English Herbal Reconstructed from Various Manuscripts* (Upsala: Ludequist, 1950),157-158.

[36] Gabrielle Hatfield, *Encyclopedia of Folk Medicine; Old World and New World Traditions* (Santa Barbara, CA: ABC-CLIO, 2004), 48.

[37] Korin Miller, "What to Know About Using Gripe Water for Colic and Tummy Trouble," *The Bump*, 2021, accessed 11 May 2022, www.thebump.com/a/gripe-water.

[38] Uscinski, "Recipes for Women's Healthcare in Medieval England," Appendix D. 26 recipes for lactation call for fennel.

[39] Maud Grieve, *A Modern Herbal,* II, 831-832.

make no mention of its effect on lactation.[40] However, vervain turns up in 51 MERWH recipes, in a variety of complaints and in 16 recipes for lactation, which indicates that a lot of people believed in its efficacy.[41] Usually combined with fennel and some liquid – either the juice of the vervain itself, wine, or water – vervain drunk "often" will give a woman "milk enough."[42] As is the case for fennel, modern clinical studies have shown that vervain contains therapeutic elements, such as antioxidants, and breastmilk itself contains a high level of antioxidants.[43] Breastfeeding requires a lot of energy, and antioxidants, which neutralize free radicals in the body, and help the body to replenish nutrients.[44] In the 1930s, Maud Grieve's *Modern Herbal* claimed that, like fennel, vervain had a reputation for its health benefits, which include aiding fevers, the eyes, and being a good galactagogue, and in 2020, La Leche League was still recommending it.[45]

[40] *The Alphabet of Galen,* trans. Everett, 317; Frisk*, A Middle English Translation of* Macer Floridus de Virius Herbarum, 169-172; Hildegard of Bingen, *Hildegard von Bingen's Physica,* trans. Throop, 75. *Agnus Castus* does not include vervain.

[41] Uscinski, "Recipes for Women's Healthcare in Medieval England," Appendix D.

[42] Ashmole 1438, fol. 23: "For a woman Þat faileth mylke take the iuse of vervayne or of fenell and drynke it ofte and sche shall have mylke ynowge;" Uscinski, "Recipes for Women's Healthcare in Medieval England," Appendix D.

[43] Pawel Kubica, et al., "*Verbena officinalis* (Common Vervain) – A Review of the Investigations of This Medically Important Plant Species," *Planta Medica* 86 (2020), 1241-57, at 1245-51. The full list of properties and benefits include: antioxidant effect, antibacterial effect, antifungal activity, anti-inflammatory effect, local analgesic effect, anticonvulsant, anxiolytic, and sedative effects, sleep promoting activity, neuroprotective effect, antidepressant effect, cardiovascular effects, antiproliferative and anticancer effect, acceleration of wound healing, gastroprotective properties, and prevention against spread of dangerous insect-borne diseases. For verbena having a reputation as a galactagogue but with no clinical studies to support this claim, see: "Vervain," in *Drugs and Lactation Database (LacMed)* (Bethesda, MD: National Library of Medicine, 2006, updated 2021), accessed 3 February 2021, www.ncbi.nlm.nih.gov/books/NBK501852/; Sevda Yuksel, et al., "Oxidant and Antioxidant Status of Human Breast Milk During Lactation Period," *Dairy Science and Technology,* 95 (2015), 295-305.

[44] "Understanding Antioxidants," *Harvard Medical School: Harvard Health Publishing,* 1 Jan. 31 2019, accessed 1 June 2022, www.health.harvard.edu/staying-healthy/ understanding-antioxidants#app; "When Breastfeeding, How Many Calories Should Moms and Babies Consume?" *NIH US Department of Health and Human Services,* 31 Jan. 2017), accessed 1 June 2022, www.nichd.nih.gov/health/topics/breastfeeding/conditioninfo/calories.

[45] Grieve, *A Modern Herbal, Volume II,* 832; Frank J. Nice and Mary Francell, "Selection and Use of Galactagogues," *La Leche League,* 26 June 2020, accessed 2 June 2022, www.llli.org/selection-and-use-of-galactagogues-2/.

The last botanical ingredient of our lactation recipe, lettuce, (*Lactuca sativa* or *Lactuca virosa*) could be a whole host of leafy plants, such as spinach, which is occasionally referred to as "wild lettuce."[46] Hildegard has three different lettuces in her *Physica:* domestic lettuce (*latich*), prickly lettuce (*lactuca agrestis*), and wild lettuce (*wilde latich*), with domestic lettuce being the only variety she considered suitable for eating.[47] Common lettuce (*Lactuca sativa*) does have many therapeutic benefits to recommend it: it is high in fiber, iron, folate, and Vitamin C, and has anti-inflammatory properties. Red lettuces have higher phenolic compounds than green lettuces, which act as antioxidants and reduce the incidence of certain chronic diseases.[48] And, of course, leafy greens are frequently recommended for a healthy lifestyle today, as they were recommended for humoral regulation in the Middle Ages. Some herbal texts claim that *Lactuca virosa,* or wild lettuce, resembles a weak opium and is often used as a mild sedative and a pain reliever.[49] Both *Agnus Castus* and *Macer Floridus* recommend it as a galactagoue.[50] Modern *Lactuca virosa* is a bitter type of lettuce and looks more like a dandelion than a head of lettuce, but in medieval recipes without visual aids or descriptions, there is no knowing which lettuce variety was meant or chosen. Modern audiences, too, recognize the health benefits of various types of leafy greens. But dietary trends vary – in the United States, the popularity of kale has dropped from its mid-2014 high, whereas romaine consumption is up –

---

[46] Grieve, *A Modern Herbal,* II, 761-762. Spinach is in the Middle English Dictionary; "endive (n.)," and "spinache (n.)," *Middle English Compendium* (University of Michigan, 2000, revised 2018), accessed 3 February 2021, https://quod.lib.umich.edu /m/middle-english-dictionary/dictionary/MED13703/track?counter=1&search_id=5433264, https://quod.lib.umich.edu/m/middle-english-dictionary/dictionary/MED4221 5/track?counter=9&search_id=5433264.

[47] Hildegard of Bingen, *Hildegard von Bingen's* Physica, trans. Throop, 48-49. Prickly lettuce (*Lactuca serriola*) is related to common lettuce. Wild lettuce's binomial name is *Lactuca virosa.* Hildegard says that prickly lettuce is a weed and can be injurious (though good for an ass that has pain in its stomach, or a person who has scrofula) and that wild lettuce may be used to quench a person's lust.

[48] Moo Jung Kim, et al., "Nutritional Value, Bioactive Compounds and Health Benefits of Lettuce (*Lactuca satvia* L.)," *Journal of Food Composition and Analysis* 49 (2016), 19-34, at 19; Derong Lin, et al., "An Overview of Plant Phenolic Compounds and Their Importance in Human Nutrition and Management of Type 2 Diabetes," *Molecules* 21, no.10 (2016), 1374.

[49] Grieve, *A Modern Herbal,* I, 476-478.

[50] Brodin, *Agnus Castus,* 172; Frisk, *A Middle English Translation of* Macer Floridus de Viribus Herbarum, 90.

leafy greens, especially the dark varieties, are touted for their high vitamin content and nutritional benefit.[51] In MERWH, lettuce is recommended in 25 recipes, primarily for lactation, but also soreness in the breast, for uterine and menstrual complaints, and during childbirth.[52] We do not have sufficient evidence to know which plant was chosen when making any of these recipes, but the benefits of all these varieties were largely understood in both medieval and modern contexts. Healthline, an online provider of health and medical articles with over 200 million views per month, mentions twenty-three foods, including dark leafy greens, fennel and fennel seed, and the catch-all categories fresh fruits and vegetables, plant and animal protein sources, and high-quality fats.[53] Hilary Jacobson, a popular lactation consultant approved by the La Leche League, recommends fennel, vervain, and lettuce in her book, *Mother Food,* to promote lactation.[54]

Beyond their nutritional content, fennel, lettuce, and vervain also have been found to contain calming, sedative properties.[55] Medieval

---

[51] Amanda Mull, "The Kale Crazy Might Be Ending: The Saddest Leafy Green," *The* Atlantic, 30 September 2019, www.theatlantic.com/health/archive/2019/09/why-kale/599041/; Lin Yan, "Dark Leafy Vegetables," USDA Agricultural Research Service, accessed 20 May 2022, www.ars.usda.gov/plains-area/gfnd/gfhnrc/docs/news2013/dark-green-leafy-vegetables/.

[52] Uscinski, "Recipes for Women's Healthcare in Medieval England", Appendix D.

[53] Timmons, "Galactagogues: 23 Foods That Increase Breast Milk;" see also "About," *Healthline,* accessed 2 February 2021, https://www.healthline.com/about.

[54] Hilary Jacobson, *Mother's Milk: A Breastfeeding Guide with Lactogenic Foods and Herbs – Build Milk Supply, Boost Immunity, Lift Depression, Detox, Lose Weight, Optimize a Baby's IQ, and Reduce Colic and Allergies* (Ashland, OR: Rosalind Press, 2004), 8, 21, 146.

[55] A. Allen and Gabrielle Hatfield, *Medicinal Plants in Folk Tradition: An Ethnobotany of Britain and Ireland* (Portland: Timber Press, 2004); Grieve, *A Modern Herbal, Volume I and II,* 293-97, 831-32; See also: Michelle A. Kominiarek, "Nutritional Recommendations in Pregnancy and Lactation," *The Medical Clinics of North America* 100, no. 6 (2016): 1199-1215; Katherine D. McManus, "Should I Be Eating More Fiber?" *Harvard Medical School* (Harvard Health Publishing, 2019), accessed 2 February 2021, www.health.harvard.edu/blog/should-i-be-eating-more-fiber-2019022115927; "Listing of Vitamins," *Harvard Medical School* (Harvard Health Publishing, 2009, updated 2020), accessed 2 February 2021, www.health.harvard.edu/staying-healthy/listing_of_vitamins; "Recommended Daily Allowances and Adequate Intakes, Vitamins," *National Institute of Health,* accessed 2 February 2021, www.ncbi.nlm.nih.gov/books/NBK56068/table/summarytables.t2/?report=objectonly; "Zinc Fact Sheet for Health Professionals," *National Institute for Health* (2020), accessed 4 February 2021, https://ods.od.nih.gov/factsheets/Zinc-HealthProfessional/#en2; Afshan Abbas, et al., "The Fennel, Foeniculum vulgare

medical tradition and therapeutics centered around care of the entire person, and both rest and attention to one's emotional state were understood to have a significant effect on the body.[56] This is not news to most people today, either. Certainly, a mother's stress level and exhaustion do play a role in inhibiting breastmilk production. Mothers of infants in ICUs who experienced decreased breastmilk experienced 63 per cent more milk after one week of relaxation techniques that reduced their anxiety.[57] Foods that contain anti-inflammatory properties can also have a real impact on maternal mental health and consequently the experience of breastfeeding.[58]

Fennel, vervain, and lettuce are the true botanical stars of the medieval lactation recipes, with wine, milk, and butter often appearing in conjunction, either to make the remedy taste appealing, as part of the medical benefit – or perhaps both.[59] Classical medical tradition heralded

---

incorporated diet shows anxiolytic potential: A pre-clinical study," *Pakistan Journal of Pharmaceutical Sciences* 32, no. 4 (2019), 1813-19; Hae Dun Kim, et al., "Sleep-inducing effect of lettuce (*Lactuca sativa*) varieties on pentobarbital-induced sleep," *Food Science Biotechnology* 26, no. 3 (2017), 807-14; Kubica, et al., "*Verbena officinalis* (Common Vervain), 1245-1251; Ranjana Das and Chiranjib Bhattacharjee, "Lettuce," in *Nutritional Composition and Antioxidant Properties of Fruits and Vegetables*, ed. Amit K. Jaiswal (Cambridge, MA: Academic Press Elsevier, 2020), 143-57.

56 Peregrine Horden, "A Non-Natural Environment: Medicine without Doctors and the Medieval European Hospital," in *The Medieval Hospital and Medical Practice,* ed. Barbara S. Bowers (Burlington: Ashgate, 2007), 133-46, at 134-37, 139.

57 Stephen D. K. Feher, et al., "Increasing Breast Milk Production for Premature Infants With a Relaxation/Imagery Audiotape," *Pediatrics* 83, no. 1 (1989): 57-60, here 57. The most commonly self-reported reasons that women stop breastfeeding center around concerns about infant nutrition and satisfaction and the mother's perception of insufficient milk supply – though work-life reasons and low income may also play a role; Ruowei Li, et al., "Why Mothers Stop Breastfeeding: Mothers' Self-Reported Reasons for Stopping During the First Year," *Pediatrics* 122, no. 2 (2008), 569-76, at 569, 571-72.

58 Kathleen Kendall-Tackett, "A new paradigm for depression in new mothers: the central role of inflammation and how breastfeeding and anti-inflammatory treatments protect maternal mental health," *International Breastfeeding Journal* (2007), accessed 2 June 2022, https://rdcu.be/cOQCw.

59 While wine was not produced widely in medieval England, there was a steady demand for it, beyond its links to elite and religious culture. There were vineyards in England from the eleventh to the fifteenth centuries, but "their produce was modest and not necessarily of a high quality; Woolgar, *The Culture of Food in England*, 52-55. As early as the twelfth-century, it was imported from Rouen, and later Bordeaux and Gascony, and its tunnage was almost consistently in the tens of thousands; Melitta Weiss Adamson, *Food*

the many therapeutic benefits of wine.[60] In Greek medicine, wine was utilized for the betterment of the sick in a variety of remedies, many of which were related specifically to women.[61] Many remedies take the form of drinks, either because of their palatability alone, their therapeutic properties, or because of the influence of the Hippocratic belief that medicines were better received in drink than in food.[62] With its capacity to cool fevers and serve as a purgative, wine was used extensively in the Middle Ages as well, both medicinally and as part of nutritional management, what Latin physicians termed *regimen*.[63]

---

in Medieval Times (Westport, Connecticut: Greenwood Press, 2004), 50; Susan Rose, *The Wine Trade in Medieval Europe, 1000-1500* (New York: Bloomsbury Publishing, 2011), 67-68; Tim Ulwin, *Wine and the Vine: An Historical Geography of Viticulture and the Wine Trade* (New York: Routledge, 1991, 1996), 184. One tun of wine was approximately equal to 250 gallons. Wine imports took a dive in between 1346-1348 due to war and plague; Rose, *The Wine Trade in Medieval Europe,* xvi, 67; Ronald Edward Zupko, *British Weights and Measures: A History from Antiquity to the Seventeenth Century* (Madison, WI: University of Wisconsin Press, 1977), 30. Adamson notes that wine was a drink common to both higher and lower classes in the Iberian Peninsula, France, and Italy.

[60] Hippocrates warned that too much wine could cause a head- or stomachaches. Galen cautioned that wine could adversely affect the liver, spleen, and upper chest. He remarks that wine is "naturally warming" and would heal any part of the body suffering from cold. He tells his readers how to use wine in various medicinal capacities, both edible and topical, and what the types of wine are appropriate for which constitutions; Everett, *The Alphabet of Galen*, trans. Everett, 371-73; Hippocrates, "Regimen in Acute Diseases," in *Hippocratic Writings,* ed. G. E. R. Lloyd, trans. J. Chadwick and W. N. Mann (London: Penguin Books, 1978, 1983), 186-205, at 195, 199-200; Jacques Jouanna, "Wine and Medicine in Ancient Greece," in *Greek Medicine from Hippocrates to Galen: Selected Papers*, trans. Neil Allies, ed. Philip van der Eijk (Boston: Brill, 2012), 173-194, at 179. The ancient Egyptians also found wine to be medicinally valuable for improving coughs and gout; P. A. Norrie, "The History of Wine as a Medicine," in *Wine: A Scientific Exploration,* eds. Merton Sandler and Roger Pinder (New York: Taylor and Francis, 2003), 21-56, at 21-23.

[61] Hippocrates' *Nature of Women* prescribes wine for provoking menstruation; those women who experience red discharges should drink very little, but what they do drink should be dark, undiluted wine; Jouanna, "Wine and Medicine in Ancient Greece," 184.

[62] Hippocrates, *Hippocrates, vol. 2*, trans. W. S. H. Jones (Cambridge: Harvard University Press, 1967), 111; see also R. A. Buck, "Women's Milk in Anglo-Saxon and Later Medieval Medical Texts," *Neophilologus* 96 (2012), 467-95, at 474.

[63] The *Regimen Sanitatis* of Salerno specificies that wine, drunk in moderation, could aid in digestion; Joannes de Mediolano, *Regimen Sanitatis Salerni, Or The Schoole of Salernes Regiment of Health* (London: B. Alsop, 1649), 55-56; Norrie, "The History of Wine as a Medicine," 27.

Wine was a ubiquitous commodity in medieval England. It was a standard ingredient in culinary texts, and as a beverage, was more commonly – though not exclusively – drunk by the upper classes.[64] For those of lesser means, wine could still be within reach. Wine that had passed its prime was sold off cheaply and quickly as newer vintages were imported.[65] Wine was also sold in urban establishments by the cup, so buying a small amount for a medical concoction was certainly within reach of more than just the wealthy. Medieval expenditures on medicines tended to be higher than our own,[66] and a working-class person could have justified spending on an important recipe ingredient. Few of those offering advice to nursing women today would recommend wine as part of a lactation remedy, but you can still find Guinness recommended for its supposed breastfeeding benefits.[67]

Dairy products, like milk and butter, were also believed to have therapeutic value. *The Alphabet of Galen* discusses butter, made from cows

64 Woolgar, *The Culture of Food in England,* 53-55. At minimum, wine is used in culinary recipes 10 percent of the time, 40 percent max, and often around 20 percent. Wine use in culinary recipes peaked in the fifteenth century, where after use drops to 15 percent of recipes in the sixteenth century. Laurioux suggests that this statistic might be dubious due to manuscripts being written in verse; and so wine may have suffered due to the need to rhyme; Bruno Laurioux, *Une histoire culinaire du Moyen Âge* (Paris: Honoré Champion Éditeur, 2005), 233, 235. Even though it was available, wine could be expensive, both to produce and to consume. Voyages were long – often dangerous – and the wine did not tend to last terribly long. Aside from production costs, wine's price was driven up by various trading costs such as freight, cooperage expenses, cellarage labor, and especially war; Ulwin, *Wine and the Vine,* 188.

65 Margery James, *Studies in the Medieval Wine Trade* (New York: Clarendon Press, 1971), 7; James does not say just how cheap this wine was, but she emphasizes that the highly perishable nature of the product meant that wine dealers were eager to offload and sell what they could. Rose writes that wine hovered between 6*d.* and 8*d.* a gallon in the mid-fourteenth century. Thorold Rogers lists wine between 8*d.* and 10*d.* per two gallons in Cambridge between 1410 and 1491, respectively; James E. Thorold Rogers, *A History of Agriculture and Prices in England from the Year After the Oxford Parliament (1259) to the Commencement of the Continental War (1793), Volume III (1401-1582)* (Oxford: Clarendon Press, 1882), 510, 513.

66 Paul Freedman, *Out of the East: Spices and the Medieval Imagination* (New Haven: Yale University Press, 2008), 68-69.

67 If there are health benefits to Guinness, it seems they come from the hops, which can help produce prolactin, rather than the alcohol. As early as the 1900s, Guinness' supposed health benefits were being touted as part of a marketing campaign; Emma Bryce, "Should Breastfeeding Women Really Drink Guinness?" *LiveScience,* accessed 3 August 2021, www.livescience.com/63122-breastfeeding-moms-guinness-beer.html.

or sheep. The best butter, according to *The Alphabet*, comes from sheep, has a slightly red color, and is very fatty. This butter contains loosening properties helpful in specifically female complaints.[68] Hildegard wrote that butter was beneficial to a healthy person.[69] Lactating women were not considered to be suffering from a disease, but within the humoral tradition, the female complexion was considered colder and moister than men's, which explained both women's supposed timid temperaments, as well as their particular conditions.[70] In the *Regimen* literature as well as later medieval culinary texts, mild dishes often omitted fats, onions and spices, all items that were considered to be too hot for, and thus irritating to, a person's complexion.[71] But, for a woman seeking to balance her cold and moist complexion, these things could be helpful. Milk was considered wholesome and appears often in medical recipes, conceivably because of its humorally moderate nature and its ready availability. Both butter and milk contain essential vitamins, as well as calcium, potassium, and protein.[72] Milk, especially, is high in calcium, Vitamin D, and omega-

---

[68] Butter is helpful for vaginal pain and swelling and "similar complaints in other sensitive and delicate areas;" Everett, *The Alphabet of Galen,* trans. Everett, 175.

[69] Hildegard of Bingen, *Physica,* trans. Priscilla Throop, 83-84.

[70] Nancy G. Siraisi, *Medieval and Early Renaissance Medicine: An Introduction to Knowledge and Practice* (The University of Chicago Press, 1990), 102-103; Green and Mooney, eds., "The Sickness of Women," in *Sex, Aging, and Death in a Medieval Medical Compendium,* ed. Tavormina, 485. Galen believed that women were less perfect than men because of their cold nature; Vern L. Bullough, "Medieval Medical and Scientific Views of Women," *Viator* 4 (1973), 485-501, at 492. For other medieval remedies designed to treat women's conditions in medieval Western and Asian traditions, see also Minji Lee, "How to Treat a Woman's Cold and Porous Body: Mugwort Fumigation for Fertility in Medieval and Modern Folk Medicine of Western and Asian Cultures" and Wee Siang Margaret Ng, "The Art of Giving Birth in Middle Period China," in this volume.

[71] Terence Scully, "The Sickdish in Early French Recipe Collections," in *Health, Disease and Healing in Medieval Culture,* eds. Sheila Campbell, Bert Hall, and David Klausner (New York: St. Martin's Press, 1992), 132-40, 134-35; Johanna Maria van Winter, "Medieval Recipes for Invalid Food," in *Spices and Comfits: Collected Papers on Medieval Food* (Totnes: Prospect Books, 2007), 355-60, at 356. Scully lists wine as part of this list of items irritating to the complexion. Carole Rawcliffe mentions wine in her list of items given to hospital patients in London. Not all hospital patients were necessarily ill, however, but it was understood that the infirm stood a better chance of recovery if they were fed nourishing, plentiful, and easy foods – which in this case, included wine; Carole Rawcliffe, "Hospitals of Later Medieval London," *Medical History* 28, no. 1 (1984), 1-21, at 13.

[72] Kominiarek, "Nutritional Recommendations in Pregnancy and Lactation," 1199-1215; "Listing of Vitamins;" "Recommended Daily Allowances and Adequate Intakes, Vitamins."

3 fatty acids and is often recommended for its nutritive value, especially in online advice forums for those breastfeeding infants, even though there is little evidence that dairy positively alters the content of breastmilk.[73]

With the possible exception of wine, these ingredients have much to recommend them to the lactating mother and infant. But what about that pulverized crystal? This, too, fit into a larger framework of humoral theory, and stones were often believed to have healing properties based on their natural composition, a tradition which extends back to antiquity and forward into our own time.[74]

In the twelfth century, Hildegard of Bingen wrote that crystals were pure substances of great strength, able to cure diseases of the eyes, heart, and belly. Crystals could also reduce swelling and pain, and Hildegard recommends them for all these complaints.[75] Stones worked just like plants and food. They operated under the same logical framework of humoral theory and were utilized in many medieval medical contexts, where they were largely crushed and ingested as medicines.[76] In the modern West, there are infused teas available that claim to bring the "healing powers" of crystals into your life – but the bulk of the industry centers around topical applications and absorbing the crystals' energies

---

[73] María Achón, et al. "Effects of Milk and Dairy Product Consumption on Pregnancy and Lactation Outcomes: A Systematic Review," *American Society for Nutrition* 10, Supplement no. 2 (2019), S74-S87; Tian C., "Can Drinking Milk While Breastfeeding Help to Produce Milk?" *Parenting.firstcry.com*, 15 October 2018, accessed 17 June 2022, https://parenting.firstcry.com/articles/can-drinking-milk-while-breastfeeding-help-to-produce-more-milk/. The Mayo Clinic advises to make healthy choices in one's diet and names dairy as a protein rich food but makes no claims about dairy specifically increasing breastmilk production; "Breast-feeding Nutrition: Tips for Mom," *Mayo Clinic,* accessed 17 June 2022, www.mayoclinic.org/healthy-lifestyle/infant-and-toddler-health/in-depth/breastfeeding-nutrition/art-20046912. Some online advice forums actually say to avoid dairy because it can make the infant gassy, but Johns Hopkins says this is more of a myth; Diane Vizthum, "5 Breastfeeding Diet Myths," *Health: Johns Hopkins Medicine,* accessed 17 June 2022, https://www.hopkinsmedicine.org/health/wellness-and-prevention/5-breastfeeding-diet-myths.

[74] Harris, "Loadstones are a Girl's Best Friend," 183; Nichola E. Harris, "The Idea of Lapidary Medicine: Its Circulation and Practical Applications in Medieval and Early Modern Europe," PhD diss., (Rutgers University, 2009), 197-200; Riddle, "Lithotherapy in the Middle Ages," 39-40.

[75] Hildegard of Bingen, *Hildegard von Bingen's* Physica, trans. Throop, 153-54.

[76] Riddle, "Lithotherapy in the Middle Ages," 39-40.

by matter of proximity.[77] The crystal industry has seen a boom since the onset of the COVID-19 Pandemic, with jewelers reporting a surge in demand from customers seeking the comforting energy of quartz, amethyst, and topaz.[78] The healing properties of stones can be found in New Age lapidary literature, available for purchase online, as well as in the corner pharmacy, in sunscreens and vitamin supplements and cosmetics.[79] While the therapeutic value of some of these claims may be disputed, lithotherapy has not gone away.

The expectation that someone might be helped by ingesting crystals could have had a real effect on a woman's physical state via her mental one, an idea rooted in modern science, in the placebo effect and expectancy theory. Placebos have been shown to have beneficial effects, by what scholars have called the "altering [of] the therapeutic environment."[80] The expectation that a drink containing crystals would

---

[77] Amethyst Crystal Tea, accessed 20 May 2022, https://www.crystalvaults.com/shop-crystals/420001/; Colleen McCann, "8 Crystals for Better Energy," *Goop*, accessed 31 May 2022, https://goop.com/wellness/spirituality/the-8-essential-crystals/; Muang' Akili Tugmakvu, "Who Was Marcel Vogel? From IBM Researcher to a Crystal Healer," *Medium*, 22 December 2021, accessed 31 May 2022, https://medium.com/broader insights/who-was-marcel-vogel-a9430f8c11e3.

[78] Alexandra Cheney, "Why the Renewed Interest in Crystals? The Pandemic," *The New York Times*, 26 January 2022, https://www.nytimes.com/2022/01/26/fashion/jewelry-crystals-jacquie-aiche-beverly-hills-california.html. This renewed interest has no doubt worsened the inhumane conditions of many miners; Tess McClure, "Dark Crystals: the Brutal Reality Behind a Booming Wellness Craze," *The Guardian*, 17 September 2019, accessed 31 May 2022, www.theguardian.com/lifeandstyle/2019/sep/17/healing-crystals-wellness-mining-madagascar.

[79] Harris, "The Idea of Lapidary Medicine," 198-200.

[80] Mayberg et al. begin by saying that there is "little debate as to the power of the placebo effect;" Helen S. Mayberg, et al., "The Functional Neuroanatomy of the Placebo Effect," *The American Journal of Psychiatry* 159, no. 5 (2002), 728-37, at 728 and 734; see also: Nicholas Humphrey, "Great Expectations: the Evolutionary Psychology of Faith-Healing and the Placebo Effect," in *The Mind Made Flesh: Essays from the Frontiers of Psychology and Evolution* (New York: Oxford University Press, 2002), 255-88; Daniel E. Moerman, *Meaning, Medicine, and the 'Placebo Effect'* (Cambridge: University of Cambridge Press, 2002), 7-22. Preliminary neuroimaging studies on patients administered inert medicines have shown activation in the same brain centers that non-placebo medicines also triggered, instigating the same analgesic responses; Fabrizio Bendetti et al., "Neurobiological Mechanisms of the Placebo Effect," *The Journal of Neuroscience* 25, no. 45 (2005): 10390-402, at 10393. On medieval placebo effects, see: Judith Wilcox and John M. Riddle, "Qustā ibn Lūqā's Physical Ligatures and the Recognition of the Placebo Effect, With an Edition and Translation," *Medieval Encounters* 1:1 (1995), 1-50.

promote lactation could have itself triggered a neural chain reaction that ultimately caused the bodily response sought by the recipe.[81] And belief in lapidary medicine does still exist: crystals are endorsed by the British Flower and Vibrational Essences Association, which claims that, through their vibrations, crystals have real strengthening, supportive, and empowering effects.[82] Healthline echoes this sentiment, noting that American adults are increasingly turning to complementary and alternative medicines,[83] either because they see no harm in trying or they have been persuaded – by their own experience or others' – that these things really do work.

Medieval recipes and modern, despite their different theoretical underpinnings, overlap in their recommendations, and the benefits for promoting breastmilk production were – and are – potentially many. There are a few drugs, sold under the brand names of Reglan and Motilium, that have been shown in a clinical setting to increase breastmilk production.[84] In the United States, Reglan, which is a form of

[81] Howard Brody, "Ritual, Medicine, and the Placebo Response," in *The Problem of Ritual Efficacy,* eds. William S. Sax, Johannes Quack and Jan Weinhold (New York: Oxford University Press, 2010), 151-69, at 155.

[82] The British Flower and Vibrational Essence Therapy Association (BFVEA), *Welcome to the Website of the British Flower and Vibrational Essences Association* (2020), accessed 4 February 2021, www.bfvea.com/. Cancer Research U.K. has a section on essence therapy, including crystals, and though they are careful to point out that essences to not prevent, control, or cure cancer, many people do claim to find essences helpful and they provide some short advice on using essences safely. "Essence Therapy," (2019), accessed 4 February 2021, www.cancerresearchuk.org/about-cancer/cancer-in-general/treatment/complementary-alternative-therapies/individual-therapies/essence-therapy.

[83] Emily Rekstis, "Healing Crystals 101," medically reviewed by Debra Rose Wilson (2018, updated 2019), accessed 4 February 2021, www.healthline.com/health/mental-health/guide-to-healing-crystals.

[84] Jennifer Ingram, et al., "Metoclopramide or domperidone for increasing maternal breast milk output; a randomised controlled trial," *Archives of Disease in Childhood-Fetal and Neonatal Edition,* 97:4 (2012): F241-F245, at F241; "Reglan (Metoclopramide Hydrochloride) NDA #017862, Injectable; Injection," *Drugs @FDA-Approved Drugs,* accessed 31 January 2021, www.accessdata.fda.gov/scripts/cder/daf/index.cfm?event=overview.process&ApplNo=017862. For the latest label insert for Reglan, see: "Reglan (Metoclopramide Hydrochloride) NDA #017854, Tablet; Oral, Labeling-Package Insert, SUPPL-62, 08/29/2017," *Drugs @FDA-Approved Drugs,* accessed 31 January 2021, https://www.accessdata.fda.gov/scripts/cder/daf/index.cfm?event=overview.process &ApplNo=017854; "FDA Talk Paper: FDA Warns Against Women Using Unapproved Drug, Domperidone, to Increase Milk Production," *U.S. Food and Drug Administration,* 18

metoclopramide, is approved by the Food and Drug Administration (FDA) only for nausea, migraines, and gastroparesis. When it is used for lactation, it is off-label. Motilium is a form of domperidone. It is not approved for use in the United States, while in Canada and the United Kingdom it is similarly used off-label as a galactagogue. Modern women, like medieval women, continue to seek out remedies for a common concern. Most clinical studies on fennel, vervain, and lettuce are inconclusive; however, the interest is there.[85] The community network site Reddit has over 70,000 members in its r/Breastfeeding forum, and the r/beyondthebump forum has fifty-five conversations on breastfeeding with hundreds of comments.[86] We may never know if a medieval remedy "worked" by modern medical criteria, but we do not need to in order to understand the commonality between medieval and modern medical practice.

III. Recipes for the Breast and for Lactation

Medieval recipes for women's breasts are often related to breastmilk production or cessation, although many also deal with sores, aches, and abscesses as well as issues related to size and texture. Women's breasts were the subject of many medieval concerns, several of which were addressed in the recipe collections, and these recipes represent a

---

April 2016, accessed 31 January 2021, https://www.fda.gov/drugs/information-drug-class/fda-talk-paper-fda-warns-against-women-using-unapproved-drug-domperidone-increase-milk-production; Kent, Prime, and Garbin, "Principles for Maintaining or Increasing Breast Milk Production," 117; see also Eliza Shapiro, "Breastfeeding Pills' Risky Results," *The Daily Beast*, 7 August 2021, updated July 13, 2017, accessed 31 January 2021, https://www.thedailybeast.com/breastfeeding-pills-risky-results; "Domperidone General Information," *Canadian Breastfeeding Foundation,* accessed 31 January 2021, www.canadianbreastfeedingfoundation.org/induced/domperidone_general.shtml.

[85] Katarzyna Budzynska et al., "Systematic Review of Breastfeeding and Herbs," *Breastfeeding Medicine* 7:6 (2012), 489-503, at 497, 499-500; Antonio Alberto Zuppa, et al., "Safety and Efficacy of Galactagogues: Substances that Induce, Maintain, and Increase Breast Milk Production," *Journal of Pharmaceutical Science* 1:2 (2010), 170-71; see also Alessandra N. Bazzano et al., "Health Provider Experiences with Galactagogues to Support Breastfeeding: A Cross-Sectional Survey," *Journal of Multidisciplinary Healthcare* 9 (2016), 623-30.

[86] r/breastfeeding, *Reddit,* accessed 2 February 2021, www.reddit.com/r/breastfeeding/; r/beyondthebump, *Reddit,* accessed 2 February 2021, www.reddit.com/search/?q=breastfeeding%20r%2Fbeyondthebump.

significant portion of women's complaints and conditions related specifically to them.[87]

The majority of lactation recipes (approximately 84 percent of total recipes for conditions of the breast in MERWH) are designed to address a deficiency in milk or to stimulate its production.[88] Though there was some debate over when an infant should begin breastfeeding, Hippocratic tradition considered the lactating woman to be in a healthy state.[89] In addition to the physical benefits, breastfeeding can serve social and psychological functions, such as bonding between mother and child or require the employment of a wet nurse.[90] Several recipes for lactation appear to indicate that they were meant for wet nurses, such as these:

> [F]or the nurse Þ(a)t wolde yeve mylke. Take vervane & drynke it w(i)t wyght wyne or fenel & ete letuse and buttre and drynke wyne w(i)t fenel seed or take cristal & breke it & make powd(er) Þ(er)of and drynke it wyth mylke. [91]

---

87 There are 184 recipes out of a total 1960 in MERWH (or 9.4%), which deal with the complaints and conditions of women's breasts, such as aches, sores, pains, inflammation, swelling and conditions related to size and texture. There are 93 recipes (or 4.7%) which deal with lactation. Three of these recipes have a stated intention of being both for the breasts and lactation; Kristin Uscinski, "Recipes for Women's Healthcare in Medieval England," PhD diss., (Fordham University, 2017), Appendix D. See also Belle Tuten, "Care of the Breast in the Late Middle Ages," in *Gender, Health and Healing, 1250-1550,* ed. Sara Ritchey & Sharon Strocchia (Amsterdam: Amsterdam University Press, 2020), 119-38.

88 In MERWH, there are 59 recipes that address milk insufficiency and 19 that address milk deficiency. In addition to these 78 recipes, there are 4 which address a clogged duct and one which addresses thick milk; Uscinski, "Recipes for Women's Healthcare in Medieval England," Appendix D.

89 Helen King, "Motherhood and Health in the Hippocratic Corpus: Does Maternity Protect Against Disease?" *Mètis Anthropologie des Mondes Grecs Anciens* 11 (2013), 51-70, at 62. According to humoral theory, after birth, the blood that had been nourishing the fetus was sent to the breasts where it then was turned into breastmilk; Buck, "Women's Milk in Anglo-Saxon and Later Medieval Medical Texts," 476. Soranus did not believe newborn infants should receive their mother's milk until twenty days after birth, whereas Avicenna should begin right away; Soranus, *Soranus' Gynecology*, trans. Temkin, 88-89; H.D. Modanlou, "Avicenna (AD 980 to 1037) and the Care of the Newborn Infant and Breastfeeding," *Journal of Perinatology* 28 (2008), 3-6, at 5.

90 Avner Giladi, "Breast-feeding in Medieval Islamic Thought," *Journal of Family History* 23, no. 2 (1998), 108-109. Though Avner's article focuses mostly on the Islamic world, he does address practices in medieval Europe as well.

91 Trinity College Cambridge O.1.13, fol. 170v. This fifteenth-century recipe from Trinity College Cambridge MS O.1.13 appears in a miscellany that includes treatises on herbs, husbandry and the zodiac, as well as medical and culinary recipes.

> [For the nurse that would give milk. Take vervain and drink it with white wine or fennel; and eat lettuce and butter; and drink wine with fennel seed; or take crystal and break it and make it into a powder and drink [the powder] with milk.]
>
> For a noirse Þat defauteÞ melke. Þe norissh Þat defauteÞ mylke shal ete ofte or drynke fenel or Þe iuse; so shal she haue mylke y-nowe.[92]
>
> [For a nurse that lacks milk. The nurse that lacks milk shal eat often or drink fennel or the juice. So shall she have milk enough.]

Different versions of this recipe indicate that it could be used by either a wet nurse or any breastfeeding mother. In recipes for lactation, "woman" is used more than twice as often as "nurse."[93] This could be an indication of an interchangeable vocabulary, where "nurse" may have meant either "nursing mother" or wet nurse, although these were uncommon in England. Proof-of-age inquests (legal documents that include men's recollections of the events surrounding the births of heirs to crown lands) show that it was customary for the English gentry and nobility to be wet-nursed from the late twelfth through the late fifteenth centuries, but there is not as much evidence for widespread practice of wet nursing in medieval England as there was in Southern Europe.[94] The

---

[92] Frisk, *A Middle English Translation of* Macer Floridus de Virius Herbarum, 88.

[93] In MERWH, approximately 54 (18%) of lactation recipes refer to women and nurses, respectively. The remainder of the recipes for lactation (27%) either refer generally to the breast or it is unclear if the "she" in question is intended as "nurse" or "woman;" Uscinski, "Recipes for Women's Healthcare in Medieval England," Appendix D.

[94] Becky R. Lee, "A Company of Women and Men: Men's Recollection of Childbirth in Medieval England," *Journal of Family History* 27, no. 2 (2002), 92-100, at 97. See also: Christiane Klapisch-Zuber, "Blood Parents and Milk Parents: Wet-nursing in Florence, 1300-1530," in *Women, Family and Ritual in Renaissance Italy,* trans. Lydia Cochrane (Chicago: University of Chicago Press, 1985), 132-64, at 143; Rebecca Lynne Winer, "The Mother and the *Dida* [Nanny]: Female Employers and Wet Nurses in Fourteenth-Century Barcelona," in *Medieval and Renaissance Lactations: Images, Rhetorics, Practices,* ed. Jutta Gisela Sperling (New York: Routledge, 2013), 55-78; Debra Blumenthal, "'*With My Daughter's Milk*': Wet Nurses and the Rhetoric of Lactation in Valencian Court Records," in *Medieval and Renaissance Lactations,* ed. Sperling, 101-14. Barbara Hanawalt calls information on nursing in England "elusive": Barbara Hanawalt, *The Ties That Bound: Peasant Families in Medieval England* (Oxford: Oxford University Press, 1986), 56. This is similar to what

"Book on the Conditions of Women" in *The Trotula* ensemble devotes two paragraphs to the selection of a wet nurse.[95] This same book does not include recipes for difficulty in lactation, perhaps because the task had been outsourced.[96] Other recipes that use the word "nurse" when referencing lactation are not of Mediterranean origin.[97]

It is not difficult to see why medieval women were concerned with breastfeeding: it was the most logical – and cost-effective – way of feeding their children.[98] Religious rhetoric and imagery of the Virgin Mary breastfeeding the Baby Jesus reinforced the ideal nature of the practice.[99] The English theologian Thomas de Chobham went so far as to call women who refused to breastfeed their own children cruel and neglectful; it was, he wrote, why God gave women breasts in the first place.[100] Modern scientific studies have confirmed the many health benefits of breastfeeding – from positive effects on infants' immune systems to possible defenses later in life against obesity, heart disease,

---

Klapisch-Zuber found for Florentine families; except that in Florence, wet-nurse hiring and weaning decisions were assumed by men, whereas in England this was a task shared by men and women. Wet-nursing existed further down the social ladder in Southern Europe; see Klapisch-Zuber, "Blood Parents and Milk Parents," 143.

[95] Green, ed. and trans., *The* Trotula, 84-85.

[96] One recipe for pain in the breasts caused by lactation is provided in "Treatments for Women;" Recipe 50.178; see also Green, ed. and trans., *The* Trotula, 104. This recipe does not refer to the woman as a nurse.

[97] These recipes come from Bodleian Ashmole 1443, BL Add 34210, Add 37786, Sloane 3550, MC 878, RCP 411 and TCC O.1.20.

[98] Medieval women are further validated by modern archaeological evidence which shows that infant skeletal growth was on par with modern levels; Simon Mays, "The Effects of Infant Feeding Practices on Infant and Maternal Health in a Medieval Community," *Childhood in the Past* 3, no. 1 (2010): 63-78. The women themselves seemed to have suffered from depressed bone mineral density, which was a result of their breastfeeding.

[99] Carolyn Walker Bynum, "The Body of Christ in the Later Middle Ages: A Reply to Leo Steinberg," in *Fragmentation and Redemption: Essays on Gender and the Human Body in Medieval Religion* (New York: Zone Books, 1992), 86-87, 101-14; Jutta Gisela Sperling, "Introduction," in *Medieval and Renaissance Lactations*, 1-20: 4-5; Rebecca Totaro, "Mother London and the *Madonna Lactans* in England's Plague Epic," in *Medieval and Renaissance Lactations,* 154-55.

[100] "Quod ex eo patet quod gentiles lacte ferarum filios suos fecerunt nutriri ut exinde feritatem contraherent. Crudelior autem est omni fera mulier que fetum quem genuit nutrire contemnit. Pavit eum in utero sanguine menstruo, et nunc nutrire negligit lacte divinitus dato. Ideo enim deus mammas mulieri dedit et lac in eis nasci precepit, ut inde prolem suum educaret;" Thomas de Chobham, *Thomas de Chobham Summa Confessorum,* ed. F. Broomfield (Paris: Analecta Mediaevalia Namurcensia, 1963), 465.

and allergies.[101] A Google search for "mommy blogs + breastfeeding + best" returns over 18 million results. The author of the site *The Badass Breastfeeder* discusses how she struggled to breastfeed her son and that with the help of a board-certified lactation consultant, she was soon "exclusively breastfeeding" and "felt like a million dollar badass."[102] There is considerable pressure on modern women to breastfeed their children, but the many social, psychological, and economic pressures mean they often choose formula. For those who adopt or rely on a surrogate, there is no choice. And for most medieval women, breastfeeding was not a choice. Premodern women did not have many good alternatives to breastmilk, and many of those children who could not be breastfed died.[103] If possible, medieval children were commonly breastfed until the age of two,[104] which left a generous amount of time for lactation issues to arise. The recent infant formula shortage in the United States only highlights how critical having an alternative to breastfeeding can be and how devastating it is when those alternatives do not exist.[105]

When issues did arise, medieval women had a variety of options for care. The generally uncomplicated nature of English recipes for lactation, their rather ordinary ingredients, and the essential nature of breastfeeding show us the ways in which medieval women were involved in both the

---

[101] American College of Pediatrics, "Policy Statement: Breastfeeding and the Use of Human Milk," *Pediatrics* 115, no. 5 (2005): 496-506; see also Jane Allen and Debra Hector, "Benefits of Breastfeeding," *NSW Public Health Bulletin* 16, no. 4 (2005), 42-46, at 43.

[102] Abby Theuring, "About," *The Badass Breastfeeder,* accessed 4 February 2021, www.thebadassbreastfeeder.com/about/. Dianne Cassidy, IBCLC and Abbey Theuring also have a podcast ("The Badass Breastfeeding Podcast") with 6 available episodes from December 28, 2020 to February 1, 2021; *The Badass Breastfeeding Podcast,* accessed 4 February 2021, https://podcasts.apple.com/us/podcast/badass-breastfeeding-podcast /id1268282458.

[103] Carla Cevasco, PhD, Twitter post, 11 May 2022, 7:40pm, accessed 31 May 2022, https://twitter.com/Cevasco_Carla/status/1524534926430904320?s=20&t=gdQdNX Kl6hUArulRGSzRAQ; Laura Earls, "The Solution to Formula Shortage Isn't Calling for More Breastfeeding," *The Washington Post*, 18 May 2022, www.washingtonpost.com /outlook/2022/05/18/solution-formula-shortage-isnt-calling-more-breastfeeding/.

[104] Jennifer Ward, *Women in Medieval Europe, 1200-1500* (New York: Longman, 2002), 57-58.

[105] Christina Szalinski, "America Is Grappling with a Baby Formula Shortage. Here's How to Navigate It," *The New York Times Wirecutter*, 27 May 2022, www.nytimes.com/ wirecutter/blog/baby-formula-shortage-what-to-do/.

supply and demand of medical care and how they made choices over their own healthcare, in much the same way they do today.

IV. Conclusion

A first reaction to the subject of medieval medical recipes is the demand to know all the bizarre things people used to do in the pursuit of health – such as the ingestion of powdered crystals – perhaps to feel better about our progress or at the very least to be entertained. We tend to laugh at this type of cure while entertaining the possibility that botanical items could have had a measurable therapeutic effect. No doubt in medieval medical recipes there are methods and ingredients that raise a modern eyebrow, but botanicals are the primary *materia medica* of women's recipes, and plant-based, and "natural" remedies are considered by many today to be efficacious medicines.[106] The lactation recipes discussed here are predominantly based on easily accessible ingredients and incorporate scholastic and folkloric rationales. The same can be said for modern galactagogues. It is impossible to replicate medieval medical recipes with a confident measure of exactness, but it is possible to investigate whether the elements deemed medicinally valuable in medieval England could have had a positive effect on recipe users' health. The repetition of certain cures across collections in the fifteenth century and the continuation of many of these same remedies today demonstrate a perception of efficacy and tell us a good deal about the landscape of women's healthcare in both medieval England and the modern world.

[106] Anne Van Arsdall, "Challenging the 'Eye of Newt' Image of Medieval Medicine," in *The Medieval Hospital and Medical Practice*, ed. Barbara S. Bowers (Aldershot: Ashgate, 2007), 195.

THE ART OF GIVING BIRTH IN MIDDLE PERIOD CHINA

Wee-Siang Margaret Ng*

What does it take to prepare for childbirth? The thirteenth-century medical author Chen Ziming 陳自明 (fl. ca. 1237-1271) answered this question in the form of a list. What was in this list of items? An apparently eclectic assortment of medicines and household materials. Starting with medicine, there were seven types of medicinal *san* 散 (powdered formulas), three types of *wan* 丸 (pills), two types of *dan* 丹 (elixirs), and several types of roots commonly used in medicinal formulas. Other household materials include alcohol, vinegar, the urine of a little boy, kitchen implements, containers, soap, candles, and a stool. (See full list and translation in Appendix I). The household items were listed after the medicines, with the last few items used for light source (lamp wick, matchstick, torch, etc.) The author did not provide any explanation on the logic for the order of the items listed. No instructions were provided on why, how, and when the fifty-four items listed were to be used. The author assumed that anyone who read the list knew what those items were, when, and perhaps even how those items should be used. The names of the items provide some clues to intended uses, and the lack of instructions speaks perhaps to widely known uses of these medicines and everyday materials. Some of the items, such as lamp wicks, are common household materials and were easy to procure. Others, such as the medicines, were perhaps not so easy to gather and required time and

* Department of History, College of Wooster.

effort to assemble. The origins of some of these items also remind us of the difference between what is local, and what might also be from a larger regional network of materials, goods, and practices circulating in Middle Period China. The midwives, or other women assisting in birth, were the users and were likely also tasked with gathering the items on the list. Their ability to decide when to deploy which pill or when to give the smoked plum to the parturient was based on their experience and skills. The most skillful of midwives and women practitioners were the arbitrators of the art of giving birth.

The ubiquitous nature of childbirth does not preclude changing discourses and new medical innovations. Childbirth, therefore, makes an excellent topic of historical inquiry. This essay examines this momentous event. While discourses and medical technologies take much time to shift and transform, the act of giving birth occupies a short time in a woman's life, and yet leaves profound and long-term effects on the parturient and her marital and natal families. In Middle Period China (ca.100-1500 CE), birth required ample preparation because of the speed of how things could go quickly and occasionally horribly wrong, with the lives of the parturient and her child hanging by a thread. How did a household in Middle Period China prepare for the arrival of a new family member?[1] To answer this question, I examine Chen Ziming's *Furen daquan liangfang* (Comprehensive Compendium of Good Formulas for Women), the most authoritative work on women's medicine in the Middle Period.[2] With an entire *juan* (similar to a "chapter") sixteen devoted to the month prior to childbirth, Chen Ziming highlighted the importance of preparation for birth. In section ten of *juan* sixteen of his twenty-four

[1] I use Middle Period instead of "medieval" to reflect the trends in Chinese historiography. The "middle period" in Chinese history currently refers to the post-Han dynasty period, from about 100 CE to about 1500 CE. This covers many dynasties, including prominent ones like the Tang (618-907), Song (960-1279), Yuan (1271-1368) and a part of the Ming dynasty (1368-1644). See John Chaffee, "Middle Period China," *Oxford Bibliographies*, www.oxfordbibliographies.com/view/document/obo-9780199920082/obo-9780199920082-0003.xml.

[2] Chen Ziming 陳自明 (fl. ca. 1237-1271), *Furen daquan liangfang* (Comprehensive Compendium of Good Formulas for Women), compiled in 1237, preface dated 1271, Modern critical edition of Yuan dynasty Qinyou shutang edition (Beijing: Beijing tushuguan chubanshe, 2005). Thereafter referred to as *FRDQLF*. See Wee-Siang Margaret Ng, "Male Brushstrokes and Female Touch," (PhD dissertation, McGill University, 2013), on the history of Chen Ziming and *Furen daquan liangfang*.

juan book, *Furen daquan liangfang*, Chen provided a long list of items to prepare. Yet from the list, we know very little about what actually went on in the birthing chamber or who used the items listed.

Based on extant sources, literate women in Middle Period China did not write about their birth experiences and midwives left no writings.[3] Women did not write about childbirth possibly because they did not need to, hinting at the existence of a thriving oral tradition. Much of what we know comes from the ink of men such as Chen Ziming, a Southern Song (1127-1279 CE) dynasty physician and professor of medicine, who was meticulous in his instructions on the preparation in the month prior to giving birth. Chen provided a wide range of practices and formulas from different regions of China in his hefty collection. Unlike the thick descriptions we might see in contemporary anthropological birth stories, the medical texts written by male authors contain sparse information and these medical works were not written for training women practitioners. Chen was writing for other men, and perhaps women and families who had access to his works. In Chen's time and for most of imperial China, giving birth took place in woman-only spaces.[4] I read the persistent male authorial voice as men's attempts to comprehend and make sense of what they did not know and found hard to manage: the bodies of women and the process of childbirth.[5] We know that men were not in the birthing room from numerous sources and Chen Ziming carefully noted

---

[3] On women's literacy and writing in the Song period, see Patricia Ebrey, *The Inner Quarters: Marriage and the Lives of Chinese Women in the Sung Period* (Berkeley: University of California Press, 1993); and on literacy of women in imperial China, see Grace Fong, *Herself An Author: Gender, Agency and Writing in Late Imperial China* (Honolulu: University of Hawaii Press, 2008).

[4] This should not be construed as a form of "oppression" by men in premodern China, as described by twentieth century intellectuals and contemporary political pundits eager to paint a simplistic picture of premodern gender relations. The question of why men wrote extensively, while women, especially those highly educated and literate, did not, would require a lengthier analysis in a separate essay. For now, we have very few medical works written by women in premodern China, especially in the area of childbirth and women's medicine, most of the extant works were written men. However, based on close reading of male-authored sources, there are many traces of various oral traditions, particularly in skills which were more tactile.

[5] My inspiration came from a monograph on writing about women's sexuality in middle period China: Cheng Hsiao-wen, *Divine, Demonic and Disordered: Women Without Men in Song Dynasty China* (Seattle: University of Washington Press, 2021). In the introduction, Cheng wrote, "this is a book on what we do not know about women."

that fact. The absence of men in the birthing chamber was ameliorated by the authority men like himself asserted through the provision of advice on how families could choose the right midwife, whose expertise could save the lives of both parturient and the baby. The midwife's knowledge was embodied, which meant that the midwife's ability to utilize her skills and techniques at the opportune time could not always be textualized or even described. I call that embodiment a form of art, subtly preserved through the oral tradition and apprenticeship for fellow women. Not only for us today, but also for any not privy to oral transmission and knowledge about the details of the craft of midwives, to get a glimpse of that embodiment, we have to rely on male-authored medical writings, which recorded the skills and expertise, which I call "the art" of giving birth. Chen's record of women practitioners' skills provides us with materials to understand how complex the process of giving birth was and why it could be referred to as "the art." The authority of the men came from their writing about the art of giving birth as well as discoursing on the form of the art, which they were unable to fully experience.

The art of giving birth, like other forms of art, involved intuitive knowledge used in a timely way to bring forth life. This art was creative, and it was a type of response to something alive, dynamic, and changing. To practice this type of art was to know "Heaven's Way," as described in the writings of Zhuangzi (fl. 390-319 BCE), an early thinker from the Zhou period (ca.1046-256 BCE). Zhuangzi's story spoke to the difficulty of describing the art wielded by the artisan and craftsperson, whose skills were embodied. The passage from the classic, *Zhuangzi* (named after the purported author), exemplifies that art by which the artisan performs the work of chiseling a wheel.

> Wheelwright Bian said, "Your servant looks at it from the point of view of his own business. When I chisel a wheel, if I hit too softly, it slips and won't bite. If I hit too hard, it jams and won't move. Neither too soft nor too hard—I get it in my hand and respond with my mind. But my mouth cannot put it into words. There is an art to it.[6]

[6] Paul Kjellberg, translated, "Chapter Thirteen: Heaven's Way," *Zhuangzi*, in *Readings in Classical Chinese Philosophy*, ed. Philip Ivanhoe and Bryan W. van Norden (Indianapolis: Hackett Publishing, 2005, 2nd edition), 244-245.

"Chapter Thirteen: Heaven's Way." *Zhuangzi.*

In the passage, the craftsperson, wheelwright Bian, explained to Duke Huan that, as an artisan, Bian could describe where he would chisel, but could not say exactly how much force to exert. The author of *Zhuangzi*, through the figure of Wheelwright Bian, described expertise as embodied. Here the author was also questioning the adoption of a rigid plan to respond to a situation which was dynamic, requiring practitioners to have skillsets that would enable them to interact and react in order to respond to the needs of the moment.[7] Giving birth in Middle Period China could hardly be planned. We might have a little more control when the choice to give birth today with a Caesarean section operation at an appointed time could perhaps be scheduled around and after the due date. For premodern women, the moment of birth was unscheduled, unstructured, and unconstrained by the needs or expectations of the parturient and the family. Such unpredictable and sometimes urgent situations required expertise. The knowledge of when to apply such skills remained in the hands (literally) of midwives and those who assisted in birth. Like wheelwright Bian, their knowledge of how to manage birth remains difficult to put into words but their skills had to be called upon at any moment.

The application of this intuitive knowledge – deciding when and how to apply or use relevant skills – took place in a women-only space for most of premodern China.[8] The use of this art was practical and depended on the needs of individuals as they developed through an often lengthy and complicated process. Such practical aspects of childbirth were hard to theorize. Childbirth resisted attempts at rationalization and theorizing by male medical authors who were re-constructing structured knowledge in the Song dynasty (960-1279 CE). Medical authors were incorporating elements of contemporary philosophical discourse into their writings on women's medicine, such as the *wuyun liuqi* 五運六七

[7] Much ink has been spilled on Zhuangzi's ideas of spontaneity and expertise. See Wim De Reu, "How to Throw A Pot: The Centrality of the Potter's Wheel in the *Zhuangzi*," *Asian Philosophy* 20.1 (2010), 43-66.

[8] On the history of gendered spaces see Patricia Ebrey, *The Inner Quarters: Marriage and the Lives of Chinese Women in the Sung Period* (California: University of California Press, 1993), and Xu Man, *Crossing the Gate: Everyday Lives of Women in Song Fujian (960-1279)* (Albany: SUNY Press, 2016).

(five circulatory phases and six influences) popular in *Yijing* studies.[9] In fact, the art of giving birth was being written about precisely because Song scholars wanted to write about different aspects of science.[10] Here, I cite Nathan Sivin's definitions of science as "different modes of exploration"[11] through processes to understand patterns and principles of change and transformation. Many Song intellectuals reviewed and commented on classics from earlier periods, reorganizing and rewriting their observations of the systematic patterns of nature's principles (*li* 理). Although they used the same language to discuss these principles as had been developed in the Zhou period, the Song scholars were in fact rewriting and expanding the science of their world described with *qi* 氣, *yin-yang* 陰陽 and *wuxing* 五行 (Five Phases). However, childbirth would prove to be "particularly resistant to modes of knowing of the sort easily codified in print."[12] The "art" of giving birth as reflected in the title of the chapter captures the difficulty associated with recording the practice despite medical knowledge produced, and highlights the "display, application and expression" of skills possessed by the women practitioners.[13] This was an art form which required embodied knowledge, not just a step-by-step set of instructions on how to do something. The art described should be placed alongside, not in contrast to, the science which was being produced in the same period.

[9] Ng, "Male Brushstrokes and Female Touch," 186, see also Catherine Despeaux, "Ch4: The System of the Five Circulatory Phases and the Six Seasonal Influences (*wuyun liqi*), a Source of Innovation in Medicine under the Song (960-1279)," in *Innovations in Medicine*, ed. E. Hsu, (Cambridge: Cambridge University Press, 2001), 121-65. On the history of astrocalendrical system and the sexagenary system, see Nathan Sivin, *Granting the Seasons: The Chinese Astronomical Reform of 1280* (New York: Springer, 2009).

[10] On the history of science and issues of calling Chinese intellectual inquiry "science," see Benjamin Elman, *A Cultural History of Modern Science in China* (Cambridge, MA: Harvard University Press, 2006), Joseph Needham, *Science in Traditional China* (Cambridge, MA: Harvard University Press, 1981), Shigeru Nakayama and Nathan Sivin, edited, *Chinese Science: Explorations of an Ancient Tradition* (Cambridge, MA: MIT Press, 1973).

[11] Sivin, ed., "Preface," *Chinese Science*, xi-xxxvi.

[12] Charlotte Furth, *A Flourishing Yin: Gender in China's Medical History, 960-1665* (Berkeley: University of California Press, 1999), 99.

[13] "Art" also denotes having skills to do something as a result of knowledge or practice, or the practical application of a particular type of knowledge, learning or technical skill. See "art, n.1". *OED Online.* March 2023. Oxford University Press. https://www-oed-com.ezproxy.library.astate.edu/view/Entry/11125?rskey=uaP2YK&result=1&isAdvanced=true (accessed March 26, 2023).

I examine this "art" embodied by women practitioners through the analysis of *juan* sixteen devoted to the process of preparing for birth. The entire *juan* sixteen contains eleven subsections (*lun*) on the care of the parturient in the month prior to birth. These include advice and admonitions, recipes for making the fetus "slippery" and easier to birth, birth charts (*chantu* 產圖) based on astronomical placement, and chants for ritual cleansing and appeasement of ancestors, deities, and malevolent spirits. Then there is the long list. I have focused on the list in section ten and talismans in section eleven of *juan* sixteen titled *Zuoyue* 坐月, literally "sitting month." This list, described at the start of this chapter, consists of numerous items, assembled with no obvious thread or instructions. That lack of organization at first sight tells us something about the women practitioners assisting in birth. A modern reader of this list might have no idea how those items were used. It is possible that the male medical authors and their readers knew or had heard of the items. A closer reading of this list as a historical source, which is vastly different from other types of sources which might have instructions, stories or historical actors, tells us about the women who practiced the art of giving birth. The most skilled midwives would know what those items were and how to use them at the opportune time in childbirth.

I have chosen to examine two items from the list to illustrate the art of giving birth and make some preliminary connections between Middle Period medicine and today's general or popular uses. I will first examine a pill called *Lizhong wan* 理中丸 (Center-regulating pill). Its name is attached to a formula found in other medical works of the same time and subsequent periods. The pill has a long history which goes back to the eastern Han period (25-220 CE), and features in the history of pharmaceutics.[14] The other item is a talisman, which is pictorial and associated with less textual material, or none at all. Both pills and talismans existed as material culture in the Middle Period and are still used today, but in different circumstances. The Center-regulating pill is no longer prepared for childbirth but does exist as a common medicine one can purchase in a store or online. The birth hastening talisman is

[14] Zhao Zhongzhen and Xue Changli, *Illustrated Chinese Medicinal Formulae* (Hong Kong: Chung Hwa Book Co., 2005), 7, 68, 75-76. On contemporary pharmacological studies, see Ning Zhao, et al. "Effects on Neuroendocrinoimmune network of Lizhong Pill in the reserpine induced rats with spleen deficiency in traditional Chinese medicine," *Journal of Ethnopharmacology* 133 (2011): 454-459.

downloadable from the internet and can be purchased from temples and other religious specialists, especially Daoist practitioners. Their inclusion in the Middle Period medical works provides a snapshot of that moment, and hints at the users and practitioners who took care to prepare them. The continued existence and common use of the pill and talisman today provides interesting insights into continuities in medical practices and our persistent anxieties with birth, life, and death.

I. *Lizhong wan* 理中丸 *(Center-Regulating pill)*

Among the medicines included in the list, the *wan*, or prepared pills particularly warrant an examination. These were and still are very common medicines in Asia and among diasporic Chinese communities outside of Asia. Many households would have had these pills, ready to be deployed for common ailments, as we might have bottles of Tylenol in our medicine cabinets in North America. Take the *Lizhong wan* 理中丸 (Center-regulating pill) as an example. This formula contains four ingredients:

- Ginseng (Ginseng Radix et Rhizoma, *Ren Shen* 人參)
- Dried Ginger (Zingiberis Rhizoma, *Gan Jiang* 乾薑)
- Licorice (Glycyrrhizae Radix et Rhizoma Praeparata cum Melle, *Zhi Gan Cao* 甘草)
- White Atractylodes Rhizome (Atractylodis Macrocephalae Rhizoma, *Bai Zhu* 白朮)

Lizhong wan was not a new medicine in the Song dynasty. Its origin was established in the Song period as a formula in a third-century work, *Shanghan zabinglun* 傷寒雜病論 (Treatise on Cold Damage and Miscellaneous Disorders) by Zhang Ji (also known as Zhang Zhongjing, ca. 150-219? CE). Its revival in the Song period was in part due to the imperially-issued medical publication, *Taiping huimin hejiju fang* 太平惠民和濟局方 (Formulary of the Pharmacy Service for Benefiting the People Under the Era of Great Peace),[15] which reintroduced this formula to

[15] For extensive research on Song government publications, see various works of Asaf Goldschmidt, "Commercializing Medicine or Benefiting People: The First Public

medical authors and into the medical marketplace through government dispensaries.[16] It became widely known and possibly easily made or procurable.

However, to use the *Lizhong wan*, Song-era midwives needed to know what the ingredients were, how they acted in combination with each other, and what type of effects the ingredients should bring about. The midwife had to decide that this pill was preferable to another on the list of twelve medicines. If the midwife or the women in the household were to make this pill or the rest of the medicines on the list, they had to learn or know something about the composition of the pill, how the different ingredients should be processed and made into the pill, including storage, labeling and when to use the medicine.

According to contemporary Chinese medical works, this formula "regulates *yang qi* of the Spleen and Stomach, which occupies the middle burner, hence the name *zhong* (middle)."[17] Although its primary use is to regulate the middle burner (*zhongjiao*) from *qi* deficiency, characterized by "watery stools, nausea and vomiting, occasional thirst, loss of appetite, abdominal pain and a pale tongue with a white coating and a submerged, thin pulse," its other important use is to treat bleeding.[18] Bleeding here was associated with middle *yang* deficiency and manifests as nosebleed, vomiting of blood, excessive menstrual blood, bleeding from the rectum

---

Pharmacy in China." *Science in Context* 21:3 (2008), 311-50. On *shanghan lun* or Cold Damage disease history, see Marta Hanson, *Speaking of Epidemics in Chinese Medicine: Disease and the Geographic Imagination in Late Imperial China* (London: Routledge Press, 2011).

[16] On Song government's public pharmacy, see A. Goldschmidt, *Evolution of Chinese Medicine: Song Dynasty, 960-1200* (London: Routledge Press, 2009), 123-30.

[17] In Chinese medical physiology, the organ systems are categorized as bowels and viscera. Viscera includes the heart, lung, spleen, liver, and kidney, all of these produce qi, blood, and fluids. The six bowels include the stomach, small intestine, large intestine, bladder, gallbladder, and triple burner, all of these handle food and discharge waste. The triple burner consists of three parts, including the upper, middle, and lower burners, all hollow and link to other organ system parts. Nigel Wiseman and Andrew Ellis, *Fundamentals of Chinese Medicine* (Brookline, MA.: Paradigm Publications, 1996), 51-52, 74-75. Volker Scheid, et al., *Chinese Herbal Medicine: Formularies and Strategies* (Eastland Press, 2009), 257-258 on Lizhong wan. The Burner here refers to the Triple Burner or *Sanjiao* 三焦, which is a part of the Chinese medical organ system in the body cavity. The Triple Buner is one of the six hollow organ system (fu) and was first theorised in the medical classic, *Nanjing* 難經 (The Classic of Difficult Issues), *juan* 31, and also in *Suwen* (Inner Classic of the Yellow Emperor), in *linglan midian lun.*

[18] Volker Scheid et al., *Chinese Herbal Medicine*, 257.

and various types of internal bleeding. The blood described in this symptom pattern is pale blood, accompanied by cold extremities (hands and legs), ashen complexion, pallid tongue, and a frail pulse.[19] It is also used to treat pain which is mild and chronic, and not acute pain. Physicians have argued for centuries over the nature of the chief ingredient of this formula. Despite the lack of agreement over the main ingredient, the formula remained the basis for a number of new formulas. For example, *Fuzi lizhong wan* includes ingredients such as *Fuzi* 附子 (aconite root, *radix aconiti praeoarata*) to increase the potency of the *Lizhong wan*. *Sijunzi tang* 四君子湯 (Four Gentlemen Decoction), one of the most famous decoctions from early modern and late imperial China to today, uses these same basic three ingredients of ginseng, atractylodis, and licorice, while the dried ginger is replaced by *fuling* 茯苓 (poria).[20] The similar ingredients in these two common medicines suggest widespread knowledge of and accessibility of some ingredients in the Middle Period.

However, the art of using the pill at the opportune time fell on the midwives. These women would have needed to know the basic indications of this pill and decide when to use *Lizhong wan* instead of another pill, e.g., *Baoqi san* (*Qi* guarding powder). If none of these could be procured, purchased, or made before the parturient gave birth, the midwives had to make the medicines. They would need to be able to recognize the ingredients in simple formulas. Which part of the root or plant should be used and how much to include was based on the constitution of the parturient. The art of using the right amount at the right time required skills. Today, *Lizhong wan* is widely used as an over-the-counter medicine in the Sinosphere where Chinese medicine is practiced as well as where diasporic Asian communities thrive.[21] It is most commonly used by Chinese medical practitioners as a liquid

[19] Scheid, et al., *Chinese Herbal Medicine*, 258.

[20] See Fuzi lizhong wan, *Taiping huimin hejiju fang*. See also Volker Scheid et al., *Chinese Herbal Medicine*, 309-311, for Four Gentlemen Decoction. Fuling 茯苓 (poria) is a subterranean fungus that grows on the roots of pine trees.

[21] Liu Chang-xiao, "Overview on Development of ASEAN traditional and herbal medicines," *Chinese Herbal Medicines* 13 (2021): 441-450. On Lizhong wan in ethnopharmacology, see Ning Zhao et al., "Effects on Neuroendocrinoimmune network of Lizhong Pill in the reserpine induced rats with spleen deficiency in traditional Chinese medicine," *Journal of Ethnopharmacology* 133 (2021): 454-459.

decoction, but it has also been made into pills and is sold by several different pharmaceutical companies. In the textbook used by modern practitioners and students of Chinese medicine, *Lizhong wan* is used to treat different types of illness patterns associated with yang deficiency caused by Coldness invading the abdomen area or the middle burner. Specific signs and symptoms used by clinicians include abdominal distention or pain, and other blood deficiencies. It has been used for the treatment of biomedically defined disorders, including abdominal pain and diarrhea, and an assortment of problems marked by bleeding.[22] Given its usefulness today for such a wide range of symptoms, why did medical authors like Chen Ziming include the pill in the list and how did a midwife deploy the medicine? These unanswered questions suggest the dynamic nature of the art of giving birth in Middle Period China.

The other item from the list I wish to examine is the Birth Hastening talisman. These talismans were pictorial representations or expressions of the legitimation of power invested by the gods to their representatives on earth and were usually used together with incantations or spells. They served to manifest cosmic energies and orders from gods or were used to keep certain deities or gods under control.[23] Also called *fu* 符, talismans were written documents and texts associated with Daoism, and were protective in nature. A talisman was a tool used if there was a birth complication, which could be interpreted as the manifestation of the wrath of an angry god in the space where birth was taking place.

Like the history of Chinese *materia medica*, the history of talismans is complex, and tied to the rise and fall of various schools of Daoism.[24] Talismans and diagrams (such as the birth charts mentioned above) utilized "a combination of patterns found in nature and highly archaic forms of writing."[25] The characters were often drawn with curved lines resembling cloud patterns, suggesting celestial beings floating from

[22] Scheid, et al., *Chinese Herbal Medicine,* 257-61.

[23] Catherine Despeux, translated by Livia Kohn, "Chapter 17: Talismans and Diagrams," *Daoism Handbook*, ed. Livia Kohn (Leiden: Brill, 2004), 498-500.

[24] The main schools include the Celestial School (Tianshi) founded by Zhang Daoling in the Han dynasty (221 BCE-206 CE), followed by the Numinous Treasure School (Lingbao) and the Highest Clarity (Shangqing) School in the fourth century CE. For a brief history of Daoism, see Pregadio, Fabrizio, "Religious Daoism," *The Stanford Encyclopedia of Philosophy* (Fall 2020), Edward N. Zalta (ed.), https://plato.stanford.edu/archives/fall2020/entries/daoism-religion/.

[25] Catherine Despeux, "Chapter 17: Talismans and Diagrams," 533-36.

heaven. These stylized, geometrical patterns and symbolic signs were drawn in combination to create the representation of forces of the universe and the words which controlled them. Besides the material item itself, there were rituals associated with drawing and application or use of these talismans. The rituals needed to take place at an appropriate time selected from auspicious dates, while matching the function and elements on the talisman. Besides paper, some talismans were drawn in the air, in the sand or in blood, depending on the occasion and context of their use.[26] The production and utilization of these talismans spoke to yet another form of art which responded not only to dynamic changes of nature but also to the unpredictable gods and spirits. There were many ways to use different talismans. In rituals, they were burned as a contract with the celestial beings, invoking their assistance. Talismans were also used to exorcise demons, eliminate malevolent forces, stabilize a situation and obtain the protection of gods and deities. Talismans were used in treatment for illnesses and epidemics, as well as in immortality cultivation.[27]

In Chen Ziming's section ten of *juan* sixteen, talismans were listed as an item to procure. In section eleven, the author provided pictorial representations of eighteen of the actual talismans for hastening birth. The author advised that some of these talismans should be written with *zhusha* 朱砂 (cinnabar) and pasted on the inner northern wall of the room where birth would take place. When the parturient was about to give birth and started to crouch on the straw, the talisman should be poked with a needle and burned over the lamp in the room. One should avoid the ashes from the burning talisman from flying around. Then the ash of the burnt talisman should be mixed with warm water and the parturient woman would be asked to consume that mixture. All these talismans were for use during difficult births and specific ones were used for malpresentations of various sorts. For example, the talismans in column B (Appendix II) are used for *hengchan* 橫產 (horizontal birth) and for the placenta which could be stuck after birth. In column E, the author advised that these should be prepared before the first day of the final month of pregnancy, written with black ink on the bottom of the parturient's shoe insert, and then hidden in the straw under which the

[26] Despeux, "Chapter 17: Talismans and Diagrams," 533-36.
[27] Despeux, "Chapter 17: Talismans and Diagrams," 535.

parturient would give birth. The family member charged with this was supposed to do this secretly, without anyone knowing.[28] The secrecy was emphasized in part due to the need to maintain the potency of the talisman and also to preserve the art only among those who knew and practiced it.[29]

The family had to prepare these talismans, but it was the midwife who decided which ones to use, depending on malpresentation during complicated births. The inclusion of what the talismans looked like could also signal the male medical author's desire to caution families against charlatans whose talismans were not efficacious or were simply scribblings. Perhaps Chen Ziming was also trying to educate midwives and the women in the birthing chambers because they needed to know something about these talismans, with some minimal understanding of the different types of cloud script and their associated deities, and schools.[30]

In the Middle Period, especially in the Song dynasty, there were new Daoist liturgical movements which incorporated the practice of using talismans and other Daoist elements to manage plagues and other social upheavals. The southern plague deity cults were particularly popular,

---

[28] Chen Ziming, *juan* sixteen, *Furen daquan liangfang.*

[29] Michel Strickmann, *Chinese Magical Medicine* (Stanford, California: Stanford University Press, 2002), 174-75 on secrecy as the key to the potency of the talisman. The ritual to create the talismans had to be performed in secret, after the ritual specialist had performed ritual cleansing and fasting. The method of how to produce the talisman and the timing of when the talisman was used were all subject to secrecy. There is a tension here since the male medical author is advising for this to be performed and everyone thus know that someone was going produce the talisman and locate it in the birthing chamber. In other words, this was an open secret.

[30] For various works on talismans and their association with the mantic arts (*shushu* 數), see the bibliographies in the works of Despeux and Fabrizio. The most important writings include Jonathan Chaves, "The Legacy of Ts'ang Chieh: The Written Word as Magic." *Oriental Art* 23.2 (1977), 200-15; John Lagerway, "The Oral and the Written in Chinese and Western Religions," in *Religions and Philosophie in Ostasien, Festschrift für Hans Steininger,* ed. Jean-Pierre Vernant, 275-86 (Paris: Gallimard, 1986); Jacques Gernet, "Aspects et fonctions psychologique de l'écriture," in *L'intelligence de la Chine, le social et le mental*, ed. Jacques Gernet, 361-79 (Paris: Gallimard, 1994); Léon Vandermeersch, "La langue graphique chinoise," *Etudes sinologiques* (1994), 235-76. Christine Mollier, *Buddhism and Taoism Face to Face: Scripture, Ritual, and Iconographic Exchange in Medieval China* (Honululu: University of Hawai'i Press, 2008). See also Grégoire Espesset, "A case study on the evolution of Chinese religious symbols from talismanic paraphernalia to Taoist liturgy," *Bulletin of the School of Oriental and African Studies* 78.3 (October 2015), 493-514.

with the apotheosis of Marshal Wen, who became the plague-quelling deity Wen Qiong in the thirteenth century.[31] The art of producing and deploying talismans to deflect demonic attacks at crucial points of one's life would continue to be important in subsequent periods of history. Their existence was not incommensurate with shifting discourses in science, technology, and medicine. As demonstrated by Luis F.B. Junqueira, talismans and occult healing have survived and thrived, especially at the local and popular level, despite the predominance of Western science and biomedicine in twentieth and twenty-first century China. [32] Junqueira traces the history of talismanic healing from Republican China and presents a story of how Chinese mantic art practitioners created and formed a market for their work despite working in secrecy. These healers utilized various new media like printing presses to print cheap manuals, widely circulated newspapers, and other informal publications to continue their work.

Talismans are available today throughout southern China, Fujian, and Guangdong, and in Southeast Asia, including Singapore, Malaysia, and Indonesia, where large parts of the population associate or identify with the tradition, and seek out the practitioners who write and supply such talismans. I have included a modern computer-designed birth-hastening talisman (Appendix II, Talisman B) in bright yellow, a color associated with the robes of Daoist priests who routinely produce these for sale in temples in Taipei and Singapore. The continued use of talismans for protection during childbirth suggests the parturient's need for objects, in this case ritual objects, for an important and transformative life event.

Both the *Lizhong wan* and birth-hastening talismans were items prepared by midwives with expertise that enabled them to decide when and how to use these two different materials. The textual tradition associated with the development of *materia medica* and formulary medical literature provide a rich textual history of the *Lizhong wan* pill. The talismans' lack of dense textual tradition did not render them obsolete, but instead gave the religious or ritual specialists more flexibility on the transmission and production. New technologies, such as mass media and

---

[31] Paul Katz, *Demon Hordes and Burning Boats: The Cult of Marshal Wen in Late Imperial China* (Albany: SUNY Press, 1995).

[32] Luis Fernando Bernardi Junqueira, "Revealing Secrets: Talismans, Healthcare and the Market of the Occult in Early Twentieth-Century China," *Social History of Medicine* 34:4 (2021), 1068-93.

the internet, have made these items from the Middle Period easily available. However, these changes also coincided with the loss of the art of giving birth as embodied and practiced by midwives. The erosion of the authority of the midwife in China, a twentieth-century phenomenon, was in part the result of the preference for medicine from the West introduced by medical missionaries and the vilification of the profession of midwifery and its association with infanticide.[33]

Giving birth was a woman-centered event, but most of our textual sources concerning it were recorded by men for most of Chinese history. Male medical authors produced almost all the knowledge we have today on premodern childbirth in China, despite being entirely absent in the birthing chambers. Unlike their counterparts in some areas of early modern Europe, where male accoucheurs gradually replaced female midwives, in both China and Europe, men dominated the production of knowledge on women's health issues.[34] But in terms of practice, men did not venture into the birthing chambers in China. This tension between practice and textual knowledge did not diminish the importance of obstetrical works published and disseminated in Middle Period China and more broadly throughout East Asia. These medical works written by men have allowed me to make several observations about the importance of the midwives and their practice, which I argue was really an art. What little male medical authors knew about how to give birth came from their most important interlocutors, the women in the birthing chambers such as the parturient or the midwives. These medical works are records of women practitioners and their practice. But not very useful for women. These were lists, consisting of names of formularies, household goods and materials, and prayers, spells, and incantations. There were no

---

33 See Tina Phillips Johnson, *Childbirth in Republican China: Delivering Modernity* (Lanham, Maryland: Lexington Books, 2011). On the politics of infanticide and midwives, see Anne Waltner, "Infanticide and Dowry in Ming and Early Qing China," *Chinese Views of Childhood* (Honolulu: University of Hawaii Press, 1995), 201-205. David Mungello David, *Drowning Girls in China: Female Infanticide since 1650* (Lanham, MD: Rowman & Littlefield, 2008). On the work of midwives after 1949, see Fang Xiaoping, *Barefoot Doctors and Western Medicine in China* (Boydell & Brewer, University of Rochester Press, 2012).

34 Adrian Wilson, *The Making of Man-Midwifery: Childbirth in England, 1660-1770* (Cambridge, Mass.: Harvard University Press, 1995); Nina Gelbart, *The King's Midwife: A History and mystery of Madame du Coudray* (Berkeley, CA: University of California Press, 1998); Monica H. Green, *Making Women's Medicine Masculine: The Rise of Male Authority in Pre-Modern Gynaecology* (Oxford: University of Oxford Press, 2008).

instructions on how to use these things. Women practitioners embodied the knowledge of how and when to use these materials or things effectively. Yet, one could also read these lists of things a household had to prepare for birth from the Middle Period as the loss of the art of giving birth.

Appendix I

Chen Ziming (fl. ca. 1237-1271), *Furen daquan liangfang* 婦人大全良方 (Comprehensive Compendium of Good Formulas for Women), compiled in 1237, preface dated 1271.
Modern critical edition of Yuan dynasty Qinyou shutang edition (Beijing: Beijing tushuguan chubanshe, 2005).

Juan 卷 16: *Zuoyue* 坐月 (Sitting Month Topic)
Section Ten: Materials and medicine to prepare a month before birth 入月預備藥物第十

[*medicines*]

1. Baoqi san 保氣散 (Qi guarding powder)
2. Foshou san 佛手散 (Hand of the Buddha powder)
3. Zhiqiao san 枳殼散 (Bitter orange powder)
4. Shenqing wan 神寢丸 (Deity sleep pill)
5. Yubaipi san 榆白皮散 (White elm bark powder)
6. Baosheng wan 保生丸 (Protecting life pill)
7. Cuisheng dan 催生丹 (Hastening birth elixir)
8. Heishen san 黑神散 (Black deity powder)
9. Dasheng san 大聖散 (Great sage powder)
10. Huaruishi san 花蕊石散 (Stone flower stamen powder)
11. Heilong dan 黑龍丹 (Black dragon elixir)
12. Lizhong wan 理中丸 (Center-regulating pill)

[*talismans*]

13. Cuisheng fu 催生符 (Hastening birth talisman)

[*materia medica and common household items*]

14. Shengdi huang 生地黃 (Chinese foxglove, *Rehmannia glutinosa*)

15. Qianghuo 羌活 (notopterygium Root, *Notopterygium incisum*)
16. Kuizi 葵子 (muskroot, like Semiaquilegia Root, *Semiaquilegiae Radix*)
17. Huanglian 黃連 (Chinese Goldthread Rhizome, *Coptis chinensis*)
18. Zhuru 竹茹 (bamboo shavings, *Bambusae Caulis in Taenias*)
19. Wumei 烏梅 (smoked plum, *Mume Fructus*)
20. Cixiong shiyan 雌雄石燕 (cyrtiospirifer sinensis, fossil shell of Spirifer)
21. Gancao 甘草 (Liquorice/ licorice root, *Glycyrrhizae Radix et Rhizoma*)
22. Haima 海馬 (Kellogg's Seahorse, *Hippocampus*)
23. Maxian tie 馬銜鐵 (bit of a horse bridle)
24. Zaozi 棗子 (jujube, *Jujubae Fructus*)
25. Chenpi 陳皮 (tangerine peel, *Citri Reticulatae Pericarpium*)
26. Jiangqian 薑錢 (good amount of giner)
27. Heidou 黑豆 (black soy bean, glycines Semen Atrum)
28. Baimi 白蜜 (white or churned honey)
29. Wuhui jiu 無灰酒 (wine without lime (calcium oxide))
30. Tongzi xiaobian 童子小便 (little boy's urine)
31. Haocu 好醋 (good vinegar)
32. Baimi 白米 (white rice)
33. Jianyao lu 煎藥爐 (stove/ furnace for decocting medicine, possible portable)
34. Diaozi 銚子 (a wide pan with a long handle)
35. Zhuzhou shaping 煮粥沙瓶 (a stone vessel for cooking porridge)
36. Lüyao mian 濾藥帛 (cotton sieve for straining medicine)
37. Cutan peng 醋炭盆 (container for heating charcoal for vinegar fumes)
38. Xiaoshi 小石（一、二十顆）(one to twenty pieces of little stones)
39. Tangping 湯瓶 (vessel for holding hot liquid)
40. Ruanying tan 軟硬炭 (soft and hard charcoal)
41. Gancai mao 乾柴茅 (dry firewood reed or rush)

42. Ruan shuifu 暖水釜 (kettle or cauldron which can keep water warm)
43. Xi'er feizhao 洗兒肥皂 (soap for washing the child)
44. Toufa 頭發 (hair from the head, presumably from the father)
45. Duan qimian ji jiandao 斷臍綿及剪刀（斷臍本不用刀，只用帛裹臍下，齒嚙斷）(cotton thread for cutting the umbilical cord and scissors) (do not use a knife to sever the umbilical cord, only use silk to wrap the umbilical cord, bite with one's teeth to sever)
46. 乾蓐草 (dry straw mattress)
47. Wojiaoyi 臥交椅 (folding chair)
48. Ruanhou zhan 軟濃氈 (soft dense felt material)
49. Denglong 燈籠 (lantern)
50. Huoba 火把 (fire torch)
51. Jiaojing 繳巾 (long piece of cloth for wrapping)
52. Youzuo 油燭 (oil for burning or candle)
53. Fazhu 發燭 (fire starter, like a matchstick)
54. Dengxin 燈心 (lamp wick)

Appendix II

Juan 卷 16, *Zuoyue* 坐月 (Sitting Month)
Section 11: Efficacious Talismans to Hasten Birth
催生靈符第十一.

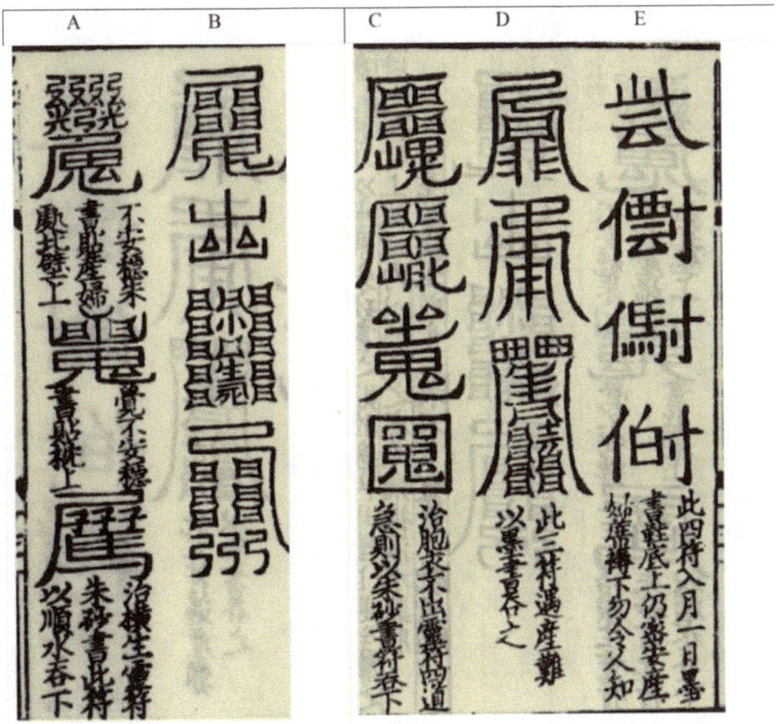

Section eleven. *Furen daquan liangfang*, *juan* 16.

Contemporary talismans

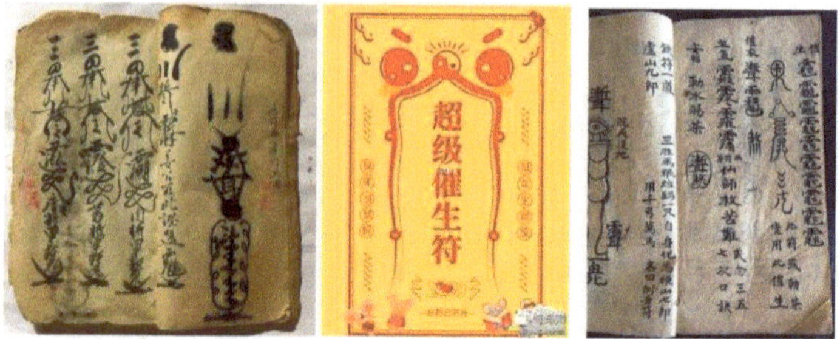

A B C

A. A talismanic magic manuscript from https://www.sgss8.com/tpdq/18830901/3.htm.
B. Hastening birth talisman for 2020. https://www.sgss8.com/tpdq/18830901/
C. Page from talismanic manuscript. http://www.kfzimg.com/sw/kfzimg/1261/ea56394e9fbc8055_b.jpg

Table 1. *Lizhong wan* 理中丸 (Center Regulating Pill)

Dried ginger (Zingiberis Rhizoma, Gan Jiang 乾薑) - Warms the spleen and stomach - Disperses cold - Assists yang qi to inhibit yin	Ginseng (Ginseng Radix et Rhizoma, Ren Shen 人參) - Tonifies the middle burner - Replenish qi - Supplements the spleen
Bai Zhu/White Atractylodes Rhizome (Atractylodis Macrocephalae Rhizoma, Bai Zhu 白朮) - Promotes the function of the spleen - Eliminate dampness	Licorice (Glycyrrhizae Radix et Rhizoma Praeparata cum Melle, Zhi Gan Cao 甘草) - boost qi - supplements the spleen - harmonizes the actions of other herbs - relieves urgency and stops pain

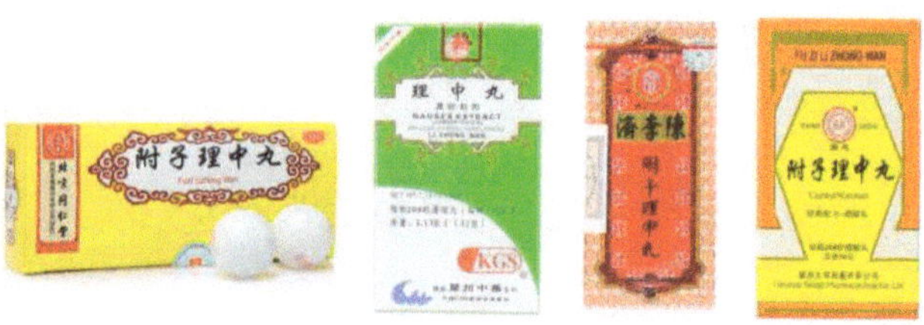

Different brands of *Lizhong wan* today (Public Domain Internet images)

BIBLIOGRAPHY

Manuscripts

Cambridge, Cambridge University Library, Taylor-Schechter 16.288

Cambridge, Trinity College, MS O.1.13
Cambridge, Trinity College, MS O.1.20

Cambridge, Magdalene College MS 878

London, British Library, MS Additional 34210
London, British Library, MS Additional 37786
London, British Library, MS Sloane 3550

London, Royal College of Physicians, MS 411

London, Wellcome Library, MS MSL 133

Mainz, Stadtarchiv Mainz, 33/1
Mainz, Stadtarchiv Mainz, 33/3

Montreal, Letter from M. Sa'eed to William Osler, October 19, 1916. William Osler Letter Index, McGill University Library, CUS417/39.80, https://osler-letters.library.mcgill.ca/record/cus417-3980

Oxford, Bodleian Library, MS Ashmole 1443
Oxford, Bodleian Library, MS Ashmole 1447

Paris, Bibliothèque Nationale de France, MS lat. 7065
Paris, Bibliothèque Nationale de France, MS lat. 17817

Modern Fictional Literature

Ashley, Mike, ed. *The Mammoth Book of More Historical Whodunits.* New York, NY: Carroll and Graf, 2001.

Clare, Alys. *The Rufus Spy.* London: Severn House, 2018.

——. *The Winter King.* Sutton: Severn House Publishers, 2013.

Coleridge, Samuel Taylor. *The Rime of the Ancient Mariner.* London: Sampson Low, Son & Co., 1857.

Conan Doyle, Arthur. *The New Annotated Sherlock Holmes*, ed. Leslie S. Klinger. New York, NY: Norton and Company, 2005.

Doherty, Paul. *Candle Flame.* Sutton: Severn House Publishers, 2014.

Eco, Umberto. *The Name of the Rose.* New York, NY: Harcourt Brace & Co., 1983.

Franklin, Ariana. *Mistress of the Art of Death.* New York, NY: G.P. Putnam and Sons, 2007.

——. *The Serpent's Tale.* New York, NY: G.P. Putnam and Sons, 2008.

Gellis, Roberta. *A Mortal Bane.* New York, NY: Tor Books, 1999.

Gordon, Noah. *The Physician.* New York, NY: Simon & Schuster, 1986.

Grace, C.L. *The Book of Shadows.* New York, NY: Minotaur Press, 1996.

——. *A Maze of Murders.* New York, NY: St. Martin's Minotaur, 2003.

Gregory, Susanna. *An Unholy Alliance.* New York, NY: St. Martin's Press, 1997.

——. *A Plague on Both Your Houses.* New York, NY: St. Martin's Press, 1998.

Hargla, Indrek. *Apothecary Melchior and the Mystery of St. Olaf's Church.* Translated by Adam Cullen. London: Peter Owens, 2015.

——. *Apothecary Melchior and The Ghost of Rataskaevu Street.* Translated by Christopher Moseley. London: Peter Owen Publishers, 2016.

Jecks, Michael. *The Leper's Return.* London: Headline Books, 1998.

——. Review of *The Leper's Return.* Goodreads, November 16, 2011. https://www.goodreads.com/review/show/236174512.

Jordan, Robert. *The Eye of the World.* New York: Tor Books, 1990.

——. *The Shadow Rising.* Tor Books, 1992.

——. *Lord of Chaos.* Tor Books, 1994.

——. *A Crown of Swords.* Tor Books, 1996.

Martin, George R.R. *A Dance with Dragons.* New York, NY: Bantam Books, 2011.

The Medieval Murderers. *The Tainted Relic.* London: Simon and Schuster, 2005.
Moore, Christopher. *Lamb: The Gospel According to Biff, Christ's Childhood Pal.* New York, NY: William Morrow, 2004.
Parker, I.J. *The Rashomon Gate.* New York, NY: St. Martin's Press, 2002.
Penman, Sharon Kay. *The Queen's Man.* London: Henry Holt, 1996.
Peters, Ellis. *Dead Man's Ransom.* New York, NY: Mysterious Press, 1997.
——. *The Devil's Novice.* New York, NY: Mysterious Press, 1983.
——. *The Leper of St. Giles.* New York, NY: Mysterious Press, 1995.
——. *A Morbid Taste for Bones.* New York, NY: Mysterious Press, 1994.
——. *Monk's Hood.* New York, NY: Mysterious Press, 1992.
——. *The Pilgrim of Hate.* New York, NY: Mysterious Press, 1997.
——. *The Sanctuary Sparrow.* New York, NY: Mysterious Press, 1995.
——. *The Virgin in the Ice.* New York, NY: Mysterious Press, 1995.
Robb, Candace. *The Apothecary Rose.* New York, NY: St. Martin's Press, 1993.
——. *The Lady Chapel.* New York, NY: St. Martin's Press, 1995.
——. *A Trust Betrayed.* New York, NY: Mysterious Press, 2002.
Roe, Caroline. *An Antidote for Avarice.* New York, NY: Berkley Publishing, 1999.
——. *Cure for a Charlatan.* New York, NY: Berkeley Prime Crime, 1999.
——. Solace for a Sinner. New York, NY: Berkeley Prime Crime, 2000.
Royal, Priscilla. *Forsaken Soul.* Scottsdale, AZ: Poisoned Pen Press, 2008.
Sansom, C.J. *Dissolution.* New York, NY: Penguin Books, 2003.
Sayers, Dorothy L. *Strong Poison.* New York, NY: Avon Books, 1967.
Silvers, Laury. *The Lover: A Sufi Mystery.* Kindle Direct Publishing, 2019.
——. *The Jealous: A Sufi Mystery.* Kindle Direct Publishing, 2020.
Tiraboschi, Roberto. *The Apothecary's Shop: A Novel of Venice 1118 A.D.* Translated by Katherine Gregor. New York, NY: Europa Editions, 2017.
Tolkien, J.R.R. *The Hobbit.* London: George Allen & Unwin, 1937.
——. *The Fellowship of the Ring.* London: George Allen & Unwin, 1954.
——. *The Two Tower.* London: George Allen & Unwin, 1954.
——. *The Return of the King.* London: George Allen & Unwin, 1955.
Van Gulik, Robert. *The Lacquer Screen.* New York, NY: Charles Scribner & Sons, 1972.
——. *The Haunted Monastery and the Chinese Maze Murders.* New York, NY: Dover Press, 1977.

Audiovisual Media

Akroyd, Dan, Anne Beatts, Tom Davis, et al., writers. *Saturday Night Live.* Season 3, episode 18, "Theodoric of York, Medieval Barber." Featuring Steven Martin. Aired April 22, 1978.

Butchard, Stephen, screenplay writer (based on Bernard Cornwell, *The Saxon Stories*). *The Last Kingdom.* Aired 2015-22 on the BBC.

Cherones, Tom, dir. *Seinfeld.* Season 2, episode 8, "The Heart Attack". April 25, 1991 on NBC.

Fuqua, Antoine, dir. *King Arthur.* 2004; Buena Vista Pictures.

Gilliam, Terry, and Terry Jones, dir. *Monty Python and the Holy Grail.* 1975; EMI Films.

Glatter, Lesli Linka, dir. *House.* Season 4, episode 8, "You Don't Want to Know." Aired November 20, 2007, on Fox.

Hirst, Michael, writer. *Vikings.* Aired 2013-20 on the History Channel.

"Histories and Lore: Greyscale and the Stone Men." *Game of Thrones* DVD special feature. HBO, 2016.

Der Medicus (*The Physician*): dir. Philipp Stölzl, starring Tom Payne, Ben Kingsley, Stellan Skarsgård, Olivier Martinez, and Emma Rigby. Universal Pictures, 2013.

Mylod, Mark, dir. *Game of Thrones.* Season 5, episode 3, "High Sparrow," April 26, 2015, on HBO.

——. *Game of Thrones.* Season 5, episode 4, "Sons of the Harpy," May 3, 2015, on HBO.

Podeswa, Jeremy, dir. *Game of Thrones.* Season 5, episode 5, "Kill the Boy," May 10, 2015, on HBO.

Reynolds, Kevin, dir. *Tristan and Isolde.* 2006; 20th Century Fox.

Scott, Ridley, dir. *Kingdom of Heaven.* Los Angeles: 20th Century Fox, 2005.

Theakston, Graham, dir. *Cadfael.* Season 1, episode 1. "One Corpse Too Many," May 29, 1994, on ITV.

U2. "One," *Achtung Baby*, Island Records, 1992.

Wellington, David, dir. *Knightfall.* Season 2, episode 4, "Equal Before God." April 15, 2019, Netflix.

Exhibitions and Websites

"10 Foods to Nourish Breastfeeding Moms." *Mom365,* https://www.mom365.com/baby/breastfeeding/10-foods-to-nourish-breastfeeding-moms.

"A Brief History." *The International Society for the Study of Medievalism*, www.medievalisms.org/about.

"About." *Healthline.* https://www.healthline.com/about.

Amethyst Crystal Tea. https://www.crystalvaults.com/shop-crystals/420001/.

"The Archive of 'A Song of Ice and Fire' Lore. So Spake Martin." *The Citadel.* https://www.westeros.org/Citadel/SSM/Entry/1165.

Barnhouse, Lucy. "The Pestilential Premodern? Going Digital with the Medieval." *EuropeNow*, Dec. 2020. www.europenowjournal.org/2020/12/07/the-pestilential-premodern-going-digital-with-the-medieval/.

Bichell, Rae Ellen. "Iconic Plague Images Are Often Not What They Seem." *NPR Goats and Soda*, August 18, 2017. https://www.npr.org/sections/goatsandsoda/2017/08/18/542435991/those-iconic-images-of-the-plague-thats-not-the-plague.

"Breast-feeding Nutrition: Tips for Mom." *Mayo Clinic.* https://www.mayoclinic.org/healthy-lifestyle/infant-and-toddler-health/in-depth/breastfeeding-nutrition/art-20046912.

The British Flower and Vibrational Essence Therapy Association (BFVEA): *Welcome to the Website of the British Flower and Vibrational Essences Association* (2020): https://www.bfvea.com/.

Bryce, Emma. "Should Breastfeeding Women Really Drink Guinness?" *LiveScience,* www.livescience.com/63122-breastfeeding-moms-guinness-beer.html.

Canadian Breastfeeding Foundation. "Domperidone General Information," https://www.canadianbreastfeedingfoundation.org/induced/domperidone_general.shtml, accessed 31 January 2021.

Cassar-Uhl, Diana. "Feeding the New Mother," La Leche League International, https://www.llli.org/feeding-the-new-mother/.

Cassidy, Dianne, IBCLC, and Abbey Theuring. "The Badass Breastfeeding Podcast," 6 episodes, December 28, 2020 to February 1, 2021. https://podcasts.apple.com/us/podcast/badass-breastfeeding-podcast/id1268282458.

Cevasco, Carla, PhD. *Twitter* post, 11 May 2022, 7:40 pm. https://twitter.com/Cevasco_Carla/status/1524534926430904320?s=20&t=gdQdNXKl6hUArulRGSzRAQ, accessed 31 May 2022.

Chaffee, John. "Middle Period China." *Oxford Bibliographies.* www.oxfordbibliographies.com/view/document/obo-9780199920082/obo-9780199920082-0003.xml.

Cheney, Alexandra. "Why the Renewed Interest in Crystals? The Pandemic." *NYTimes* (26 January 2022): www.nytimes.com/2022/01/26/fashion/jewelry-crystals-jacquie-aiche-beverly-hills-california.html.

Die Chroniken des Bruder Cadfael, http://www.cadfael.de/html/es-s-quest.html.

Common Sense Media. https://www.commonsensemedia.org/

"Crazy Potions and Nasty Nostrums: Six Bizarre Medieval Medicines," *History on the Net,* https://www.historyonthenet.com/crazy-potions-and-nasty-nostrums-six-bizarre-medieval-medicines.

Croop, Kari. *The Last Kingdom* – TV Review, *Common Sense Media,* www.commonsensemedia.org/tv-reviews/the-last-kingdom.

Dawkins, Richard, et al. "The Minds Boggle," The Guardian 16 May 2005. https://aeon.co/essays/is-debunking-more-about-the-truth-teller-than-the-truth.

Deya, K.N. "The enduring legacy of Ibn Sina's work on contagions." *The Business Standard* 26 April 2020, www.tbsnews.net/panorama/enduring-legacy-ibn-sinas-work-contagions-73987.

"Domperidone General Information." *Canadian Breastfeeding Foundation,* www.canadianbreastfeedingfoundation.org/induced/domperidone_general.shtml.

Drugs and Lactation Database (LacMed) (Bethesda, MD: National Library of Medicine, 2006, updated 2021): www.ncbi.nlm.nih.gov/books/NBK501852/.

"조선궁중여성." https://terms.naver.com/.

Earls, Laura. "The Solution to Formula Shortage Isn't Calling for More Breastfeeding," *The Washington Post* (18 May 2022): https://www.washingtonpost.com/outlook/2022/05/18/solution-formula-shortage-isnt-calling-more-breastfeeding/.

Emoto, Masaru. https://masaru-emoto.net/en.masaru/.

——. https://hado.com/ihm/.

Esh, "9 Horrifying & Weird Medieval Medical Practices," *Medium.com,* 16 January 2021, https://medium.com/lessons-from-history/9-horrifying-weird-medieval-medical-practices-8188901ae45.

"Essence Therapy." (2019): https://www.cancerresearchuk.org/about-cancer/cancer-in-general/treatment/complementary-alternative-therapies/individual-therapies/essence-therapy.

Ferguson, Maggie. "How Does it Really Feel to Be Lonely?" *The Economist. 1843: Stories of an Extraordinary World.* February/March 2018. www.1843magazine.com/features/in-solitude-what-happiness.

"Foods to Eat While Breastfeeding: A Healthy, Well-balanced Diet is Key." *The Cleveland Clinic* (11 October 2021): https://health.clevelandclinic.org/breastfeeding-diet/.

"Game of Thrones' Westeros Is Really Just Britain and An Inverted Ireland." Brilliant Maps. March 7, 2015. https://brilliantmaps.com/westeros/.

Gilbert, T. "Vikings Come Ashore in a New Light." *The New York Times.* 22 April 2013. https://www.nytimes.com/2013/02/24/arts/television/vikings-struggles-come-to-life-in-history-channels-series.html?searchResultPosition=1.

Green, Monica H. "Who/What Is Trotula?" January 6, 2020 www.academia.edu/41537366/WHO_WHAT_IS_TROTULA_2020.

Greuter, W. "Compositae (pro parte majore)." *Compositae. Euro+Med Plantbase - the information resource for Euro-Mediterranean plant diversity*, ed. W. Greuter and E. von Raab-Straube. www.bgbm.org/euroPlusMed/PTaxonDetail.asp?UUID=30F7AED4-1BAC-4C46-A86D-ECC7A13DF924.

Gruber, Christiane. "The Arts of Protection and Healing in Islam: Water Infused with Blessing." Ajam Media Collective, May 6, 2021. https://ajammc.com/.

Heo Jun. "Donguibogam." 한의학고전 DB. www.mediclassics.kr/books/8.

Ifft Decker, Sarah, and Abigail Agresta. "Cadfael." *Media-eval Podcast* August 24, 2019. https://soundcloud.com/user-834389367/cadfael

Ingram, Jennifer, et al. "Metoclopramide or domperidone for increasing maternal breast milk output; a randomised controlled trial." *ADC Fetal and Neonatal* (December 5, 2011): F241-F245.

The Islamic Information: All About Islam. https://theislamicinformation.com/.

Kendall-Tackett, Kathleen. "A new paradigm for depression in new mothers: the central role of inflammation and how breastfeeding and anti-inflammatory treatments protect maternal mental health." *International Breastfeeding Journal* (2007): https://rdcu.be/cOQCw.

King, Helen. "Why I Wasn't Excited About the Medieval Remedy That Works Against MRSA." *The Conversation* (9 April 2015): https://theconversation.com/why-i-wasnt-excited-about-the-medieval-remedy-that-works-against-mrsa-39719.

The Last Kingdom Wiki. https://the-last-kingdom.fandom.com/wiki/The_Last_Kingdom_Wiki.

"Leprosy (Hansen's disease)." World Health Organization, last modified May 10, 2021, www.who.int/news-room/fact-sheets/detail/leprosy.

"Listing of Vitamins." *Harvard Medical School* (Harvard Health Publishing, 2009, updated 2020): https://www.health.harvard.edu/staying-healthy/listing_of_vitamins.

Lower, Stephen. "H_2O dot con. Water-related pseudoscience, fantasy and quackery." https://www.chem1.com/CQ/.

Mackenzie, Natalie Gingerich. "How to Eat a Healthy Breastfeeding Diet." *TheBump,* https://www.thebump.com/a/breastfeeding-diet.

Marsden, Richard. "Game of Thrones: Imagined World Combines Romantic and Grotesque Visions of Middle Ages." *The Conversation.* http://theconversation.com/game-of-thrones-imagined-world-combines-romantic-and-grotesque-visions-of-middle-ages-105141.

McCann, Colleen. "8 Crystals for Better Energy." *Goop.* https://goop.com/wellness/spirituality/the-8-essential-crystals/.

McClure, Tess. "Dark Crystals: the Brutal Reality Behind a Booming Wellness Craze." *The Guardian* (17 September 2019): https://www.theguardian.com/lifeandstyle/2019/sep/17/healing-crystals-wellness-mining-madagascar.

McManus, Katherine D. "Should I Be Eating More Fiber?" *Harvard Medical School* (Harvard Health Publishing, 2019): www.health.harvard.edu/blog/should-i-be-eating-more-fiber-2019022115927.

Middle English Compendium (University of Michigan, 2000, revised 2018): https://quod.lib.umich.edu/m/middle-english-dictionary/.

Miller, Jeff. "Jeff Miller's postage stamps." https://mathshistory.st-andrews.ac.uk/Miller/stamps/.

Miller, Korin. "What to Know About Using Gripe Water for Colic and Tummy Trouble." *The Bump* (2021): https://www.thebump.com/a/gripe-water.

A Modern Herbal by Mrs M. Grieves. www.botanical.com/botanical/mgmh/mgmh.html.

Moffett, Martha. "Cadfael's cloister." *South Florida Sun-Sentinel* Jan 1, 1995. www.sun-sentinel.com/news/fl-xpm-1995-01-01-9412270315-story.html.

"The Mother of All Pandemics: The State of Black Death Research in the Era of Covid-19." Winston Black and Lori Jones, moderators; Monica H. Green, respondent; Joris Roosen, bibliographer. 15 May 2020. Medieval Academy of America. Webinar. www.medievalacademy.org/general/custom.asp?page=PandemicWebinar.

Mudan Finn, Kavita. "Game of Thrones is Based in History—Outdated History." *The Public Medievalist.* May 2019. www.publicmedievalist.com/thrones-outdated-history/.

Mull, Amanda. "The Kale Craze Might Be Ending: The Saddest Leafy Green," *The Atlantic,* www.theatlantic.com/health/archive/2019/09/why-kale/599041/.

The National Archives, London. https://shop.nationalarchives.gov.uk/products/medicine-in-the-middle-ages-surviving-the-times.

National Library of Medicine, Renaissance Science, Magic, and Medicine in Harry Potter's World. www.nlm.nih.gov/exhibition/sciencemagicmedicine/index.html.
https://shop.nationalarchives.gov.uk/products/medicine-in-the-middle-ages-surviving-the-times.

National Library of Medicine. "Native Voices." www.nlm.nih.gov/nativevoices/index.html.

Nice Frank J. and Mary Francell. "Selection and Use of Galactagogues." *La Leche League* (26 June 2020): https://www.llli.org/selection-and-use-of-galactagogues-2/.

Ogden, Emily. "Debunking Debunked." Aeon, August 12, 2019. https://aeon.co/essays/is-debunking-more-about-the-truth-teller-than-the-truth.

"Overview." *Healthy Kitchens, Healthy Lives.* www.healthykichens.org/overview.

Pregadio, Fabrizio. "Religious Daoism." *The Stanford Encyclopedia of Philosophy* (Fall 2020 Edition): Edward N. Zalta (ed.): https://plato.stanford.edu/archives/fall2020/entries/daoism-religion.

"The Real Medieval History Behind Of 'Game of Thrones.'" *WBUR Radio Boston.* April 15, 2019. www.wbur.org/radioboston/2019/04/15/game-of-thrones.

"Recommended Daily Allowances and Adequate Intakes, Vitamins." *National Institute of Health.* www.ncbi.nlm.nih.gov/books/NBK56068/table/summarytables.t2/?report=objectonly.

Rekstis, Emily. "Healing Crystals 101," medically reviewed by Debra Rose Wilson (2018, updated 2019): www.healthline.com/ health/mental-health/guide-to-healing-crystals.

"Robert Jordan: The Name Behind the Wheel," excerpted from *Locus Magazine.* March 2000. *LocusMag Archive Page.* www.locusmag.com/2000/Issues/03/Jordan.html.

"Rulers of the Realm." San Diego Comic Con. July 2014. www.youtube.com/watch?v=lUCz3c6-akU.

Schoppert, Stephanie. "8 Medical Practices from Medieval Times That Will Turn Your Stomach." *History Collection.* 16 March 2017. https://historycollection.com/medieval-medical-practices-sure-turn-stomach/.

Shapiro, Eliza. "Breastfeeding Pills' Risky Results." *The Daily Beast* (August 7, 2021, updated July 13, 2017): www.thedailybeast.com/breastfeeding-pills-risky-results.

"STANBIS (STannard's ANnotated Bibliographical Information System):" University of Kansas Libraries, Spencer Research Library, 1952-1988. https://archives.lib.ku.edu/repositories/3/resources/ 3443.

Stevenson, Angus, ed. *Oxford Dictionary of English* (Oxford, 2010), www.oxfordreference.com/view/10.1093/acref/9780199571123.001.0001/m_en_gb0832630

Szalinski, Christina. "America Is Grappling with a Baby Formula Shortage. Here's How to Navigate It." *NYTimes Wirecutter* (27 May 2022): https://www.nytimes.com/wirecutter/blog/baby-formula-shortage-what-to-do/.

Tasci, Ufuk Necat. "How Ibn Sina's work became a guiding light for scientists facing contagion," *TRT World* 15 April 2020, www.trtworld.com/magazine/how-ibn-sina-s-work-became-a-guiding-light-for-scientists-facing-contagions-35440.

"Theodoric of York, Medieval Barber." *Saturday Night Live* Season 3, Episode 18. NBC, 22 April 1978.

Theuring, Abby. "About." *The Badass Breastfeeder,* www.thebadass breastfeeder.com/about/.

Tian C., "Can Drinking Milk While Breastfeeding Help to Produce Milk?" *Parenting.com* (15 October 2018): https://parenting.firs tcry.com/articles/can-drinking-milk-while-breastfeeding-help-to-produce-more-milk/.

Tibble, Steve. "Medieval Strategy? The Great 'Leper Conspiracy' of 1321." Yale University Press Blog, September 11, 2020. https://yalebooks.yale.edu/2020/09/11/medieval-strategy-the-grea t-leper-conspiracy-of-1321.

Timmons, Jessica. "Galactagogues: 23 Foods That Increase Breast Milk," medically reviewed by Valinda Riggins Nwadike, MD, Ph.D., *Healthline,* www.healthline.com/health/parenting/galactagogues#Yo ur-breastfeeding-diet.

Tugmakvu, Muang'Akili. "Who Was Marcel Vogel? From IBM Researcher to a Crystal Healer," *Medium* (22 December 2021): https://medium.com/broaderinsights/who-was-marcel-vogel-a9430f8c11e3.

"Understanding Antioxidants." *Harvard Medical School: Harvard Health Publishing* (1 January 31 2019): www.health.harvard.edu/staying-healthy/understanding-antioxidants#app.

United States Food and Drug Administration. "Reglan (Metoclopramide Hydrochloride) NDA #017854, Tablet; Oral, Labeling-Package Insert, SUPPL-62, 08/29/2017." *Drugs @FDA-Approved Drugs,* https://www.accessdata.fda.gov/scripts/cder/daf/index.cfm?event =overview.process&ApplNo=017854.

——. "Reglan (Metoclopramide Hydrochloride) NDA #017862, Injectable; Injection." *Drugs @FDA-Approved Drugs,* www.access data.fda.gov/scripts/cder/daf/index.cfm?event=overview.process& ApplNo=017862.

——. "FDA Talk Paper: FDA Warns Against Women Using Unapproved Drug, Domperidone, to Increase Milk Production." *U.S. Food and Drug Administration* (04/18/2016): www.fda.gov/drugs/information-drug-class/fda-talk-paper-fda-warns-against-women-using-unapprov ed-drug-domperidone-increase-milk-production.

University of Rochester Medical Center (NY: Rochester, 2021). https://www.urmc.rochester.edu/.

V., Isabelle. "Lupus." May 9, 2017. www.sante-sur-le-net.com/maladies/maladies-auto-immunes/lupus/.

Vikings Wiki. https://vikings.fandom.com/wiki/Vikings_Wiki

Vizthum, Diane. "5 Breastfeeding Diet Myths," *Health: Johns Hopkins Medicine.* www.hopkinsmedicine.org/health/wellness-and-prevention/5-breastfeeding-diet-myths.

Waxman, Olivia B. "Game of Thrones Effect Seen in Medieval Studies Scholarship." *Time Magazine* July 14, 2017. https://time.com/4837351/game-of-thrones-real-medieval-history/.

Wenger, Adam. "11 Old Medical Treatments That Will Make Your Stomach Turn. Including Heroin for Kids!" *Healthline* (1 September 2017): https://www.healthline.com/health/old-medical-treatments-make-your-stomach-turn.

"When Breastfeeding, How Many Calories Should Moms and Babies Consume?" *NIH US Department of Health and Human Services* (31 January 2017): www.nichd.nih.gov/health/topics/breastfeeding/conditioninfo/calories.

Yan, Lin. "Dark Leafy Vegetables." USDA Agricultural Research Service. https://www.ars.usda.gov/plains-area/gfnd/gfhnrc/docs/news-2013/dark-green-leafy-vegetables/.

"Zinc Fact Sheet for Health Professionals," *National Institute for Health* (2020): https://ods.od.nih.gov/factsheets/Zinc-HealthProfessional/#en2.

Primary Sources in Print

Albucasis on Surgery and Instruments, ed. M.S. Spink and G.L. Lewis. Berkeley: University of California Press, 1973.

The Alphabet of Galen: A Critical Edition of the Latin Text with English Translation and Commentary, ed. and trans. Nicholas Everett. Toronto: University of Toronto Press, 2012.

Annotations de M. Laur. Joubert, sur toute la chirurgie de M. Gui de Chauliac. Lyon: Estienne Micheand, 1585.

Armstrong, Regis J., J. A. Wayne Hellmann, and William J. Short, eds. *Francis of Assisi: Early Documents — The Saint.* New York, NY: New City Press, 1999.

Assises de la Haute Cour, Recueil des Historiens des Croisades, Lois: Assises de Jérusalem ou Recueil des ouvrages de Jurisprudence composés pendant le XIIIe siècle dans les Royaumes de Jérusalem et de Chypre. Vol.1. Paris: Imprimerie Royale, 1841.

Aubertus Miraeus [Albert le Mire]. *Opera diplomatica et historica...: Codex donationum piarum.* 2nd edition. Brussels: Francis Foppens, 1723.

Babcock, Robert Gray. *The Well-Laden Ship. Egbert of Liège.* Dumbarton Oaks Medieval Library, Book 25. Cambridge, MA: Harvard University Press, 2013.

Berthollet, Jean. *Histoire de l'institution de la Fête-Dieu avec la vie des bienheureuses Julienne et Eve, toutes deux originaires de Liège.* Liège: Jacques-Antoine Gerlach, 1781.

Bocellin, Pierre. *Practique sur la matiere de la contagieuse et infective maladie de lepre.* Lyon: n.p., 1540.

Brodin, Gösta, ed. *Agnus Castus: A Middle English Herbal Reconstructed from Various Manuscripts.* Upsala: Ludequist, 1950.

Bruno da Longoburgo. *Chirurgia magna.* In: *Cyrurgia Guidonis de cauliaco. Et Cyrugia Bruni, Theodorici, Rogerij, Bertipalie, Lanfranci.* Venice: Bonetus Locatelli, 1498.

Chen Ziming 陳自明 (fl. ca. 1237-1271). *Furen daquan liangfang* (Comprehensive Compendium of Good Formulas for Women): compiled in 1237, preface dated 1271, modern critical edition of Yuan dynasty Qinyou shutang edition. Beijing: Beijing tushuguan chubanshe, 2005.

De Renzi, Salvatore, et al., eds. *Collectio Salernitana.* 5 vols. Naples: Filiatre-Sebezio, 1852-1859.

Dolaeus, Johannes. *Encyclopaedia chirurgica rationalis : in qua omnes affectus externi corpus humanum unquam invasisse observati … pertractantur.* Frankfurt: Knoch, 1689.

Egbert von Lüttich, *Fecunda Ratis*, ed. Ernst Voigt. Halle: Max Niemeyer Verlag, 1889.

Eggers, Will. "Selected Episodes on Healing and Disability from the Vulgate Bible - Matthew, Mark, Luke, and John," in *Medieval Disability Sourcebook: Western Europe,* ed. Cameron Hunt McNabb, 113-37. New York: punctum books, 2020.

Frisk, Gösta, ed. *A Middle English Translation of* Macer Floridus de Viribus Herbarum. Lundequistka: University of Bokhandein, 1949.

Galen. "On the Powers of Foods: Book 2," trans. Mark Grant, *Galen on Food and Diet* (New York: Routledge, 2000): 109-153.

Gilbertus Anglicus. *Compendium medicine.* Lyon: Portonaris, 1510.

Hafenreffer, Samuel. *Nosodochium: in quo cutis, eique adhaerentium partium, affectus omnes, singulari methodo, et cognoscendi et curandi fidelissime traduntur.* Ulm: Balthasar Kuehnen, 1660.

Henry of Huntingdon. *Anglicanus ortus: A Verse Herbal of the Twelfth Century.* Edited and translated by Winston Black. Toronto: Pontifical Institute of Mediaeval Studies, 2012.

Hildegard of Bingen. *Hildegard von Bingen's* Physica*: The Complete English Translation of Her Classic Work on Health and Healing.* Translated by Priscilla Throop. Rochester, VT: Healing Arts Press, 1998.

—. *Causes and Cures.* Translated by Priscilla Throop. Charlotte: MedievalMS, 2006.

—. *Scivias.* Translated by Columba Hart and Jane Bishop. Mahwah: Paulist Press, 1990.

Hippocrates, *Hippocrates*, trans. W. S. H. Jones. Cambridge: Harvard University Press, 1967.

Hippocrates. "Regimen in Acute Diseases," in *Hippocratic Writings,* ed. G. E. R. Lloyd, trans. J. Chadwick and W. N. Mann (London: Penguin Books, 1978, 1983): 186-205.

Ingrassia, Giovanni Filippo. *De tumoribus praeter naturam Tomus primus.* Naples: n.p., 1562.

Joannes de Mediolano, *Regimen Sanitatis Salerni, Or The Schoole of Salernes Regiment of Health.* London: B. Alsop, 1649.

Lanfranc, *Practica seu ars completa totius cyrurgie.* Venice: Bonetus Locatelli, 1498.

Laws of the Alamans and Bavarians, trans. T. J. Rivers. Philadelphia, 1977.

Leges Alamannorum, ed. J. Merkel, MGH Leges 3. Hanover, 1863.

Lemnius, Levinus. *De habitu et constitutione corporis.* Antwerp: Guilielmus Simonis, 1561.

Liber Guilielmi Placentini de Saliceto in scientia medicinali qui Summa conservationis et curationis appellatur Cyrugia. Venice, printer unknown, 1489.

The Life of Ibn Sina. A Critical Edition and Annotated Translation, ed. And trans. William E. Gohlman. Albany: SUNY Press, 1974.

Macer Floridus 'De viribus herbarum' una cum Walafridi Strabonis, Othonis Cremonensis et Ioannis Folcz' carminibus similis..., ed. L. Choulant. Leipzig: Leopold Voss, 1832.

Malory, Thomas. *Le Morte d'Arthur.* New York, NY: Heritage Press, 1955.

Manardo, Giovanni. *Epistolae medicinales diversorum authorum, nempe, Ioannis Manardi...* Lyon: n.p., 1557.

McVaugh, Michael R., ed. *Guigonis de Cauliaco (Guy de Chauliac) Inventarium sive Chirurgia magna.* Leiden: E.J. Brill, 1987.

Migne, Jacques-Paul, ed. *Patrologiae Latinae cursus completus* 207. Paris: Garnier, 1855.

"Miraculum auctore Aegidio Aureaevallensi," in *Gesta Episcoporum Leodiensium. Monumenta Germaniae Historica* SS 25, ed. Georg Heinrich Pertz. Hanover: Hahn, 1880.

Pagel, Julius, ed. *Die Chirurgie des Heinrich von Mondeville (Hermondaville).* Berlin: Hirschwald, 1892.

Platearius, Matthaeus. *Circa instans. Text und Kommentar*, ed. Hans Wölfel. Berlin, 1939.

Renier de Saint-Laurent (d. 1188). *Vita Evraclii.* In: *Monumenta Germaniae Historica* SS 20, ed. Georg Heinrich Pertz, 561-65. Hanover: Hahn, 1868.

Soranus, *Soranus' Gynecology*, trans. Owsei Temkin (Baltimore: The Johns Hopkins University Press, 1956.

Thomas de Chobham, *Thomas de Chobham Summa Confessorum,* ed. F. Broomfield. Paris: Analecta Mediaevalia Namurcensia, 1963.

The Trotula: An English Translation of the Medieval Compendium of Women's Medicine, ed. and trans. Monica H. Green. Philadelphia: University of Pennsylvania Press, 2001.

Turner, Daniel. *De morbis cutaneis: a treatise of diseases incident to the skin.* The third edition Revised and very much Enlarged. London: R. and J. Bonwicke, 1726.

Usama ibn Munqidh. *The Book of Contemplation: Islam and the Crusades*, trans. Paul M. Cobb. London: Penguin, 2008.

Vigo, Giovanni. *Prima pars practice in chirurgia: Practica in arte chirurgica copiosa Ioannis de Vigo.* Lyon: Vincent de Portonariis, 1519.

Wallis, Faith, ed. *Medieval Medicine: A Reader.* Toronto: University of Toronto Press, 2010.

William of Tyre. *Chronicon*, ed. R.B.C. Huygens. Vol 2. Turnhout: Brepols, 1986.

Zhuangzi, "Heaven's Way," trans. Paul Kjellberg. In: *Readings in Classical Chinese Philosophy*, ed. Philip Ivanhoe and Bryan W. van Norden. 2nd edition (Indianapolis: Hackett Publishing, 2005), 244-5.

Secondary Literature

Abaza, Mona. *Debates on Islam and Knowledge in Malaysia and Egypt.* London: Routledge, 2002.

Abbas, Afshan, et al., "The Fennel, Foeniculum vulgare incorporated diet shows anxiolytic potential: A pre-clinical study," *Pakistan Journal of Pharmaceutical Sciences,* 32:4 (2019): 1813-19.

Abrahamian, Ervand. *Iran Between Two Revolutions.* Princeton University Press, 1982.

—. *A History of Modern Iran.* Cambridge University Press, 2008.

Achón, María et al. "Effects of Milk and Dairy Product Consumption on Pregnancy and Lactation Outcomes: A Systematic Review," *American Journal of Clinical Nutrition,* 46:2 (1987): 74-87.

Adamson, Melitta Weiss. *Food in Medieval Times.* Westport, Connecticut: Greenwood Press, 2004.

Adamson, Peter, ed. *Interpreting Avicenna: Critical Essays.* Cambridge, 2013.

Afnan, Soheil M. *Avicenna: His Life and Works.* George Allen & Unwin, 1958.

Afshar, Ahmadreza. "Honoring Avicenna, the Great Persian Physician on the World's Postage Stamps," *Archives of Iranian Medicine* 13:5 (2010): 447-53.

Agrimi, Jole, and Crisciani, Chiara. "Charity and Aid in Medieval Christian Civilization," in *Western Medical Thought from Antiquity to the Middle Ages*, ed. Mirko D. Grmek , 170-96. Cambridge, MA: Harvard University Press, 1998.

Albin, Andrew et al., eds., *Whose Middle Ages? Teachable Moments for an Ill-Used Past.* New York, NY: Fordham University Press, 2019.

Allen, A. and Gabrielle Hatfield, *Medicinal Plants in Folk Tradition: An Ethnobotany of Britain and Ireland.* Portland: Timber Press, 2004.

Allen, Jane and Debra Hector, "Benefits of Breastfeeding," *NSW Public Health Bulletin* 16:4 (2005): 42-46.

Altschul, Nadia. *Politics of Temporalization: Medievalism and Orientalism in Nineteenth-Century South America.* University of Pennsylvania Press, 2020.

American College of Pediatrics, "Policy Statement: Breastfeeding and the Use of Human Milk," *Pediatrics* 115:5 (2005): 496-506.

Amster, Ellen. *Medicine and the Saints: Science, Islam, and the Colonial Encounter in Morocco, 1877-1956.* Austin: University of Texas Press, 2013.

Arnott, Robert, Stanley Finger, and C. U. M. Smith, *Trepanation: History, Discovery, Theory*. Lisse: Swets & Zeitlinger, 2003.

Banham, D. and C. Voth, "The Diagnosis and Treatment of Wounds in the Old English Medical Collections: Anglo-Saxon Surgery?" in *Wounds and Wound Repair in Medieval Culture,* ed. Larissa Tracy and Kelly DeVries, 153-74. Leiden: Brill, 2015.

Barber, Malcolm. "Lepers, Jews and Moslems: The Plot to Overthrow Christendom in 1321," *History* 66:216 (1981): 1-17.

—. "The Order of Saint Lazarus and the Crusades." *Catholic Historical Review* 80 (1994): 439-56.

Barnes, Linda L. *Needles, Herbs, Gods, and Ghosts: China, Healing and the West to 1848.* Cambridge: Harvard University Press, 2009.

Barnhouse, Lucy. "Languages of Experience: Translating Medicine in MS Laud Misc. 237," in *New Approaches to Disease, Disability, and Medicine in Medieval Europe*, ed. Erin Connelly and Steffi Künzel, 94-108. Oxford: Archaeopress, 2018.

Barzilay, Tzafrir. *Poisoned Wells: Accusations, Persecution, and Minorities in Medieval Europe, 1321-1422.* Philadelphia, PA: University of Pennsylvania Press, 2022.

Bazell, Dianne M. "Strife among the Table-fellows: Conflicting Attitudes of Early and Medieval Christians toward the Eating of Meat." *Journal of the American Academy of Religion* 65:1 (1997): 73-99

Bazzano, Alessandra N., et al., "Health Provider Experiences with Galactagogues to Support Breastfeeding: A Cross-Sectional Survey," *Journal of Multidisciplinary Healthcare,* 9 (2016): 623-30.

Beccaria, Augusto. *I Codici di medicina del periodo presalernitano (secoli IX, X e XI)*. Rome: Edizioni di Storia e Letteratura, 1956.

Bendetti, Fabrizio et al., "Neurobiological Mechanisms of the Placebo Effect," *The Journal of Neuroscience* 25:45 (2005): 10390-402.

Biddick, Kathleen. *The Shock of Medievalism.* Durham, NC: Duke University Press, 1998.

Bille, Mikkel. "Seeking Providence through Things: The Word of God versus Black Cumin," in *An Anthropology of Absence: Materializations of*

Transcendence and Loss, ed. Mikkel Bille et al., 167-84. New York: Springer, 2010.

Binder, M., J. Eitler, J. Deutschmann, et al., "Prosthetics in Antiquity—An Early Medieval Wearer of a Foot Prosthesis (6th Century AD) from Hemmaberg/Austria," *International Journal of Paleopathology* 12 (2016): 29-40.

Black, Winston. *The Middle Ages: Facts and Fictions*. Santa Barbara, CA: ABC-CLIO, 2019.

——. "Review: *La 'Practica' de Plateario: Edición Crítica, Traducción y Estudio*," *Speculum* 93:3 (2018): 895-97.

Blumenthal, Debra. "'*With My Daughter's Milk*': Wet Nurses and the Rhetoric of Lactation in Valencian Court Records," in *Medieval and Renaissance Lactations: Images, Rhetorics, Practices,* ed. Jutta Gisela Sperling, 101-14. Farnham: Ashgate, 2013.

Boddy, Janice. *Wombs and Alien Spirits: Women, Men, and the Zār Cult in Northern Sudan*. Madison: University of Wisconsin Press, 1989.

Boyarin, Shamma. "The New Metal Medievalism: Alexander the Great, Islamic Historiography and Nile's 'Iskander Dhul Kharnon'," in *Medievalism and Metal Music Studies: Throwing Down the Gauntlet*, ed. Ruth Barratt-Peacock and Ross Hagen, 81-91. Bingley, UK: Emerald Publishing, 2019.

Bowen, John. *Muslims through Discourse: Religion and Ritual in Gayo Society*. Princeton, NJ: Princeton University Press, 1993.

Brears, Peter. *Cooking and Dining in Medieval England.* Devon: Prospect Books, 2008.

Brenner, Elma. *Leprosy and Charity in Medieval Rouen*. Woodbridge: Boydell and Brewer, 2015.

Brenner, Elma and François-Olivier Touati, eds. *Leprosy and Identity in the Middle Ages: From England to the Mediterranean*. Manchester: Manchester University Press, 2021.

Brigliardi, Stefa: "The 'Scientific Miracles of the Qur'an': Map and Assessment," in *Islamic Studies Today: Essays in Honor of Andrew Rippin*, ed. Majid Daneshgar and Walid A. Saleh, 248-63. Leiden: Brill, 2017.

Brodman, James W. *Charity and Religion in Medieval Europe*. Washington, DC: Catholic University of America Press, 2009.

Brody, Howard. "Ritual, Medicine, and the Placebo Response," in *The Problem of Ritual Efficacy,* ed. William S. Sax, Johannes Quack and Jan Weinhold, 151-69. Oxford: Oxford University Press, 2010.

Brody, Saul Nathaniel. *The Disease of the Soul: Leprosy in Medieval Literature.* Ithaca, NY: Cornell University Press, 1974.

Brown, Catherine. "In the Middle." *Journal of Medieval and Early Modern Studies* 30:3 (2000): 547-74.

Brown, Ray B. and Lawrence A. Kreiser, eds., *The Detective as Historian: History and Art in Historical Crime Fiction.* Madison, WI: University of Wisconsin Press, 2013.

Brundage, James A. *Law, Sex, and Christian Society in Medieval Europe.* Chicago: University of Chicago Press, 1987.

Brunn, Stanley D. "Stamps as messengers of political transition," *Geographical Review* 101:1 (2011): 19-36.

Buck, R.A. "Women's Milk in Anglo-Saxon and Later Medieval Medical Texts," *Neophilologus* 96 (2012): 467-85.

Budzynska, Katarzyna, et al., "Systematic Review of Breastfeeding and Herbs," *Breastfeeding Medicine,* 7:6 (2012): 489-503.

Bull, Marcus. *Thinking Medieval: An Introduction to the Study of the Middle Ages.* New York, NY: Palgrave, 2005.

Bulman, William J. *Anglican Enlightenment: Orientalism, Religion and Politics in England and Its Empire, 1648-1715.* Cambridge: Cambridge University Press, 2015.

Burnett, Charles. "Manuscripts of Latin Translations of Scientific Texts from Arabic," in *Taxonomies of Knowledge: Information and Order in Medieval Manuscripts,* ed. Emily Steiner and Lynn Ransom, 80-89. Philadelphia: University of Pennsylvania Press, 2015.

Burnett, Charles and Danielle Jacquart, eds. *Constantine the African and Alī ibn Al-'Abbās Al-Magūsī: The Pantegni and Related Texts.* Leiden: Brill, 1995.

Bynum, Carolyn Walker. *Holy Feast, Holy Fast: The Religious Significance of Food to Medieval Women.* Berkeley: University of California Press, 1987.

——. "The Body of Christ in the Later Middle Ages: A Reply to Leo Steinberg," in *Fragmentation and Redemption: Essays on Gender and the Human Body in Medieval Religion* (New York: Zone Books, 1992): 79-118.

Cabré, Montserrat. "Women or Healers? Household Practices and the Categories of Health Care in Late Medieval Iberia." *Bulletin of the History of Medicine* 82:1 (2008): 18-51.

Cadden, Joan. *Meanings of Sex Difference in the Middle Ages: Medicine, Science, and Culture* Cambridge: Cambridge University Press, 1993.

Carroll, Shiloh. "Rewriting the Fantasy Archetype: George R. R. Martin, Neomedievalist Fantasy, and the Quest for Realism," in *Fantasy and Science-Fiction Medievalisms: From Isaac Asimov to A Game of Thrones*, ed. Helen Young, 59-76. Amherst, NY: Cambria Press 2015.

Caviness, Madeline H. "Feminism, Gender Studies, and Medieval Studies." *Diogenes* 57, no. 1 (February, 2010): 30-45.

Cecire, Maria Sachiko. *Re-Enchanted: The Rise of Children's Fantasy Literature in the Twentieth Century*. Minneapolis: University of Minnesota Press, 2019.

Cha, Wung-Seok, Jun-Ho Oh, Hi-Joon Park, Sang-Woo Ahn, Se-Young Hong, and Nam-Il Kim. "Historical difference between traditional Korean medicine and traditional Chinese medicine." *Neurological Research* 29 (2007): 5-9.

Chace, Jessica. "Diagnostic Medievalism: The Case of Leprosy's Stigma." *Disability Studies Quarterly* 39 (2019): https://dsq-sds.org/article/view/6410/5409.

Chance, Jane. *Tolkien the Medievalist.* London: Routledge, 2008.

Chaves, Jonathan. "The Legacy of Ts'ang Chieh: The Written Word as Magic." *Oriental Art* 23.2 (1977): 200-215.

Chazelle, Celia, Simon Doubleday, Felice Lifshitz, and Amy G. Remensnyder, eds. *Why the Middle Ages Matter: Medieval Light on Modern Injustice*. London: Routledge, 2012.

Cheng Hsiao-wen. *Divine, Demonic and Disordered: Women Without Men in Song Dynasty China.* Seattle: University of Washington Press, 2021.

Choi, Yun Kyung et al., "Association of Maternal Diet with Zinc, Copper, and Iron Concentrations in Transitional Human Milk Produced by Korean Mothers," *Clinical Nutritional Research,* 5:1 (2016): 15-25.

Chrissis, Nikolaos G., Athina Kolia-Dermitzaki, and Angeliki Papageorgiou. *Byzantium and the West: Perception and Reality (11th-15th C.)*. London: Routledge, 2019.

Clanchy, Michael T. *From Memory to Written Record.* Malden, MA: Blackwell, 1979.

——. "Parchment and Paper: Manuscript Culture 1100-1500," in *A Companion to the History of the Book*, ed. Simon Eliot and Jonathan Rose. Second Edition (Malden, MA: Wiley Blackwell, 2007): 219-233.

Clarke, Arthur C. *Profiles of the Future; an Inquiry into the Limits of the Possible.* New York: Harper & Row, 1962.

Cobb, Paul M. *Usama Ibn Munqidh: Warrior-Poet in the Age of Crusades.* Oxford: Oneworld, 2005.

Cohen, Jeffrey Jerome. "Hybrids, Monsters, Borderlands," in *The Postcolonial Middle Ages*, ed. Jeffrey Jerome Cohen (New York: Palgrave, 2000), 85-104.

Cohen, Mark R. *Poverty and Charity in the Jewish Community of Medieval Egypt.* Princeton: Princeton University Press, 2005.

Coker, Elizabeth. "Claiming the Public Soul: Representations of Qur'anic Healing and Psychiatry in the Egyptian Print Media." *Transcultural Psychiatry* 46:4 (2009): 672-94.

Coleman, Joyce. "Aural Illumination: Books and Aurality in the Frontispieces to Bishop Chevrot's *Cité de Dieu*," in *Orality and Literacy in the Middle Ages: Essays on a Conjunction and its Consequences in Honour of D.H. Green*, ed. Mark Chinca and Christopher Young, 223-52. Turnhout: Brepols, 2005.

——. *Public Reading and the Reading Public in Late Medieval England and France.* New York: Cambridge University Press, 1996.

Conn, Jennifer J. "What Can Clinical Teachers Learn from *Harry Potter and the Philosopher's Stone*?" *Medical Education* 36:12 (December 1, 2002): 1176-81.

Conover, Elizabeth Ann. "Herbal agents and over-the-counter medications in pregnancy." *Best Practice & Research Clinical Endocrinology & Metabolism* 17:2 (2003): 237-51.

Conrad, Lawrence I., Michael Neve, Vivian Nutton, Roy Porter, and Andrew Wear, eds. *The Western Medical Tradition: 800 BC to AD 1800.* Cambridge, 1995.

Crosby, Ruth. "Oral Delivery in the Middle Ages," *Speculum* 11 (1936): 88-110.

Cummings, Juliana. *Medicine in the Middle Ages: Surviving the Times.* London: Pen and Sword, 2021.

Dallal, Ahmad. *Islam, Science, and the Challenge of History.* New Haven: Yale University Press, 2010.

D'Arcens, Louise. "Medievalism: Scope and Complexity," in *The Cambridge Companion to Medievalism*, ed. Louise D'Arcens (Cambridge: Cambridge University Press, 2016), 1-13.

Das, Ranjana and Chiranjib Bhattacharjee, "Lettuce," in *Nutritional Composition and Antioxidant Properties of Fruits and Vegetables*, ed. Amit K. Jaiswal (Cambridge, MA: Academic Press Elsevier, 2020): 143-57.

Das, Shinjini. *Vernacular Medicine in Colonial India: Family, Market, and Homeopathy*. Cambridge University Press, 2019.

Date, Anand. "Sir William Osler's Arab and other Middle Eastern contacts," *The Ulster Medical journal* 60:1 (1991): 120-28.

Davis, Adam. *The Medieval Economy of Salvation: Charity, Commerce, and the Rise of the Hospital.* Ithaca, NY: Cornell University Press, 2019.

Dearnley, Elizabeth. "'Women of Oure Tunge Cunne Bettir Reede and Vnderstonde This Language': Women and Vernacular Translation in Medieval England," in *Multilingualism in Medieval Britain (c.1066-1520):* eds. Judith A. Jefferson and Ad Putter, 259-72. Turnhout: Brepols, 2013.

Delbourgo, James. "The Knowing World: A New Global History of Science," *History of Science* 57:3 (September 1, 2019): 378-81.

Demaitre, Luke. "The Clapper as 'vox miselli': New Perspectives on Iconography," in *Leprosy and Identity in the Middle Ages: From England to the Mediterranean*, ed. Elma Brenner and François-Olivier Touati (Manchester: Manchester University Press, 2021): 208-65.

——. "The Description and Diagnosis of Leprosy by Fourteenth-Century Physicians." *Bulletin of the History of Medicine* 59 (1985): 327-44.

——. *Leprosy in Premodern Medicine: A Malady of the Whole Body*. Baltimore: Johns Hopkins University Press, 2007.

——. "'Vita brevis, Ars autem prolixa': forging a medical language," in *Petrarca e la medicina. Atti del Convegno di Capo d'Orlando 27-28 giugno 2003,* ed. Monica Berté, Vincenzo Fera, and Tiziana Pesenti, 123-43. Biblioteca umanistica 8. Messina: Centro interdipartmentale di studi umanistici, 2006.

Demoulin-Auzary, Florence. "Pro sustentandis Christi pauperibus: La naissance d'un droit de l'aumône aux xiie et xiiie siècles," in *Der Einfluss der Kanonistik auf die Europäische Rechtskultur: Das Recht der Wirtschaft*, ed. David von Mayenburg, Orazio Condorelli, Franck Roumy, and Mathias Schmoekel, 73-100. Köln: Böhlau Verlag, 2016.

Despeaux, Catherine. "The System of the Five Circulatory Phases and the Six Seasonal Influences (*wuyun liqi*): a Source of Innovation in Medicine under the Song (960-1279):" in *Innovations in Medicine*, ed. E. Hsu, 121-65. Cambridge: Cambridge University Press.

Despeaux, Catherine. "Talismans and Diagrams," in *Daoism Handbook*, ed. Livia Kohn, 498-540. Leiden: Brill, 2004.

DeVries, Kelly. "Gunpowder Weaponry and the Rise of the Early Modern State," *War in History* 5:2 (1998): 127-45.

Dinshaw, Carolyn. *Getting Medieval: Sexualities and Communities, Pre- and Postmodern.* Durham, NC: Duke University Press, 1999.

Do, Choon H. "Progress of Chemistry in South Korea." *Chemistry International* 37:5-6 (2015): 4-11.

Dols, Michael W. "The Leper in Medieval Islamic Society." *Speculum* 58 (1983): 891-916.

——. "The Origins of the Islamic Hospital, Myth and Reality." *Bulletin of the History of Medicine* 91 (1987): 367-90.

Doostdar, Alireza. *The Iranian Metaphysicals: Explorations in Science, Islam, and the Uncanny.* Princeton: Princeton University Press, 2018.

Doumato, Eleanor. *Getting God's Ear: Women, Islam, and Healing in Saudi Arabia and the Gulf.* New York: Columbia University Press, 2000.

Du Cange, Charles et al., eds. *Glossarium mediae et infimae Latinitatis.* Niort: L. Favre, 1883-87.

Ebrey, Patricia. *The Inner Quarters: Marriage and the Lives of Chinese Women in the Sung Period.* California: University of California Press, 1993.

Eco, Umberto. "Dreaming of the Middle Ages," in *Travels in Hyperreality: Essays*, trans. William Weaver (San Diego: Harcourt Brace Jovanovich, 1990), 61-85.

Edbury, Peter W. and John Gordon Rowe. *William of Tyre: Historian of the Latin East.* Cambridge: Cambridge University Press, 1988.

The Egyptian Gazette (*Al-Waqa'i'a al-Misiryya*): July 22, 1954.

Ekiert, Halina, Joanna Pajor, Paweł Klin, Agnieszka Rzepiela, Halina Ślesak, and Agnieszka Szopa. "Significance of Artemisia vulgaris L. (Common Mugwort) in the History of Medicine and Its Possible Contemporary Applications Substantiated by Phytochemical and Pharmacological studies," *Molecules* 25, no. 19 (2020): 4415.

El-Tom, Abdullahi. "Drinking the Koran: The Meaning of Koranic Verses in Berti Erasure." *Africa: Journal of the International African Institute* 55:4 (1985): 414-31.

Elliott, Andrew B.R. *Remaking the Middle Ages: The Methods of Cinema and History in Portraying the Medieval World.* Jefferson, NC: McFarland and Co., 2011.

——. *Medievalism, Politics and Mass Media: Appropriating the Middle Ages in the Twenty-first Century.* Cambridge: D.S. Brewer, 2017.

Elman, Benjamin. *A Cultural History of Modern Science in China*. Cambridge, MA: Harvard University Press, 2006.

Espesset, Grégoire. "A case study on the evolution of Chinese religious symbols from talismanic paraphernalia to Taoist liturgy." *Bulletin of the School of Oriental and African Studies* 78.3 (October 2015): 493-514.

Evans, Jennifer. "Female Barrenness, Bodily Access and Aromatic Treatments in Seventeenth-Century England." *Historical Research* 87:237 (2014): 424-43.

Fahmy, Khaled. "Medicine and Power: Towards a Social History of Medicine in Nineteenth-Century Egypt." *Cairo Papers in Social Science* 23:2 (2000): 1-45

Falk, Avner. *Franks and Saracens: Reality and Fantasy in the Crusades*. New York: Routledge, 2010.

Farmer, Sharon, ed. *Approaches to Poverty in Medieval Europe: Complexities, Contradictions, Transformations, c. 1100-1500*. Turnhout: Brepols, 2016.

——. *Surviving Poverty in Medieval Paris: Gender, Ideology, and the Daily Lives of the Poor*. Ithaca, NY: Cornell University Press, 2001.

Feher, Stephen D. K., et al., "Increasing Breast Milk Production for Premature Infants with a Relaxation/Imagery Audiotape," *Pediatrics,* 83: 1 (1989): 57-60.

Finke, Laurie A. and Martin B. Shichtman. *Cinematic Illuminations: The Middle Ages on Film*. Baltimore, MD: Johns Hopkins University Press, 2007.

Fitzpatrick, KellyAnn. *Neomedievalism, Popular Culture, and the Academy: From Tolkien to Game of Thrones*. Woodbridge: Boydell and Brewer, 2019).

Fleming, Robin. "Bones for Historians: Putting the Body Back into Biography," in *Writing Medieval Biography, 750-1250: Essays in Honour of Frank Barlow*, ed. D. Bates, J. Crick, and S. Hamilton, 29-48. Woodbridge: Boydell and Brewer, 2006.

——. "Writing Biography at the Edge of History," *The American Historical Review* 114 (2009): 606-14.

Flint, Valerie J. "The Early Medieval *Medicus*, the Saint – and the Enchanter," *Social History of Medicine* 2 (1989): 127-45.

Flood, Finbarr Barry. "Bodies and Becoming: Mimesis, Mediation, and the Ingestion of the Sacred in Christianity and Islam," in *Sensational Religion: Sensory Culture in Material Practice*, ed. Sally Promey, 459-93. New Haven: Yale University Press, 2014.

Flueckiger, Joyce. *In Amma's Healing Room: Gender and Vernacular Islam in South India.* Bloomington: Indiana University Press, 2006.

Foscati, Angela. "Un'analisi semantica del termine erysipelas. Le Centuriae di Amato Lusitano nella tradizione dei testi dall'Antichità al Rinascimento," in Praxi theoremata coniungamus. *Amato Lusitano y la medicina de su tiempo,* ed. Miguel Ángel González Manjarrés, 125-43. Madrid: Guillermo Escobar, 2019.

Freedman, Paul. *Out of the East: Spices and the Medieval Imagination.* New Haven: Yale University Press, 2008.

Gabriele, Matthew and David Perry. *The Bright Ages: A New History of Medieval Europe.* New York: Harper, 2021.

Ganim, John M. "Medieval Noir: Anatomy of a Metaphor," in *Medieval Film*, ed. Anke Bernau and Bettina Bildhauer, 182-202. Manchester: Manchester University Press, 2009.

Garrido, Pablo F. *et al.* "The Lord of the NanoRings: Cyclodextrins and the Battle against SARS-CoV-2," *International Journal of Pharmaceutics* 588 (October 15, 2020), 119689.

Gaylord, Alan T. "O Rare Ellis Peters: Two Rules for Medieval Murder," in *Studies in Medievalism XX: Defining Neomedievalism(s) II*, ed. Karl Fugelso, 129-46. Woodbridge: Boydell and Brewer, 2011.

Geltner, Guy. "Healthscaping a Medieval City: Lucca's curia viarum and the Future of Public Health History." *Urban History* 40:3 (2013): 395-415.

——. "Public Health and the Pre-Modern City: A Research Agenda." *History Compass* 10:3 (2012): 231-45.

Gernet, Jacques. "Aspects et fonctions pyshcologiques de l'écriture," in *L'intelligence de la Chine, le social et le mental,* ed. Jacques Gernet, 361-79. Paris: Gallimard, 1994.

Getz, Faye. "Black Death and the Silver Lining: Meaning, Continuity, and Revolutionary Change in Histories of Medieval Plague." *Journal of the History of Biology* 24:2 (Summer 1991): 265-89.

Gibbs, Frederick W. *Poison, Medicine, and Disease in Late Medieval and Early Modern Europe.* New York: Routledge, 2019.

Giladi, Avner. "Breast-feeding in Medieval Islamic Thought," *Journal of Family History* 23:2 (1998): 107-123.

Glaze, Florence Eliza. "The Perforated Wall: The Ownership and Circulation of Medical Books in Medieval Europe, ca. 800-1200". Doctoral Dissertation, Duke University, 1999.

Glenn, Cheryl. "Medieval Literacy Outside the Academy: Popular Practice and Individual Technique," *College Composition and Communication,* 44:4 (1993): 497-508.

Glick, Thomas F. "Communication," in *Medieval Science, Technology, and Medicine: An Encyclopedia*, eds. Thomas Glick, Steven J. Livesey, and Faith Wallis, 135-39. New York: Routledge, 2005.

Goldschmidt, Asaf. "Commercializing Medicine or Benefiting People: The First Public Pharmacy in China." *Science in Context* 21:3 (2008): 311-50.

—. *Evolution of Chinese Medicine: Song Dynasty, 960-1200.* London: Routledge Press, 2009.

Grattan, John Henry Grafton, and Charles Singer. *Anglo-Saxon Magic and Medicine: Illustrated Specially from the Semi-Pagan Text* Lacnunga. Oxford: Oxford University Press, 1952.

Green, Monica H. *Making Women's Medicine Masculine: The Rise of Male Authority in Pre-Modern Gynecology*. Oxford: Oxford University Press, 2008.

—. "Medical Books," in *The European Book in the Twelfth Century*, ed. Erik Kwakkel and Rodney Thomson, 277-92. Cambridge: Cambridge University Press, 2018.

—. "Rethinking the Manuscript Basis of Salvatore de Renzi's *Collectio Salernitana*: The Corpus of Medical Writings in the 'Long' Twelfth Century," in *La Collectio Salernitana di Salvatore de Renzi*, ed. Danielle Jacquart and Agostino Paravicino Bagliani, 15-60. Florence: SISMEL, 2008.

—. "The Possibilities of Literacy and the Limits of Reading: Women and the Gendering of Medieval Literacy," in *Women's Healthcare in the Medieval West: Texts and Contexts,* 1-76. Aldershot: Ashgate, 2000.

—. "Editor's Introduction to *Pandemic Disease in the Medieval World: Rethinking the Black Death,"* in *Pandemic Disease in the Medieval World: Rethinking the Black Death,* ed. Monica Green, 9-26. Kalamazoo: ARC Medieval Press, 2015.

—. Kathleen Walker-Meikle, and Wolfgang P. Mueller. "Diagnosis of a 'Plague' Image: A Digital Cautionary Tale." *The Medieval Globe* 1 (2014): 309-25.

Grieve, Maude. *A Modern Herbal: The Medicinal, Culinary, Cosmetic and Economic Properties, Cultivation and Folk-Lore of Herbs, Grasses, Fungi,*

Shrubs and Trees with Their Modern Scientific Uses, 2 vols. New York: Dover Publications, 1971 (1931).

Grigor, Talinn. *Building Iran: Modernism, Architecture, and National Heritage under the Pahlavi Monarchs.* New York: Periscope Publishing, 2009.

——. "Recultivating 'Good Taste': The Early Pahlavi Modernists and Their Society for National Heritage," *Iranian Studies* 37:1 (2004): 17-29.

Halina, Ekiert et al. "Significance of *Artemisia Vulgaris* L. (Common Mugwort) in the History of Medicine and Its Possible Contemporary Applications Substantiated by Phytochemical and Pharmacological Studies." *Molecules* 25:19 (2020): 4415.

Hall, Harriet. "Masaru Emoto's Wonderful World of Water." *Skeptical Inquirer*, 31:6 (2007): 49-51

Hallaq, Wael B. *Restating Orientalism: A Critique of Modern Knowledge.* New York: Columbia University Press, 2018.

Hamdy, Sherine. "Blinding Ignorance: Medical Science, Diseased Eyes, and Religious Practice in Egypt," *Arab Studies Journal* 12-13 (2004/2005): 26-45.

——. *Our Bodies Belong to God: Organ Transplants, Islam, and the Struggle for Human Dignity in Egypt.* Berkeley: University of California Press, 2012.

Hamilton, Bernard. *The Leper King and His Heirs: Baldwin IV and the Crusader Kingdom of Jerusalem.* Cambridge: Cambridge University Press, 2000.

Hanawalt, Barbara. *The Ties That Bound.* Oxford: Oxford University Press, 1986.

Hanson, Marta. *Speaking of Epidemics in Chinese Medicine: Disease and the Geographic Imagination in Late Imperial China.* London: Routledge Press, 2011.

Harper, April. "Misdiagnosing Medieval Medicine: 'Magical' Muslims, Metanarrative, and the Modern Media," in *The Middle Ages in Modern Culture: History and Authenticity in Contemporary Medievalism*, ed. Karl C. Alvestad and Robert Houghton (London: Bloomsbury Academic, 2021), 58-73.

Harris, Nichola E. "The Idea of Lapidary Medicine: Its Circulation and Practical Applications in Medieval and Early Modern Europe," PhD diss., (Rutgers University, 2009).

——. "Loadstones are a Girl's Best Friend: Lapidary Cures, Midwives, and Manuals of Popular Healing in Medieval and Early Modern

England," in *The Sacred and the Secular in Medieval Healing: Sites, Objects, and Texts,* ed. Barbara S. Bowers and Linda Migl Keyser (New York: Routledge, 2016): 182-218.

Harris, Stephen J. and Bryon L. Grigsby, eds., *Misconceptions about the Middle Ages.* New York, NY: Routledge, 2001.

Harrison, Peter. *The Territories of Science and Religion.* Chicago: The University of Chicago Press, 2015.

Haskins, Charles Homer. *The Renaissance of the Twelfth Century.* Cambridge, MA: Harvard University Press, 1927.

——. "The Sicilian Translators of the Twelfth Century and the First Latin Version of Ptolemy's *Almagest*," *Harvard Studies in Classical Philology* 21 (1910): 75-102.

Hatfield, Gabrielle. *Encyclopedia of Folk Medicine; Old World and New World Traditions.* Santa Barbara, CA: ABC-CLIO, 2004.

Hayakawa, Satoshi et al. "Rembrandt's Maria Bockenolle has a butterfly rash and digital deformities: Overlapping syndrome of rheumatoid arthritis and systemic lupus erythematosus." *Medical Hypotheses* 68 (2007): 906-9.

Heinrichs, Erik A. "The Live Chicken Treatment for Buboes: Trying a Plague Cure in Medieval and Early Modern Europe." *Bulletin of the History of Medicine* 91:2 (2017): 210-32.

Heng, Geraldine. *Empire of Magic: Medieval Romance and the Politics of Cultural Fantasy.* New York: Columbia University Press, 2003.

——. *The Invention of Race in the European Middle Ages.* Cambridge, 2018.

——. "Afterword: Medievalists and the Education of Desire," in *Whose Middle Ages? Teachable Moments for an Ill-Used Past,* ed. Andrew Albin, Mary C. Erler, Thomas O'Donnell, Nicholas L. Paul, and Nina Rowe (New York: Fordham University Press, 2019), 275-90.

Holmes, Urban T. Jr. and Frederick R. Weedon. "Peter of Blois as a Physician." *Speculum* 37 (1962): 252-56.

Holsinger, Bruce. *Neomedievalism, Neoconservatism, and the War on Terror.* Chicago, 2007.

——. "Medievalization Theory: From Tocqueville to the Cold War," *American Literary History* 22:4 (2010): 893-912.

Homolka, Anita. "Die Lebensgewohnheiten der Leprakranken im Spätmittelalter," in *Aussatz—Lepra—Hansen-Krankheit: ein Menschheitsproblem im Wandel,* ed. Jörn Henning Wolf (Würzburg: Deutsches Aussätzigen-Hilfswerk, 1986): 151-62.

Horden, Peregrine. "A Non-Natural Environment: Medicine without Doctors and the Medieval European Hospital," in *The Medieval Hospital and Medical Practice,* ed. Barbara S. Bowers (Burlington: Ashgate, 2007): 133-46.

——. "What's Wrong with Early Medieval Medicine?" *Social History of Medicine* 24 (2011): 5-25.

Horn, Walter, and Ernest Born. *The Plan of St Gall: A Study of the Architecture and Economy of, and Life in, a Paradigmatic Carolingian Monastery*, 3 vols. Berkeley, 1979.

Hourani, Albert. *Arabic Thought in the Liberal Age, 1798–1939.* Oxford: Oxford University Press, 1970.

Humphrey, Nicholas. "Great Expectations: the Evolutionary Psychology of Faith-Healing and the Placebo Effect," in *The Mind Made Flesh: Essays from the Frontiers of Psychology and Evolution* (New York: Oxford University Press, 2002): 255-88.

Hunt, Tony. *The Medieval Surgery*. Woodbridge: Boydell and Brewer, 1992.

——. *Plant Names of Medieval England.* Woodbridge: D.S. Brewer, 1989.

Inhorn, Marcia. *Local Babies, Global Science: Gender, Religion, and In Vitro Fertilization in Egypt.* New York: Routledge, 2003.

Issawi, Charles. "Europe, the Middle East and the Shift in Power: Reflections on a Theme by Marshall Hodgson," *Comparative Studies in Society and History* 22:4 (1980): 487-504.

Jackson, A. V. Williams. *Persia Past and Present: A Book of Travel and Research.* Macmillan, 1906.

Jackson, Ralph. *Doctors and Diseases in the Roman Empire*. London: British Museum Publications, 1988.

Jackson, Stanley W. *Melancholia and Depression: From Hippocratic Times to Modern Times.* New Haven: Yale University Press, 1986.

Jacobs, Lesley. "Idealized Images of Wales in the Fiction of Edith Pargeter/Ellis Peters," in *Mass Market Medieval: Essays on the Middle Ages in Popular Culture*, ed. David W. Marshall (McFarland & Company, 2007), 90-101.

Jacobson, Hilary. *Mother's Milk: A Breastfeeding Guide with Lactogenic Foods and Herbs – Build Milk Supply, Boost Immunity, Lift Depression, Detox, Lose Weight, Optimize a Baby's IQ, and Reduce Colic and Allergies.* Rosalind Press, 2004.

Jacquart, Danielle. "Review: *Thirteenth- and Fourteenth-Century Copies of the* Ars Medicine*: A Checklist and Contents Description of the Manuscripts* by

Cornelius O'Boyle; *The* Articella *in the Early Press, c. 1476–1534* by Jon Arrizabalaga; *Papers of the Articella Project Meeting: Cambridge, December 1995* by Roger French," *Isis* 94:4 (2003): 717-8.

Jeanselme, E. "Comment l'Europe, au Moyen Age, se protégea contre la Lèpre." *Bulletin de la Société Française d'Histoire de la Médecine* 25 (1931): 1-155.

Jeong, Yong-Jae, et al. "A Sasang constitutional study on the Myunghyun symptom." *Journal of Sasang Constitutional Medicine* 21:1 (2009): 20-27.

Johnson, Tina Phillips. *Childbirth in Republican China: Delivering Modernity*. Lanham, Maryland: Lexington Books, 2011.

Jones, Lori and Nükhet Varlik, eds. *Death and Disease in the Medieval and Early Modern World: Perspectives from Across the Mediterranean and Beyond.* Woodbridge: Boydell & Brewer, 2022.

Jose, Laura. "Monstrous Conceptions: Sex, Madness and Gender in Medieval Medical Texts." *Comparative Critical Studies* 5:2 (2008): 153-63.

Jouanna, Jacques. "Wine and Medicine in Ancient Greece," in *Greek Medicine from Hippocrates to Galen: Selected Papers*, trans. Neil Allies, ed. Philip van der Eijk (Boston: Brill, 2012): 173-94.

Junqueira, Luis Fernando Bernardi. "Revealing Secrets: Talismans, Healthcare and the Market of the Occult in Early Twentieth-century China." *Social History of Medicine* 34:4 (2021): 1068-93.

Kalmar, Ivan. *Early Orientalism: Imagined Islam and the Notion of Sublime Power.* London: Routledge, 2012.

Katz, Paul. *Demon Hordes and Burning Boats: The Cult of Marshal Wen in Late Imperial China.* New York: SUNY Press, 1995.

Kaufman, Amy. "Medieval Unmoored," in *Studies in Medievalism XIX: Defining Neomedievalism(s) I*, ed. Karl Fugelso (Woodbridge: Boydell and Brewer, 2010), 1-11.

Keane, Webb. "On Spirit Writing: Materialities of Language and the Religious Work of Transduction." *Journal of the Royal Anthropological Institute* 19:1 (2013): 1–17.

Keller, Richard. *Colonial Madness: Psychiatry in French North Africa.* Chicago: The University of Chicago Press, 2007.

Kent, Jacqueline C. "How Breastfeeding Works," *The American College of Nurse-Midwives,* 52: 6 (2007): 564-70.

Kent, Jacqueline C., Daneille K. Prime, and Catherine P. Garbin, "Principles for Maintaining or Increasing Breast Milk Production,"

The Association of Women's Health, Obstetric, and Neonatal Nurses, 41 (2012): 114-21.

Khedimellah, Moussa. "Une version de la *ruqiya* de rite prophétique en France. Le cas d'Abdellah, imam guérisseur en Lorraine," in *Coran et talismans: Textes et pratique magiques en milieu musulman*, ed. Constant Hamès (Paris: Karthala, 2007), 385-407.

Kim, Hae Dun, et al., "Sleep-inducing effect of lettuce (*Lactuca sativa*) varieties on pentobarbital-induced sleep," *Food Science Biotechnology,* 26:3 (2017): 807-14.

Kim, James H. and Anthony R. Scialli. "Thalidomide: The Tragedy of Birth Defects and the Effective Treatment of Disease." *Toxicological Sciences* 122:1 (2011): 1-6.

Kim, Moo Jung et al., "Nutritional Value, bioactive Compounds and Health Benefits of Lettuce (*Lactuca satvia* L.):" *Journal of Food Composition and Analysis,* 49 (2016): 19-34.

Kim, Zaehi. "Reinterpretation of Ungnyeo through Eurasian Bear Worship and Mugwort and Garlic from Dangun Myth." *The Korean Folklore* 67 (2018): 31-57.

King, Helen. "The Mathematics of Sex: One to Two, or Two to One?" *Studies in Medieval and Renaissance History: Sexuality and Culture in Medieval and Renaissance Europe* 2:3 (2005): 47-58.

—. "Motherhood and Health in the Hippocratic Corpus: Does Maternity Protect Against Disease?" *Mètis Anthropologie des Mondes Grecs Anciens* 11 (2013): 51-70.

—. "Once upon a Text: Hysteria from Hippocrates," in *Hysteria Beyond Freud*, ed. Helen King, Sander L. Gilman, Roy Porter, G. S. Rousseau, and Elaine Showalter (Berkeley: University of California Press, 2020), 1-90.

Klapisch-Zuber, Christiane. "Blood Parents and Milk Parents: Wet-nursing in Florence, 1300-1530," in *Women, Family and Ritual in Renaissance Italy,* trans. Lydia Cochrane (Chicago: University of Chicago Press, 1985): 132-64.

Kominiarek, Michelle A. "Nutritional Recommendations in Pregnancy and Lactation," *The Medical Clinics of North America* 100:6 (2016): 1199-1215.

Kraidy, Marwan and Joe Khalil. *Arab Television Industries.* London: Palgrave Macmillan, 2009.

Krolikoski, Courtney A. "Kissing Lepers: Saint Francis and the Treatment of Lepers in the Central Middle Ages," in *Leprosy and Identity in the Middle Ages: From England to the Mediterranean*, ed. Elma Brenner and François-Olivier Touati (Manchester: Manchester University Press, 2021), 269-93.

——. "Malady or Miracle? The Influence of St Francis on the Perception of Leprosy in the High Middle Ages." MA Thesis, Central European University, 2011.

——. "'No More Horrified by Them': Royal Holy Women and Lepers in Twelfth- and Thirteenth-Century Hagiography," in *Living on the Edge: Transgression, Exclusion and Persecution in the Middle Ages*, ed. Delfi Nieto and Laura Miquel Milian (Berlin: De Gruyter, 2022), 59-74.

Kubica, Pawel et al., "*Verbena officinalis* (Common Vervain) – A Review of the Investigations of This Medically Important Plant Species," *Planta Medica* 86 (2020): 1241-57.

Kupper, Jean-Louis. *Notger de Liège (972-1008).* Brussels: Académie Royale de Belgique, 2015.

Kuuliala, Jenni. *Saints, Infirmity, and Community in the Late Middle Ages.* Amsterdam: Amsterdam University Press, 2020.

Laderman, Carol. "A Welcoming Soil: Islamic Humoralism on the Malay Peninsula," in *Paths to Asian Medical Knowledge*, ed. Charles Leslie and Allan Young (Berkeley, CA: University of California Press, 1992), 272-90.

Lagerway, John. "The Oral and the Written in Chinese and Western Religions," in *Religion and Philosophie in Ostasien, Festschrift für Hans Herman Schmidt*, ed. Gert Naundorf, Karl-Heinz Pohl, and Hans Hermann Schmidt (Würzburg: Königshausen und Neumann, 1985): 301-22.

Lambek, Michael. *Knowledge and Practice in Mayotte: Local Discourses of Islam, Sorcery, and Spirit Possession.* Toronto: University of Toronto Press, 1993.

Langford, Jean. *Fluent Bodies: Ayurvedic Remedies for Postcolonial Imbalances.* Durham, NC: Duke University Press, 2002.

Larrington, Carolyn. "Mediating Medieval(ized) Emotion in Game of Thrones," in *Studies in Medievalism XXVII: Authenticity, Medievalism, Music*, ed. Karl Fugelso (Cambridge: D.S. Brewer, 2018), 35-42.

Laurioux, Bruno: *Une histoire culinaire du Moyen Âge.* Paris: Honoré Champion Éditeur, 2005.

Lawrence, Ruth, and Robert Lawrence, *Breastfeeding: A Guide for the Medical Profession,* 7th edition. Maryland Heights, MO: Elsevier, 2011.

Lee, Becky R. "A Company of Women and Men: Men's Recollection of Childbirth in Medieval England," *Journal of Family History* 27:2 (2002): 92-100.

Lee, Kwang-Ok, Sun-Bok Jang, and Ji-Soo Yoo. "Content analysis of wormwood smoke (Ssukjahun) experiences in women." *Journal of East-West Nursing Research* 14:1 (2008): 68-77.

Lees, Clare A. and Gillian R. Overing. "Doing It Differently: Medieval and Contemporary," in *The Contemporary Medieval in Practice* (London: UCL Press, 2019), 1-11.

Leong, Elaine. "Collecting Knowledge for the Family: Recipes, Gender and Practical Knowledge in the Early Modern English Household," *Centaurus* 55:2 (2013): 81-103.

Lev, Efraim. "Reconstructed *materia medica* of the Medieval and Ottoman al-Sham." *Journal of Ethnopharmacology* 80:2-3 (2002): 167-79.

Li, Ruowei, et al., "Why Mothers Stop Breastfeeding: Mothers' Self-Reported Reasons for Stopping During the First Year," *Pediatrics,* 122:2 (2008): 569-76.

Lin, Derong et al., "An Overview of Plant Phenolic Compounds and Their Importance in Human Nutrition and Management of Type 2 Diabetes," *Molecules,* 21:10 (2016): 1374.

Lindsay, Edwin Ernest Christian Blake. "The Habit of Detection: The Medieval Monk as Detective in the Novels of Ellis Peters," in *Studies in Medievalism IV: Medievalism in England,* ed. Leslie J. Workman (Cambridge: D.S. Brewer, 1992), 276-89.

Lipoff, Jules B. "Greyscale—A Mystery Dermatologic Disease on HBO's *Game of Thrones,*" *JAMA Dermatology* 152, no. 8 (August 1, 2016), 904.

Liu Chang-xiao, "Overview on Development of ASEAN traditional and herbal medicines," *Chinese Herbal Medicines* 13 (2021): 441-50.

Livingston, John. "Muḥammad 'Abduh on Science." *The Muslim World* 85:3/4 (1995): 215–34

Locke, Hilary Jane. "Beyond 'Tits and Dragons': Medievalism, Medieval History, and Perceptions in Game of Thrones," in *From Medievalism to Early-Modernism: Adapting the English Past,* ed. Marina Gerzić and Aidan Norrise (New York: Routledge, 2019): 171-87.

Long, Pamela O. *Openness, Secrecy, Authorship : Technical Arts and the Culture of Knowledge from Antiquity to the Renaissance*. Baltimore: Johns Hopkins University Press, 2001.

Maccoby, Hyam. *Ritual and Morality: The Ritual Purity System and Its Place in Judaism.* Cambridge: Cambridge University Press, 1999.

Mahdizadeh, Saha and Reyhaneh Sadat Shojaei, "The involvement of Western Orientalists in cultural heritage affairs during the Pahlavi Era, Iran (1925-1979)" *Journal of Architectural Conservation* 24:3 (2018): 169-84.

Mahmood, Saba. *Politics of Piety: The Islamic Revival and the Feminist Subject.* Princeton, N.J.: Princeton University Press, 2005.

Malone, Irina Ruppo. "What's Wrong with Medievalism? Tolkien, the Strugatsky Brothers, and the Question of the Ideology of Fantasy," *Journal of the Fantastic in the Arts* 27:2 (2016): 204-24.

Mallavarapu, Ravi K. and Edwin W. Grimsley, "The History of Lupus Erythematosus." *Southern Medical Journal* 100:9 (2007): 896-8.

Marcombe, David. *Leper Knights: The Order of St Lazarus of Jerusalem in England, 1150-1544*. Woodbridge: Boydell Press, 2003.

Maréchal, Edouard. *Éracle et la fondation de la collégiale Saint Martin à Liège.* Liège: Dessain, 1894.

Matthee, Rudi. "Transforming dangerous nomads in useful artisans, technicians, agriculturalists: education in the Reza Shah period," in *The Making of Modern Iran: State and Society under Riza Shah, 1921-1941*, ed. Stephanie Cronin (Routledge, 2003): 123-45.

Matthews, David. *Medievalism: A Critical History*. Cambridge: D.S. Brewer, 2015.

Mayberg, Helen S. et al., "The Functional Neuroanatomy of the Placebo Effect," *The American Journal of Psychiatry* 159:5 (2002): 728-37.

Mays, Simon A. "A Possible Case of Surgical Treatment of Cranial Blunt Force Injury from Medieval England," *International Journal of Osteoarchaeology* 16 (2006): 95-103.

—. "The Effects of Infant Feeding Practices on Infant and Maternal Health in a Medieval Community," *Childhood in the Past* 3: 1 (2010): 63-78.

McCleery, Iona. "What Is 'Colonial' about Medieval Colonial Medicine? Iberian Health in Global Context," *Journal of Medieval Iberian Studies* 7:2 (2015): 151-175.

McGinnis, Jon. *Avicenna.* Oxford University Press, 2010.

McKay, William John Stewart. *The History of Ancient Gynæcology*. United Kingdom: Baillière, Tindall and Cox, 1901.

McKendry, Anne. *Medieval Crime Fiction: A Critical Overview*. Jefferson, NC: McFarland & Co., 2019.

McKitterick, Rosamond, ed. *The Uses of Literacy in Early Medieval Europe*. Cambridge: Cambridge University Press, 1990.

McNabb, Cameron Hunt. "Introduction," in *Medieval Disability Sourcebook: Western Europe,* ed. Cameron Hunt McNabb (punctum books, 2020), 13-20.

McVaugh, Michael. *The Rational Surgery of the Middle Ages*. Florence: SISMEL, 2006.

Meijer, Roel, ed. *Global Salafism: Islam's New Religious Movement.* New York, NY: Columbia University Press, 2009.

Melvin-Koushki, Matthew. "Is (Islamic) Occult Science Science?" *Theology and Science* 18:2 (2020): 303–24.

Metzler, Irina. "Disability in the Middle Ages and Cultural History." *WerkstattGeschichte* 65 (2013): 55-65.

——. *A Social History of Disability in the Middle Ages: Cultural Considerations of Physical Impairment.* London: Routledge, 2013.

Milani, Mohsen M. *The Making of Iran's Islamic Revolution: From Monarchy to Islamic Republic.* Second Edition. Westview Press, 1994.

Miller, Timothy S., and Nesbitt, John W. *Walking Corpses: Leprosy in Byzantium and the Medieval West.* Ithaca, NY: Cornell University Press, 2014.

Mitchell, Piers D. *Medicine in the Crusades: Warfare, Wounds, and the Medieval Surgeon.* New York: Cambridge University Press, 2004.

Modanlou, H.D. "Avicenna (AD 980 to 1037) and the Care of the Newborn Infant and Breastfeeding," *Journal of Perinatology* 28 (2008): 3-6.

Modarressi, Matin. "Philatelic Propaganda: U.S. Postage Stamps during the Cold War," *Journal of Cold War Studies* 19:3 (2017): 196-201.

Moerman, Daniel E. *Meaning, Medicine, and the "Placebo Effect".* Cambridge: University of Cambridge Press, 2002.

Mollat, Michel. *Les Pauvres au Moyen Âge: étude sociale.* Paris: Hachette, 1978.

Mollier, Christine. "Talismans," in *Divination et société dans la Chine médiévale: Étude des manuscrits de Dunhuang de la Bibliothèque nationale de*

France et de la British Library, ed. Marc Kalinowski (Paris: Bibliothèque nationale de France, 2003), 405-29.

Mommsen, Theodore E. "Petrarch's Conception of the 'Dark Ages.'" *Speculum* 17:2 (1942): 226-42.

Monaco, Francesca Roversi, ed., *Teoria e pratica medica nel basso Medioevo. Teodorico Borgognoni vescovo, chirurgo, ippiatra.* Firenze: SISMEL - Edizioni del Galluzzo, 2019.

Moore, R.I. *The Formation of a Persecuting Society: Authority and Deviance in Western Europe 950-1250.* 2nd edition. Oxford: Blackwell Publishing, 2007.

Moulinier-Brogi, Laurence. *L'uroscopie Au Moyen Age – "Lire Dans Un Verre La Nature de l'homme".* Paris: Champion, 2012.

Mudan Finn, Kavita, ed. *Fan Phenomena: Game of Thrones.* Bristol: Intellect Books, 2017.

Muhammad, Abu Al-Abbas. "Munazara Sakhina bayna al-Atibba' wa-l-'Ulama' wa-l-Mu'alajin bi-l-Qur'an al-Karim. Al-'Ilaj bi-l-Qur'an al-Karim Thabit wa Sahih wa Lakin!" *Al-Majalis*, June 26, 1990.

Mungello, David. *Drowning Girls in China: Female Infanticide since 1650.* Maryland: Rowman & Littlefield, 2008.

Murphy, Hannah. "Skin and Disease in Early Modern Medicine: Jan Jessen's De cute, et cutaneis affectibus (1601)," *Bulletin of the History of Medicine* 94 (2020): 179-234.

Nakayama, Shigeru and Nathan Sivin, eds. *Chinese Science: Explorations of an Ancient Tradition.* Cambridge, MA: MIT Press, 1973.

Needham, Joseph. *Science in Traditional China.* Cambridge, MA: Harvard University Press, 1981.

Nelson, Janet L. "The Dark Ages." *History Workshop Journal* 63:1 (2007): 191-201.

Newman, Barbara. *The Permeable Self: Five Medieval Relationships.* Philadelphia: University of Pennsylvania Press, 2021.

Ng, Wee-Siang Margaret. "Male Brushstrokes and Female Touch." PhD Dissertation, McGill University, 2013.

Nicholle, David. "Wounds, Military Surgery, and the Reality of Crusading Warfare; The Evidence of Usamah's Memoires," *Journal of Oriental and African Studies* 5 (2002): 33-46. Reprinted in *Medieval Warfare, 1000-1300,* ed. John France, 599-612. Burlington, VT: Ashgate, 2006.

Ning Zhao, et al. "Effects on Neuroendocrinoimmune network of Lizhong Pill in the reserpine induced rats with spleen deficiency in traditional Chinese medicine," *Journal of Ethnopharmacology* 133 (2011): 454-59.

Nirenberg, David. *Communities of Violence: Persecution of Minorities in the Middle Ages.* 2nd Edition. Princeton: Princeton University Press, 2015.

Norman, Robert A. "The History of Lupus Erythematosus and Discoid Lupus: From Hippocrates to the Present." *Lupus Open Access* 1:1 (2016). https://www.longdom.org/open-access/the-history-of-lupus-erythematosus-and-discoid-lupus-fromhippocrates-to-the-present-Lupus-1000102.pdf.

Norrie, P. A. "The History of Wine as a Medicine," in *Wine: A Scientific Exploration,* eds. Merton Sandler and Roger Pinder, 21-56. New York: Taylor and Francis, 2003.

Nutton, Vivian. *Ancient Medicine*, Second Edition. London: Routledge, 2013.

—. "Did the Greeks Have a Word for It? Contagion and Contagion Theory in Classical Antiquity," in *Contagion: Perspectives from Pre-Modern Societies*, ed. Lawrence I. Conrad and Dominik Wujastyk, 137-62. London: Routledge, 2017.

O'Boyle, Cornelius. *Thirteenth- and Fourteenth-Century Copies of the* Ars Medicine. Cambridge: Cambridge Wellcome Unit for the History of Medicine, 1998.

Ögenler, Oya, İsmaeil Ün, and İlter Uzel. "Medical plants used for treatment of gynecological disorders in Ottomans in the 15th century," *Journal of Complementary Medicine Research* 7:2 (2018), 171-77.

Orlemanski, Julie. "How to Kiss a Leper." *Postmedieval* 3 (2012): 142-57.

Ortner, Donald J. "What Skeletons Tell Us: The Story of Human Paleopathology," *Virchows Archiv*, 459 (2011): 247-54.

Osler, William. *The Evolution of Modern Medicine: A Series of Lecture Delivered at Yale University on the Silliman Foundation in April, 1913.* Yale University Press, 1921.

—. "Suggested Scheme for the Restoration of the Tomb of Avicenna," *Proceedings of the Royal Society of Medicine* 7 (Sect Hist Med) 1914, 280.

Pahta Päivi and Irma Taavitsainen, "Vernacularisation of Scientific and Medical Writing in Its Sociohistoric Context," in *Medical and Scientific Writing in Late Medieval English,* eds. Irma Taavitsainen and Päivi Pahta, 1-22. Cambridge: Cambridge University Press, 2004.

Palmer, Richard. "In bad odour: smell and its significance in medicine from antiquity to the seventeenth century," in *Medicine and the Five Senses*, ed. William F. Bynum and Roy Porter, 61-68. Cambridge: Cambridge University Press, 1993.

Park, Gunhyuk. "Oxidative Damage in Korean Medicine," *Antioxidants* 11:3 (2022): 600.

Park, Katharine. *Secrets of Women: Gender, Generation, and the Origins of Human Dissection*. New York: Zone Books, 2006.

——. "Medicine and Society in Medieval Europe," in *Medicine in Society: Historical Essays*, ed. Andrew Wear, 59-90. Cambridge: Cambridge University Press, 1992.

Parker, Joanne and Corinna Wagner, eds. *The Oxford Handbook of Victorian Medievalism*. Oxford: Oxford University Press, 2020.

Paxton, Frederick S. "Anointing the Sick and Dying in Christian Antiquity and the Early Medieval West," in *Health, Disease, and Healing in Medieval Culture*, ed. Sheila Campbell, Bert Hall, and David Klausner, 93-102. New York: St. Martin's Press, 1992.

Pilsworth, Clare. *Healthcare in Early Medieval Northern Italy: More to Life than Leeches?* Turnhout: Brepols, 2014.

Pomidor, Bill and Alice K Pomidor, "Essay: 'With Great Power…' The Relevance of Science Fiction to the Practice and Progress of Medicine," *The Lancet* 368, Special Issue 1: *Medicine and Creativity* (Dec 1, 2006): 13-14.

Poncelet, Albert. "Bulletin des publications hagiographiques." *Analecta Bollandiana* 23 (1904): 465-528.

Pormann, Peter E. *The Oriental Tradition of Paul of Aegina's* Pragmateia. Leiden: Brill, 2004.

Pormann, Peter E. and Emilie Savage-Smith. *Medieval Islamic Medicine*. Edinburgh, 2007.

Pugh, Tison and Angela Jane Weisl. *Medievalisms: Making the Past in the Present*. London: Routledge, 2013.

Pugh, Tison and Susan Aronstein. "Introduction: Theorizing America's Medievalisms," in *The United States of Medievalism*, ed. Tison Pugh and Susan Aronstein, 3-18. Toronto: University of Toronto Press, 2021.

Ragab, Ahmed. "Islam and Science," in *Routledge Companion to Religion and Science*, ed. James W. Haag, Gregory R. Peterson, and Michael L. Spezio, 45-57. London: Routledge, 2011.

Rampudda, M., P. Marson and G. Pasero, "Le principali tappe nella storia del lupus eritematoso sistemico – The main stages in the history of systemic lupus erythematosus." *Reumatismo* 61 (2009): 145-52.

Rasooli, Jay M. and Cady H. Allen, *The Life Story of Dr. Sa'eed of Iran: Kurdish Physician to Princes and Peasants, Nobles and Nomads*. William Carey Library, 1983, reprint of 1958 Second Edition.

Rawcliffe, Carole. *Leprosy in Medieval England.* Woodbridge: Boydell & Brewer, 2006.

——. *Urban Bodies: Communal Health in Late Medieval English Towns and Cities.* Woodbridge: Boydell Press, 2013.

——. "Hospitals of Later Medieval London," *Medical History* 28:1 (1984): 1-21.

Resnick, Irven M. *Marks of Distinction: Christian Perceptions of Jews in the High Middle Ages.* Washington, DC: Catholic University of America Press, 2012.

Reu, Wim De. "How to Throw a Pot: The Centrality of the Potter's Wheel in the Zhuangzi." *Asian Philosophy* 20:1 (2010): 43-66.

Richardson, Kristina L. *Difference and Disability in the Medieval Islamic World: Blighted Bodies.* Edinburgh: Edinburgh University Press, 2012.

Riddle, John M. "Lithotherapy in the Middle Ages: Lapidaries Considered as Medical Texts," *Pharmacy in History* 12:2 (1970): 39-50.

Rider, Catherine. "Gender, Old Age, and the Infertile Body in Medieval Medicine," in *Gender, Health, and Healing, 1250*-1550, ed. Sara Ritchey and Sharon Strocchia, 267-90. Amsterdam: Amsterdam University Press, 2020.

Ritchey, Sara. *Acts of Care: Recovering Women in Late Medieval Health.* Ithaca, NY: Cornell University Press, 2021.

Roberts, Charlotte A. *Human Remains in Archaeology: A Handbook*. York, 2012.

——. "Reflections on the bioarchaeology of leprosy and identity, past and present," in *Leprosy and Identity in the Middle Ages: From England to the Mediterranean*, ed. Elma Brenner and François-Olivier Touati, 21-44. Manchester: Manchester University Press, 2021.

——. "Surgery," in M. Lapidge, J. Blair, S. Keynes, and D. Scragg, eds., *The Wiley Blackwell Encyclopedia of Anglo-Saxon England*, Second Edition (Chichester: Wiley, 2014): 445-7.

Roberts, Charlotte A. and Jacqueline McKinley. "Review of Trepanations in British Antiquity Focusing on Funerary Context to

Explain their Occurrence," in R. Arnott, S. Finger, and C.U.M. Smith, *Trepanation: History, Discovery, Theory*, 55-78. Lisse: Swets & Zeitlinger, 2003.

Robson, James. "Magic Cures in Popular Islam." *The Muslim World* 24:1 (1934): 33–43

Rocca, Julius. "Galen and the Uses of Trepanation," in R. Arnott, S. Finger, and C. U. M. Smith, *Trepanation: History, Discovery, Theory*, 253-71. Lisse: Swets & Zeitlinger, 2003.

Rose, Susan. *The Wine Trade in Medieval Europe, 1000-1500.* New York: Bloomsbury Publishing, 2011.

Rosenberg, Charles E. "Disease in History: Frames and Framers," *The Milbank Quarterly* 67, Supplement 1 (1989): 1-15.

Rubin, Miri. *Charity and Community in Medieval Cambridge.* Cambridge: Cambridge University Press, 1988.

——. *Mother of God: A History of the Virgin Mary* New Haven: Yale University Press, 2009.

——. *The Middle Ages: A Very Short Introduction.* Oxford: Oxford University Press, 2014

Run-Ming, Y. "The Origin and Development of Chinese Acupuncture and Moxibustion." *Ancient Science of Life* 4:4 (1985): 224-28.

Ryu, Su-Noh and Sam Sik Kang, "Analysis of Available Component in Artemisiae Herba." *Korean Journal of Crop Science* 49 (2004): 169-75.

Saïd, Edward. *Orientalism.* New York: Random House, 1978.

Salama, Mohammad R. *Islam, Orientalism and Intellectual History: Modernity and the Politics of Exclusion since Ibn Khaldun.* Library of Middle East History. London: I.B. Tauris, 2011.

Savage-Smith, Emilie. "The Practice of Surgery in Islamic Lands: Myth and Reality," *Social History of Medicine* 13:2 (2000): 307-21.

Scanlon, Larry. "Introduction," *American Literary History* 22:4, "Medieval America" (Winter 2010): 715-23.

Schayegh, Cyrus. *Who Is Knowledgeable Is Strong: Science, Class, and the Formation of Modern Iranian Society. 1900-1950.* Berkeley: University of California Press, 2009.

Schedl, Barbara. *Der Plan von St. Gallen: Ein Modell europäischer Klosterkultur.* Vienna: Böhlau Verlag, 2014.

Scheid, Volker, et al. *Chinese Herbal Medicine: Formularies and Strategies.* Seattle, WA: Eastland Press, 2009.

Scott, Anne M., ed. *Experiences of Charity, 1250-1650*. Farnham: Ashgate Press, 2015.

Scully, Terence. *The Art of Cookery in the Middle Ages*. Rochester: The Boydell Press, 1995.

——. "The Sickdish in Early French Recipe Collections," in *Health, Disease and Healing in Medieval Culture,* eds. Sheila Campbell, Bert Hall, and David Klausner (New York: St. Martin's Press, 1992): 132-40.

Sezgin, Fuat. *Ḥunain Ibn Isḥāq (d. 260/873): Texts and studies*. Frankfurt am Main: Institute for the History of Arabic-Islamic Science at the Johann Wolfgang Goethe University, 1996.

Sezgin, Fuat, Māzin ʿAmāwī, Carl Ehrig-Eggert, and Eckhard Neubauer. *Muḥammad ibn Zakarīyāʾ ar-Rāzī (d. 313/925): Texts and studies*. Frankfurt am Main: Institute for the History of Arabic-Islamic Science at the Johann Wolfgang Goethe University, 1999.

Shahar, Shulamith. *Growing Old in the Middle Ages: 'Winter Clothes Us in Shadow and Pain.'* London: Routledge, 1997.

Shamekh, Ali, Ata Mahmoudpoor, and Sarvin Sanaie. "COVID-19: Is it the Black Death of the 21st century?" *Health Promotion Perspectives* 10:3 (2020), 166-167.

Sharma, Madhuri. *Indigenous and Western Medicine in Colonial India*. New Delhi: Foundation Books, 2012.

Shatzmiller, Joseph. *Jews, Medicine, and Medieval Society*. Berkeley: University of California Press, 1994.

Shoham-Steiner, Ephraim. *On the Margins of a Minority: Leprosy, Madness, and Disability Among the Jews of Medieval Europe*. Detroit: Wayne State University Press, 2014.

——. "Pharaoh's Bloodbath: Medieval European Jewish Thoughts About Leprosy," in *Jewish Blood: Reality and Metaphor in History, Religion, and Culture*, ed. Mitchell B. Hart, 99-115. London: Routledge, 2009.

Sholkamy, Hania. "Conclusion: The Medical Cultures of Egypt," in *Health and Identity in Egypt*, ed. Hania Sholkamy and Farha Ghannam, 111-28. Cairo: The Amsterdam University in Cairo Press, 2004.

Shyovitz, David. "Christians and Jews in the Twelfth-Century Werewolf Renaissance." *Journal of the History of Ideas* 75 (2014): 521-43.

Silvestre, Hubert. "Notes sur la 'Vita Evracli' de Renier de Saint-Laurent. Contribution à l'histoire littéraire du XIIe siècle Liégeois." *Revue d'histoire ecclésiastique* 44 (1949): 29-86.

Simonsohn, Shlomo. *The Jews in Sicily*, Vol. 1. Leiden: Brill, 1997.

Singer, Charles. "A Review of the Medical Literature of the Dark Ages, with a New Text of about 1110," *Proceedings of the Royal Society of Medicine* 10 (1917), 107-60.

Siraisi, Nancy G. *Avicenna in Renaissance Italy: The* Canon *and Medical Teaching in Italian Universities after 1500*. Princeton, NJ: Princeton University Press, 1987.

——. *Medieval and Early Renaissance Medicine: An Introduction to Knowledge and Practice*. The University of Chicago Press, 1990.

——. "How to Write a Latin Book on Surgery: Organizing Principles and Authorial Devives in Guglielmo da Saliceto and Dino del Garbo," in *Practical Medicine from Salerno to the Black Death*, ed. Luis Garcia-Ballester *et al.*, 37-62. Cambridge: Cambridge University Press, 1994.

——. "Avicenna and the Teaching of Practical Medicine," in Nancy G. Siraisi, *Medicine and the Italian Universities 1250-1600*, 63-78. Leiden: Brill, 2001.

Sivin, Nathan. *Granting the Seasons: The Chinese Astronomical Reform of 1280*. New York: Springer, 2009.

Skuse, Alanna. "Wombs, Worms and Wolves: Constructing Cancer in Early Modern England." *Social History of Medicine* 27 (2014), 632-48.

Smith, A.M., M.F. Picciano, and R.H. Deering, "Folate Supplementation During Lactation: Maternal Folate Status, Human Milk Folate Content, and Their Relationship to Infant Folate Status," *Journal of Pediatric Gastroenterol Nutrition,* 2:4 (1983), 622-8.

Smith, Pamela H. *The Body of the Artisan: Art and Experience in the Scientific Revolution*. Chicago: University of Chicago Press, 2004.

Smith, Pamela H., Amy R.W. Meyers, and Harold J. cool, eds. *Ways of Making and Knowing: The Material Culture of Empirical Knowledge*. Ann Arbor, MI: University of Michigan Press, 2014.

Song, Bong-Keun, Jin-Hee Won, and Sungchul Kim, "Historical medical value of *Donguibogam*," *Journal of Pharmacopuncture* 19:1 (2016): 16-20.

Spadola, Emilio. *The Calls of Islam: Sufis, Islamists, and Mass Mediation in Urban Morocco*. Bloomington and Indiana: Indiana University Press. 2014.

Sperling, Jutta Gisela. "Introduction," in *Medieval and Renaissance Lactations: Images, Rhetorics, Practices,* ed. Jutta Gisela Sperling (Farnham: Ashgate, 2013): 1-20.

Stahuljak, Zrinka. *Pornographic Archaeology: Medicine, Medievalism, and the Invention of the French Nation*. Philadelphia: University of Pennsylvania Press, 2013.

Stannard, Jerry. *Herbs and Herbalism in the Middle Ages and Renaissance.* London: Routledge, 1999.

——. "Alimentary and Medicinal Uses of Plants," in *Medieval Gardens,* ed. Elisabeth B. MacDougall, 69-92. Washington, DC: Dumbarton Oaks, 1986.

Stewart, Lily. "Leprosy, Chastity, and Desire in Medieval Hagiography." *Magistra* 27:1 (2021), 49-78.

Stobart, Anne and Susan Francia. "The Fragmentation of Herbal History: The Way Forward," in *Critical Approaches to the History of Western Herbal Medicine: From Classical Antiquity to the Early Modern Period*, ed. Anne Stobart and Anne Francia, 1-20. London: Bloomsbury, 2014.

Stock, Brian. *The Implications of Literacy: Written Language and Models of Interpretation in the Eleventh and Twelfth Centuries*. Princeton: Princeton University Press, 1983.

Storm, Daniela et al., "Revised Reference Values for Potassium Intake," *Annals of Nutrition and Metabolism,* 71:1-2 (2017), 118-24.

Strickmann, Michel. *Chinese Magical Medicine*. Stanford, California: Stanford University Press, 2002.

Strohm, Paul. "Historicity without historicism?" *postmedieval* 1 (2010): 380-91.

Suit, Natalia. *Qur'anic Matters: Material Mediations and Religious Practice in Egypt.* London: Bloomsbury Academic, 2020.

Talbot, Rob and Robin Whiteman. *Brother Cadfael's Herb Garden: An Illustrated Companion to Medieval Plants and their Uses*. Boston: Bulfinch Press, 1997.

Tan, S.Y. "Medicine in Stamps. Avicenna (980-1037): Prince of Physicians," *Singapore Medical Journal* 43:9 (2002), 445-6.

Telliel, Yunus. "Miraculous Evidence: Scientific Wonders and Religious Reasons." *Comparative Studies of South Asia, Africa, and the Middle East* 39 (2019): 528-42

Thomas, Donald E. Jr. *The Lupus Encyclopedia. A Comprehensive Guide for Patients and Families*. Baltimore, MD: Johns Hopkins University Press, 2014.

Thorold Rogers, James E. *A History of Agriculture and Prices in England from the Year After the Oxford Parliament (1259) to the Commencement of the Continental War (1793): Volume III (1401-1582).* Oxford: Clarendon Press, 1882.

"The Tomb of Avicenna." *British Medical Journal* July 25, 1914.

Tosi, Adelaide, Paola Badino, and Barbara Pezzoni. "Medical Conditions Observed in Osteoarchaeological Remains: Arthropathies, Traumatic Lesions, Tumours, Metabolic Diseases and Dental Pathologies," *Medicina Historica*, 1 (2017): 29-34.

Totaro, Rebecca. "Mother London and the *Madonna Lactans* in England's Plague Epic," in *Medieval and Renaissance Lactations: Images, Rhetorics, Practices,* ed. Jutta Gisela Sperling, 147-64. Farnham: Ashgate, 2013.

Touati, François-Olivier. "Contagion and Leprosy: Myth, Ideas, and Evolution in Medieval Minds and Societies," in *Contagion: Perspectives from Pre-Modern Societies*, ed. Lawrence I. Conrad and Dominik Wujastyk, 179-201. Aldershot: Ashgate, 2000.

—. *Maladie et Société au Moyen Age: la lèpre, les lépreux et les léproseries dans la province ecclésiastique de Sens jusqu'au milieu du XIVe siècle.* Brussels: De Boeck & Larcier, 1998.

—. "Maladies et pratiques médicales, IXe-XIVe siècle. Pierre de Blois. La transmission d'un dossier médical à un confrère," in *Sources d'histoire médiévale*, ed. Ghislain Brunel and Elisabeth Lalou, 786-88. Paris: Larousse, 1992.

Trexler, Richard C. "Charity and the Defense of Urban Elite in the Italian Communes," in *The Rich, the Well Born, and the Powerful: Elites and Upper Classes in History*, ed. Frederic Cople Jaher, 56-109. Urbana: University of Illinois Press, 1973.

Truitt, E. R. *Medieval Robots: Mechanism, Magic, Nature, and Art.* Philadelphia: University of Pennsylvania Press, 2015.

Turner, Bryan S. *Orientalism, Postmodernism and Globalism.* London: Routledge, 1994.

United States. Congress. Senate. *United States Senate Hearing of the Committee on Health, Education, Labor, and Pensions One Hundred Fifteenth Congress, Second Session. The Opioid Crisis: The Role of Technology and Data in Preventing and Treating Addiction. February 27, 2018*. S. Hrg. 115-782. Washington: U.S. Government Publishing Office, 2020.

Tuten, Belle. "Lactation and the Breast in Antiquity: Medical Authorities on Breast Health and Treatment," *Quaestiones Medii Aevi Novae* 19 (2014): 159-86.

——. "Care of the Breast in the Late Middle Ages," in *Gender, Health and Healing, 1250-1550,* ed. Sara Ritchey and Sharon Strocchia (Amsterdam: Amsterdam University Press, 2020): 119-38.

Ulwin, Tim. *Wine and the Vine: An Historical Geography of Viticulture and the Wine Trade.* New York: Routledge, 1991.

Uscinski, Kristin. "Recipes for Women's Healthcare in Medieval England," PhD dissertation, Fordham University, 2017.

Van Arsdall, Anne. "Challenging the 'Eye of Newt' Image of Medieval Medicine," in *The Medieval Hospital and Medical Practice*, ed. Barbara S. Bowers, 195-203. Aldershot: Ashgate, 2007.

——. "Rehabilitating Medieval Medicine," in *Misconceptions About the Middle Ages*, ed. Stephen J. Harris and Bryon L. Grigsby, 135-41. New York: Routledge, 2007.

van de Walle, Etienne. "Flowers and Fruits: Two Thousand Years of Menstrual Regulation," *Journal of Interdisciplinary History* 28:2 (1997): 183-203.

van Winter, Johanna Maria. "Medieval Recipes for Invalid Food," in *Spices and Comfits: Collected Papers on Medieval Food* (Totnes: Prospect Books, 2007): 355-60.

Vauchez, André. "Assistance et Charité en Occident, XIIIe -XVe Siècles," in *Domanda e consumi. Livelli e strutture (nei secoli XII-XVII):* ed. Vera Barbagli Bagnoli, 151-62. Florence: L.S. Olschki, 1978.

Ventura, Iolanda. "Medieval Pharmacy and Arabic Heritage: The Salernitan Collection *Circa Instans*," in *The Impact of Arabic Sciences in Europe and Asia*, Micrologus XXIV (Firenze: SISMEL, 2016), 339-401.

Vinea, Ana. "What is your Evidence? A Salafi Therapy in Contemporary Egypt." *Comparative Studies of South Asia, Africa, and the Middle East* 39:3 (2019): 500-12.

Virchow, Rudolf. "Historische Notizen über Lupus." *Archiv für pathologische Anatomie und Physiologie und für klinische Medizin* 32 (1865):139-43.

Voigts, Linda E. "Anglo-Saxon Plant Remedies and the Anglo-Saxons," *Isis* 70:2 (1979): 250-68.

Vongasthorn, Kathleen and Magnus Vollset. "'Our loathsome ancestors': Reinventing Medieval Leprosy for the Modern World," in *Leprosy and Identity in the Middle Ages: From England to the Mediterranean*, ed. Elma Brenner and François-Olivier Touati, 347-82. Manchester: Manchester University Press, 2021.

Voultsiadou, Eleni. "Therapeutic properties and uses of marine invertebrates in the ancient Greek world and early Byzantium." *Journal of Ethnopharmacology* 130:2 (2010): 237-47.

Waldron, Tony. *Palaeopathology*. Cambridge: Cambridge University Press, 2009.

Wallis, Faith. "The Experience of the Book: Manuscripts, Texts, and the Role of Epistemology in Early Medieval Medicine," in *Knowledge and the Scholarly Medical Traditions*, ed. D. G. Bates, 105-43. Cambridge: Cambridge University Press, 1995.

——. "Signs and Senses: Diagnosis and Prognosis in Early Medieval Pulse and Urine Texts," *Social History of Medicine* 13:2 (2000): 265-78.

Waltner, Anne. "Infanticide and Dowry in Ming and Early Qing China," in *Chinese Views of Childhood*, ed. Anne Kinney, 201-5. Honolulu: University of Hawaii Press, 1995.

Ward, Jennifer. *Women in Medieval Europe, 1200-1500*. New York: Routledge, 2016.

Ware, Rudolph. *The Walking Qur'an: Islamic Education, Embodied Knowledge, and History in West Africa*. Chapel Hill: The University of North Carolina Press, 2014.

Watt, James. "Sir Walter Scott and the Medievalist Novel," in *The Oxford Handbook of Victorian Medievalism*, ed. Joanne Parker and Corinna Wagner, 162-74. Oxford: Oxford University Press.

Weber, Jochen, and Alfred Czarnetzki. "Brief Communication: Neurotraumatological Aspects of Head Injuries Resulting from Sharp and Blunt Force in the Early Medieval Period of Southwestern Germany." *American Journal of Physical Anthropology* 114 (2001): 352-56.

Wells, Calvin. "Probable trephination of five Early Saxon skulls," *Antiquity* 48 (1974): 298-302.

Westermarck, Edward. *Ritual and Belief in Morocco*. Reprint. New York: Routledge, 2014.

Whiteman, Robin. *Brother Cadfael's Book of Days: The Material and Spiritual Wisdom of a Medieval Crusader-Monk*. London: Headline, 2000.

——. *The Cadfael Companion: The World of Brother Cadfael.* New York, NY: Mysterious Press, 1995.

Whittaker, Adam. "A Plague of Medievalism upon You All: Medievalism, Music, and the Plague," in *Studies in Medievalism XXVII: Authenticity, Medievalism, Music*, ed. Karl Fugelso, 201-26. Woodbridge: Boydell and Brewer, 2018.

Wigner, Eugene P. "Time and Effort Reports Defended," *Science* 159: 3812 (January 19, 1968): 255.

Wilcox, Judith and John M. Riddle, "Qustā ibn Lūqā's Physical Ligatures and the Recognition of the Placebo Effect, With an Edition and Translation," *Medieval Encounters* 1:1 (1995): 1-50.

Williams, David. "Medieval Movies." *The Yearbook of English Studies* 20 (1990): 1-32.

Winer, Rebecca Lynne. "The Mother and the *Dida* [Nanny]: Female Employers and Wet Nurses in Fourteenth-Century Barcelona," in *Medieval and Renaissance Lactations: Images, Rhetorics, Practices,* ed. Jutta Gisela Sperling, 55-78. Farnham: Ashgate, 2013.

Wiseman, Nigel and Andrew Ellis. *Fundamentals of Chinese Medicine.* Brookline, MA: Paradigm Publications, 1996.

Wollenberg, Daniel. *Medieval Imagery in Today's Politics.* Kalamazoo, MI: ARC Humanities Press, 2018.

Woolgar, C.M. *The Culture of Food in Medieval England, 1200-1500.* New Haven: Yale University Press, 2016.

Xu Man. *Crossing the Gate: Everyday Lives of Women in Song Fujian (960-1279).* Albany: SUNY Press, 2016.

Yoeli-Tlalim, Ronit. *ReOrienting Histories of Medicine: Encounters along the Silk Roads.* New York, NY: Bloomsbury Publishing, 2021.

Yoon, Saunjoo L., and Jeong-Hee Kim. "Factors contributing to the use of complementary and alternative medicine in rural older women with chronic pain in South Korea." *Applied Nursing Research* 26:4 (2013): 186-91.

Young, Helen and Kavita Mudan Finn. *Global Medievalism.* Cambridge: Cambridge University Press, 2022.

Yuksel, Sevda *et al.,* "Oxidant and Antioxidant Status of Human Breast Milk During Lactation Period," *Dairy Science and Technology,* 95 (2015): 295-305.

Zabrowski, Jason R. "Arab Christian Physicians as Interreligious Mediators: Abū Shākir as a Model Christian Expert," *Islam and Christian-Muslim Relations* 22:2 (2011): 186-96.

Zadeh, Travis. "An Ingestible Scripture: Qur'ānic Erasure and the Limits of "Popular" Religion," in *Material Culture and Asian Religions: Text, Image, Object*, ed. Benjamin J. Fleming and Richard D. Mann, 97-119. London: Routledge, 2014.

——. "Touching and Ingesting: Early Debates over the Material Qur'an." *Journal of the American Oriental Society* 129:3 (2009): 443-66.

Zhao Zhongzhen and Xue Changli. *Illustrated Chinese Medicinal Formulae.* Hong Kong: Chung Hwa Book Co., 2005.

Zimmerman, Michael R., Erik Trinkhaus, Marjorie Lemay, *et al.* "Trauma and Trephination in a Peruvian Mummy." *American Journal of Physical Anthropology* 55 (1981): 497-501.

Zimmerman, Susan. "Leprosy in the Medieval Imaginary." *Journal of Medieval and Early Modern Studies* 38 (2008): 559-87.

Ziolkowski, Jan. "A Fairy Tale from before Fairy Tales: Egbert of Liège's 'De puella a lupellis servata' and the Medieval Background of 'Little Red Riding Hood.'" *Speculum* 67 (1992): 549-75.

Zupko, Ronald Edward. *British Weights and Measures: A History from Antiquity to the Seventeenth Century.* Madison, WI: University of Wisconsin Press, 1977.

Zuppa, Antonio Alberto, et al., "Safety and Efficacy of Galactagogues: Substances that Induce, Maintain, and Increase Breast Milk Production," *Journal of Pharmaceutical Science,* 13:2 (2010): 162-74.

INDEX

C

D

N

O